Game/Set/Match
A Tennis Guide

Game/Set/Match
A Tennis Guide

EIGHTH EDITION

James E. Bryant

Professor Emeritus
San Jose State University

WADSWORTH
CENGAGE Learning™

Australia • Brazil • Japan • Korea • Mexico • Singapore • Spain • United Kingdom • United States

WADSWORTH
CENGAGE Learning™

Game/Set/Match: A Tennis Guide, Eighth Edition
James E. Bryant

Executive Editor: Yolanda Cossio
Development Editor: Liana Sarkisian
Assistant Editor: Kristina Chiapella
Editorial Assistant: Shannon Elderon
Media Editor: Miriam Myers
Marketing Manager: Laura McGinn
Marketing Coordinator: Jing Hu
Marketing Communications Manager: Linda Yip
Content Project Management: PreMediaGlobal
Art Director: John Walker
Manufacturing Buyer: Linda Hsu
Rights Specialist: Dean Dauphinais
Permissions Researcher: PreMediaGlobal, Plymouth, MA

Library of Congress Control Number: 2011925121

Student Edition:

ISBN-13: 978-0-8400-5360-2

ISBN-10: 0-8400-5360-6

Wadsworth
20 Davis Drive
Belmont, CA 94002-3098
USA

Cengage Learning is a leading provider of customized learning solutions with office locations around the globe, including Singapore, the United Kingdom, Australia, Mexico, Brazil and Japan. Locate your local office at **international.cengage.com/region**

Cengage Learning products are represented in Canada by Nelson Education, Ltd.

For your course and learning solutions, visit **www.cengage.com.**

Purchase any of our products at your local college store or at our preferred online store **www.cengagebrain.com.**

Instructors: Please visit **login.cengage.com** and log in to access instructor-specific resources.

Printed in the United States of America
1 2 3 4 5 6 7 15 14 13 12 11

Contents

Preface

In 1984 I wrote my first tennis book entitled *Tennis: A Guide for the Developing Tennis Player*. It was a forerunner to this eighth edition of *Game, Set, Match: A Tennis Guide*. Tennis was increasing in popularity on college campuses in 1984 and I was active in tennis, teaching an extensive number of tennis classes at the college level and playing competitive tennis. At the time there were also a number of tennis books on the market, some specific to college students learning to play tennis. What seemed to be missing was a book that included quality photographs regarding skill development, which enhanced a written explanation of how to play. The very first book was designed for the beginning and intermediate player, with photos and a written description of how to play the game, covering a total of 16 chapters. When the present day *Game, Set, Match*, 1st edition, appeared in 1986, the photos were improved, the writing focused specifically on the beginning player's skill development while recognizing that an advanced player could still profit from the content of the book, and as a result the book generated considerable interest as a college level tennis textbook.

Tennis is a highly popular sport played at all levels of skill and by people of all ages. For an individual to be successful at the game requires the development of a foundation of skills based on a learning progression process, an in-depth comprehension of the flow of the game, and an insight into the rules and ethics of play. Tennis is played at an intense level of competition by some, and in a spirit of enthusiasm by all who understand that tennis is a game meant to be enjoyed. As played today tennis is a never-ending process of learning. It is a complex game that, when played over the years, becomes surprisingly simple yet always remaining challenging.

Today, as an eighth edition, *Game, Set, Match* is still designed for the beginning player who as a novice is attempting to develop skills and knowledge in tennis. More advanced players can still use the book to review skills and strategy. And, in fact, the book is in many ways a confirmation for more advanced players that their skills are consistent with fundamental play, and that they are making progress beyond the beginner level.

This newest edition continues to provide a progressive learning experience that includes a logical presentation of skills coupled with information on how to play tennis effectively and how to play by the rules. At the beginning of each skill-oriented chapter, the most rudimentary skills are presented. Then, at the end of the chapter more advanced beginning skills are provided. Consequently, Chapters 2–4 present an advanced skill section subtitle called *Increasing Beginner Skills*. Photographs throughout the book present a beginning and a progressively more advanced visualization of various skills that add to the depth of the content and thus to the learning experience of the student. In addition, figures contribute general information and present strategies related to the game. This edition of the book is special for a variety of reasons but primarily through contributing to the game by presenting a logical progression of the skills, supplemented by photos that provide a visualization of skill, and followed by how to go about hitting a tennis ball effectively. In addition, there is a logical progression from chapter to chapter that enables the student to understand and relate to the game and the skills required to play the game.

The text is organized into twelve chapters. The first five chapters are presented in a progressive format, enabling the student to move from one skill area to another in a logical and understandable manner. Chapters 1–5 are focused totally on the fundamentals of tennis from how to hold the racket, to hitting groundstrokes, to the serve and receiving serve, to volleying, and finally to hitting overheads and lobs.

The next three chapters 6–8, are presented in a logical order to be used throughout the length of the course. They discuss mental practice and the strategies of playing both singles and doubles. Chapter 6 presents a mental aspect of the game that addresses how to cope with stress during a match, how to concentrate, and how to basically be mentally tough when playing the game. Chapters 7 and 8 are strategy chapters. Chapter 7 handles the singles aspect of the game and Chapter 8 describes how to use strategy in doubles play.

Chapter 9 is loaded with practice drills to be used throughout the length of the course. They are designed for the instructor to use in a progressive teaching sequence within the framework of presenting the various fundamental skills. They can also be used by students to practice individually, or with a partner, away from the class environment. Chapter 10 covers the various physical aspects of the game from warming up to cooling down, preventing and caring for injuries, and dealing with the physical environment. This chapter is also designed to be used throughout the instructional process, focusing on the student learning experience regarding being fit to play tennis, and becoming sensitive to the environment by avoiding injuries and responding appropriately when injured.

Chapters 11 and 12 are also developed to be used throughout the length of the course. Tennis can't be played without knowledge and practice regarding the ethics and rules of play. Chapter 11 provides information on how to behave appropriately on the tennis court and it presents coverage of the rules that are critical to the function of playing the game. Chapter 12 is, more than anything else, an informational chapter. It assists the student with information regarding tennis facilities, equipment, tournament competition, and getting started in tennis competition, along with a historical background on tennis. It is the last chapter since it has, among other things, a resource section that enables the student to find additional learning resources regarding tennis. Again, both of these chapters can be used at any point during the instruction process as a supplement to the skill development.

This is a tennis book culminating after 26 years of tennis writing experience into the most recent knowledge base for the student. This eighth edition provides quality reflected in previous editions while making sure that new, updated information, new concepts, and new ways to do things in tennis are covered. Adjustments for this edition include a return to color figures and a color enhancement of the black and white photographs including color cue words and colored directional arrows placed on the photographs. These adjustments greatly enhance the learning process for the student as written material is interfaced with the visual movement represented in photos. The self-help sections entitled *Points to Remember, Common Errors & How to Correct Them* and *Checkpoints*, with additional questions to aid the student in a self-testing setting, are found in each chapter.

There are adjustments in the written presentation to better clarify points. As an example, in Chapter 12 there is an update regarding resources, particularly with Website resources associated with tennis. And there is an extended effort to encourage students to be aware of the United States Tennis Association (USTA) and its many outreaches to college students. The USTA provides the *Code: The Player's Guide for Matches when Officials Are Not Present* in Appendix A, which contains the generally stated rules for the game. That, along with the many resources produced by the USTA, are significant contributions by the organization that are highlighted in the text. Although many of these content areas aren't new to this edition, they are critical to the learning experience of students and they enhance the instructor's ability to provide a full coverage of the game.

Game, Set, Match is a guide for the tennis player who is receiving instruction at the college level, and for the instructor to use as a tool to direct the student in that learning process. It is my hope that everyone who reads and studies the material in this book will continue to grow with the game and reap its rewards through the years.

James E. Bryant, Ed. D.

Acknowledgements

Ever since 1986, individuals have contributed to the continual development of *Game, Set, Match* as reviewers, models, and illustrators and as sources leading to a book that is as complete and accurate as possible. I want to extend a personal thank you to all who have permitted me to benefit from their knowledge and talents, which has led to the development of this book for the beginning tennis player.

Eight editions of a book require support from so many people that it is truly difficult to begin to thank all who have contributed to the development of this book. It is a given that I need to thank all of my former students, who have provided feedback and served as a true test for the practicality and applicability of the book. And for this latest edition of the book, models, including Shane Velez, Kate Hardin, Robbie Phillips, Janessa Elder, and Alex Wisner deserve much credit for their performance. Without their excellent skill level and performance the very essence of the visualization of tennis movement would be lost for the book. A thank you also goes to all the photographers who have contributed over the years, but in particular to Terrell Lloyd who provided excellent digital photos of tennis as it should be played. There were also several editors and production people who have contributed to the eight editions and for that a thank you goes to each and every one.

So with that, the eighth edition goes forward with a tremendous thank you to all who have contributed over the years.

Game/Set/Match
A Tennis Guide

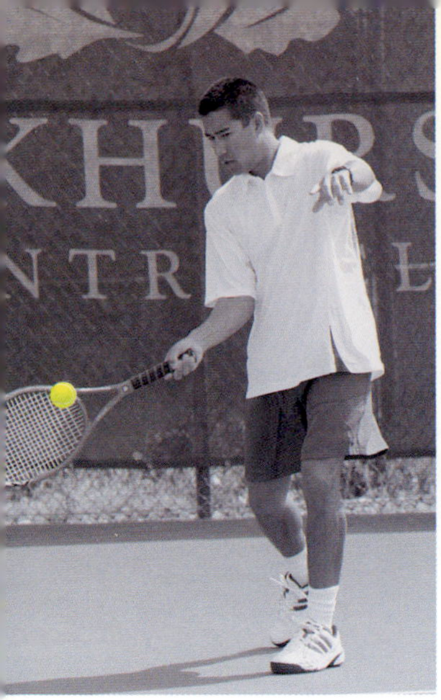

Photography by Terrell Lloyd; assisted by Anna Symonds Myers

1

Preliminaries to the Strokes in Tennis

To play tennis, a person has to know how to hold a tennis racket for each stroke and how to stand and move. Recognizing the spin of the ball, although not of immediate concern to the beginner, is extremely important as the player's skills develop. Additional needs are to comprehend racket-face control and have a feel for the ball as the racket impacts the ball. Learning how to grip and control a tennis racket and how to get ready to hit the ball must be established early in the learning experience.

Basic Tennis Grips

The tennis grip is the foundation to the execution of a specific stroke. Selecting a tennis grip that fits the stroke is a requirement for the completion of the stroke. There are two referenced points in terms of hand placement. One is the "V" formed by the thumb and index finger. The other is the location of the racket hand on the panels of the racket grip (Figure 1.1) (Photo 1.1).

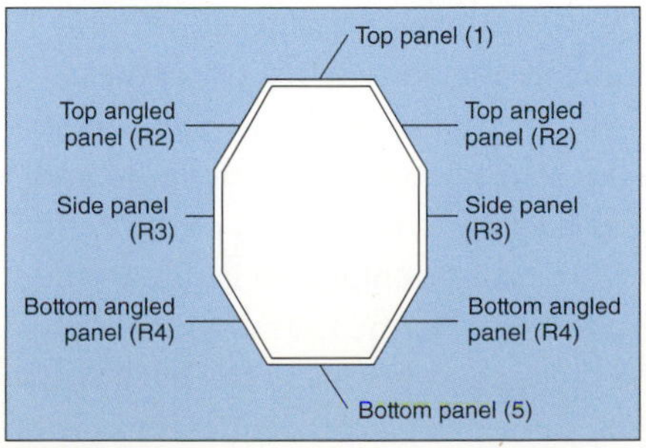

FIGURE 1.1 Panels of racket grip.

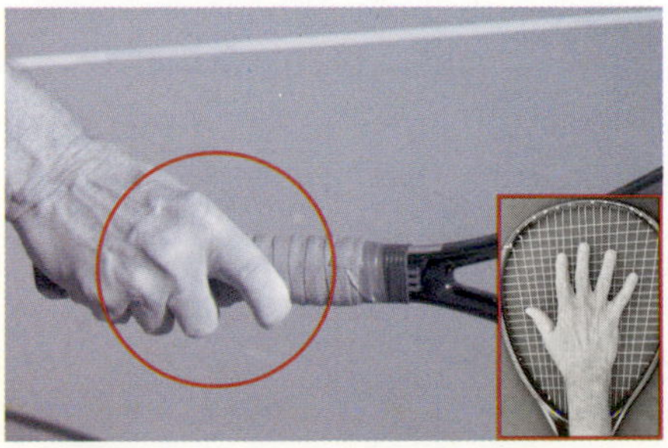

PHOTO 1.1 "Trigger-finger" position.

Photography by Virginia Bryant

Eastern Forehand Grip

The *eastern forehand grip*, a universally used grip designed for executing the forehand groundstroke, is also called the "shake hands" grip. Place your racket hand on the strings of the racket, and bring your hand straight down to the grip (Photo 1.1). The heel of your racket hand will rest on the side panel (R3) (Figure 1.1). As your hand takes the racket grip, your fingers will be spread along the length of the racket grip, with the index finger spread the farthest in a "trigger finger" style, providing control (Photo 1.2). The thumb will be situated on the back side of the racket, and the thumb and four fingers will form a "V" on the racket grip. The "V" points to the racket shoulder when the player holds the racket in front at a right angle to the body (Photo 1.3).

Eastern Backhand Grip

The *eastern backhand grip* is a conventional backhand grip used

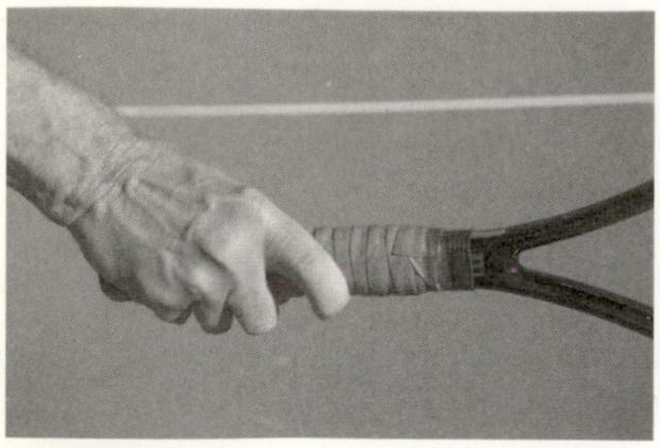

Photography by Virginia Bryant

PHOTO 1.2 Eastern forehand grip (side view).

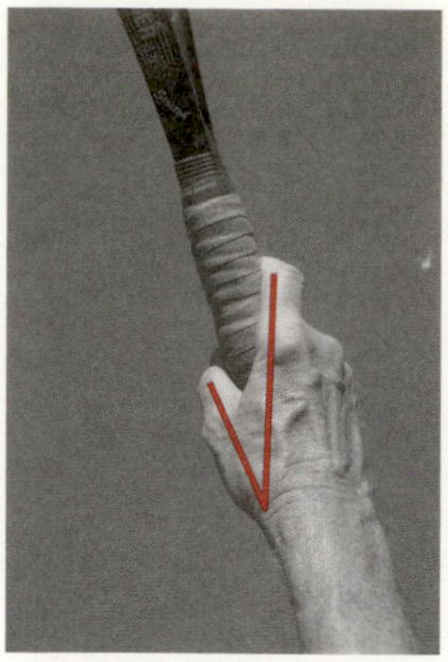

Photography by Virginia Bryant

PHOTO 1.3 Eastern forehand grip (top view).

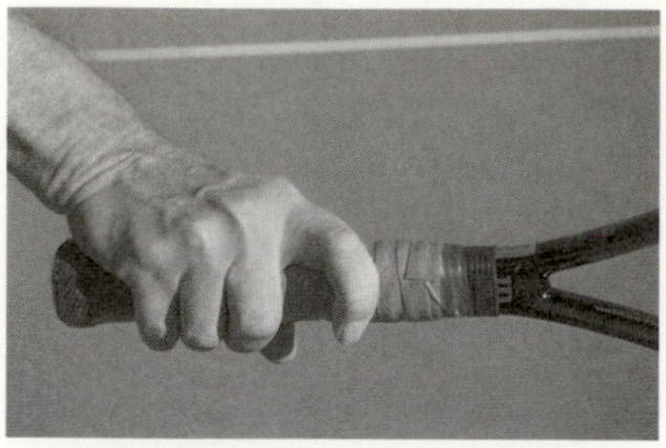

Photography by Virginia Bryant

PHOTO 1.4 Eastern backhand grip (front view).

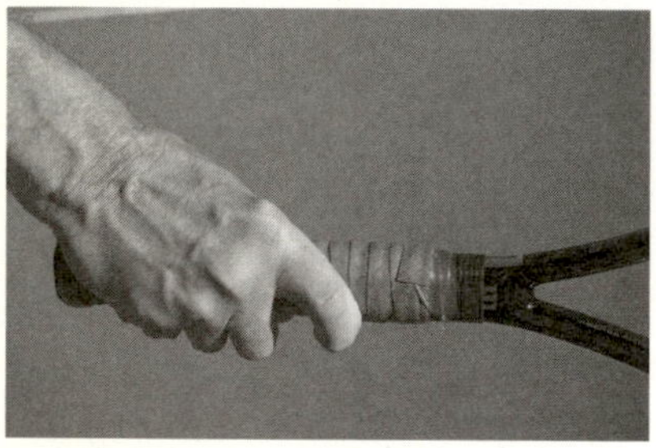

Photography by Virginia Bryant

PHOTO 1.5 Eastern backhand grip (side view).

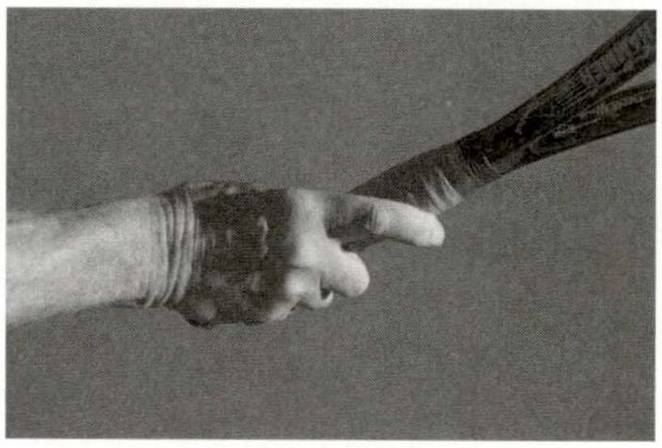

Photography by Virginia Bryant

PHOTO 1.6 Forehand–backhand continental grip (back view).

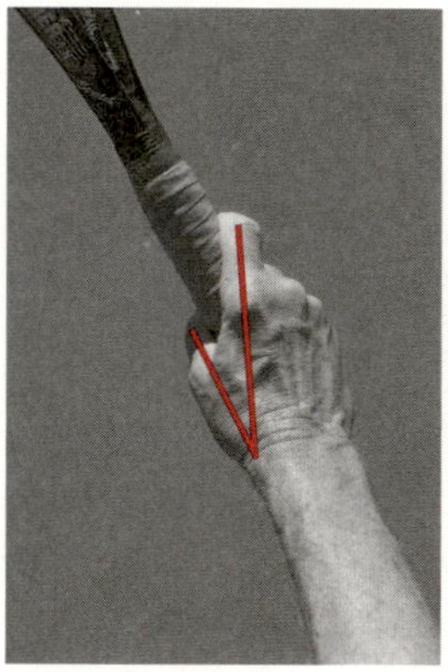

Photography by Virginia Bryant

PHOTO 1.7 Forehand–backhand continental grip (top view).

extensively in tennis (Photos 1.4 and 1.5). From the eastern forehand grip, roll your hand over the top of the racket grip and place your thumb diagonally across the rear plane of the racket grip. The heel of your racket is now on the top of the racket. From this position you should be able to see all four knuckles of the racket hand when holding the racket perpendicular to the body. When the racket is held in front of the body, the "V" formed by the thumb and fingers will point to the nonracket shoulder.

Continental Grip

The *continental grip* is used to hit either a backhand or forehand shot and as a grip for both volley shots and serves (Photos 1.6 and 1.7). It differs from the eastern forehand and backhand grips in that the hand is placed midway between the positioning of the two eastern grips. The heel of the racket hand is positioned between the top panel (1) and top angled panel (R2) (Figure 1.1). The "V" formed by the thumb and fingers points to the middle or center of the body halfway between the racket and nonracket sides of the body when the racket is held in front of the body. The subtle difference between the forehand and the backhand placement of the hand for the continental grip is that in the forehand grip the thumb grasps the racket grip, whereas in the backhand the thumb is placed diagonally across the back of the grip.

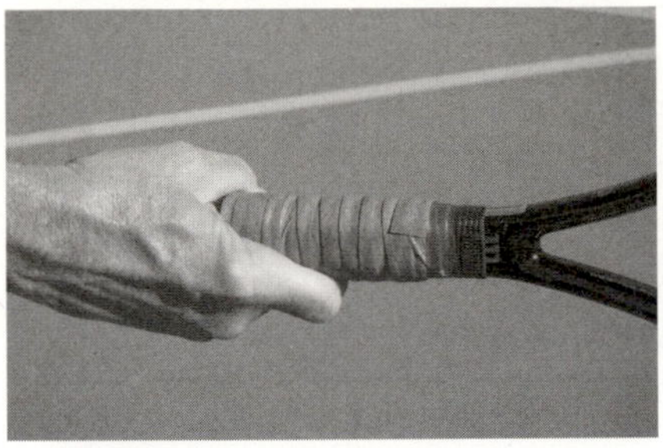

Photography by Virginia Bryant

PHOTO 1.8 Semi-western forehand grip (back view).

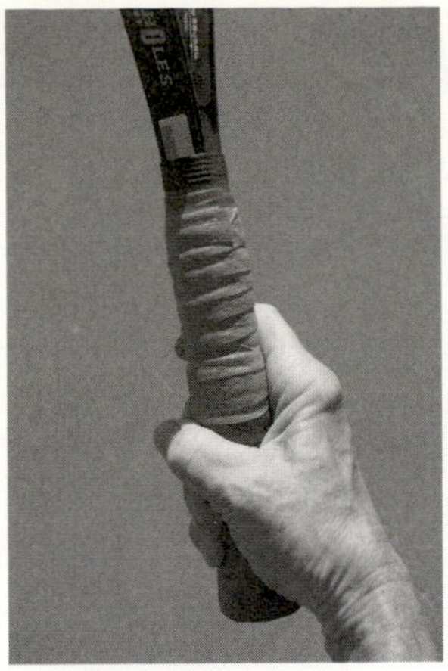

Photography by Virginia Bryant

PHOTO 1.9 Semi-western forehand grip (top view).

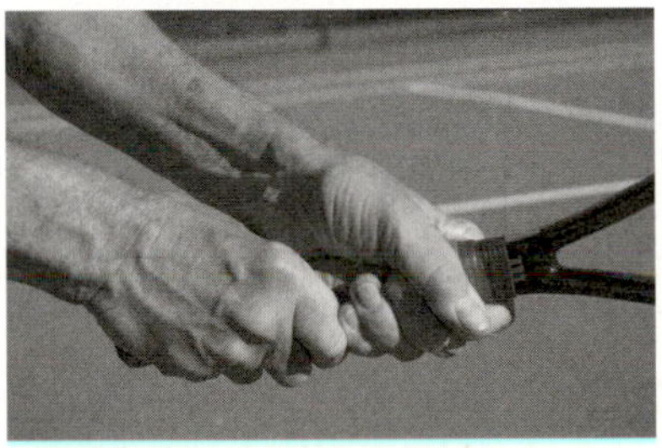

Photography by Virginia Bryant

PHOTO 1.10 Two-hand backhand grip (front view).

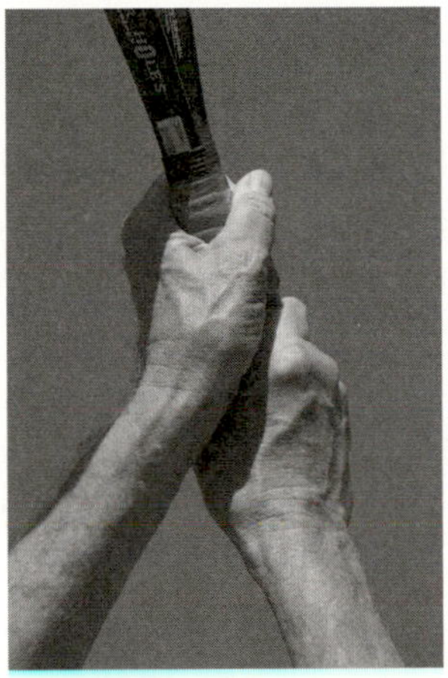

Photography by Virginia Bryant

PHOTO 1.11 Two-hand backhand grip (top view).

"V" formed by the thumb and fingers, when the racket is held in front of the body, points beyond the racket shoulder.

Two-Hand Backhand Grip

The *two-hand backhand grip* (Photos 1.10 and 1.11) has become quite popular. It is achieved when the dominant hand grasps the racket grip in a continental or eastern backhand grip, with the non-dominant hand butted above that grasp in an eastern forehand grip. To execute the stroke, the two-hand backhand grip must be a snug fit of two hands working together. Some players use a two-hand forehand grip, but this grip is not popular and thus is not considered necessary as a choice of grips for the beginning player.

Selecting the Proper Grip

Selecting a grip is based on the stroke used. Eastern forehand grips are used for the forehand groundstroke. The eastern backhand grip is used for the backhand groundstroke and for special serves. The continental grip is used for groundstrokes, volleys, overheads, and serving. The continental grip has the added advantage of requiring little in the way of grip adjustment for different strokes; consequently, the strokes are disguised when using this grip. The *semi-western forehand* is used with success when hitting topspin forehand groundstrokes.

Players who seek both power and control for their backhand groundstroke often select the two-hand backhand grip. This grip requires the player to cover more distance on a court to reach shots hit wide.

Semi-Western Forehand Grip

The *semi-western forehand grip* (Photos 1.8 and 1.9) is often the forehand groundstroke grip of choice of highly skilled players and of developing players who are taught to impart exaggerated topspin when hitting forehand groundstrokes. This grip also is used by those who pick up a tennis racket for the first time and start to play.

The grip is best achieved by laying the racket on the court and picking it up naturally. The heel of the hand will line up with the bottom angled panel (R4) (Figure 1.1). The

POINTS to REMEMBER

GRIP

1. Keep the fingers spread on the racket grip, with the index finger serving as a "trigger finger" for all grips except the two-hand backhand grip, where only the bottom hand uses a "trigger finger."
2. Be aware of the location of the "V" in relation to the racket and nonracket shoulders.
3. Grasp the racket firmly when assuming a grip.
4. Understand the subtle differences between grips and the purpose for each.

COMMON ERRORS & HOW TO CORRECT THEM *(Grip)*

The Error	What Causes the Error	To Correct the Error
Lack of control of the racket	Grasping the racket in a fist-like position.	Make sure the fingers are spread along the racket grip with a trigger finger.
Mis-hitting a ball or poor execution.	Grip is too tight.	Relax the grip. Grasp the racket firmly, not tightly.
Racket turns in hand.	Grip is too loose.	Tighten the grip. Grasp the racket firmly, not tightly. Check grip size. If the grip is too small, the racket will turn in the hand when hitting a return shot with high velocity.

To answer the question of *what grip to use for what stroke*, players who intend to stay at the baseline and hit groundstrokes typically should use the eastern forehand and backhand grip. An alternative to using the eastern backhand grip when hitting from the baseline is to use a two-hand backhand grip for backhand groundstrokes. When you are serving, the continental grip will provide control, accuracy, and power for an effective service. As a beginner, you may be more comfortable using the eastern forehand grip for the serve. As soon as possible, though, you should switch to the continental grip.

Going to the net to play a volley shot requires reaction and timing, which means that the grip should not be changed much for a forehand or a backhand volley. In other words, you should use a continental grip for play at the net.

Types of Strokes

As an introduction to strokes in tennis, a definition of the various strokes should enable better understanding of the basic skills of the game. *Groundstrokes* are either forehand or backhand.

Groundstrokes

The basic *forehand groundstroke* (Photo 1.12) is hit from the baseline following the bounce of the ball. The stroke is executed with a swinging action that produces a flat, no-spin (actually, most flat shots have a small amount of topspin) movement to the ball.

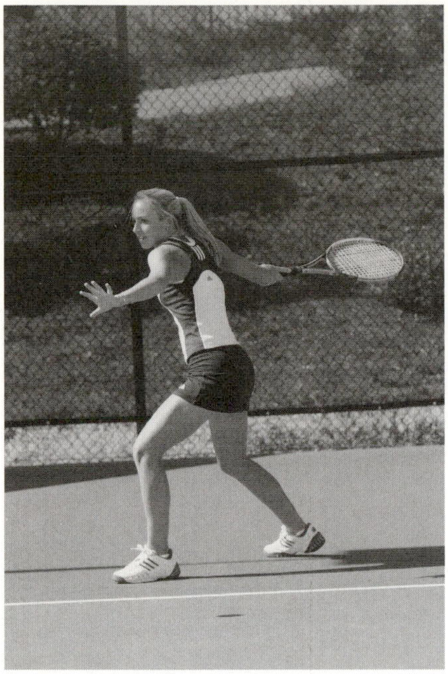

PHOTO 1.12 Forehand groundstroke follow-through.

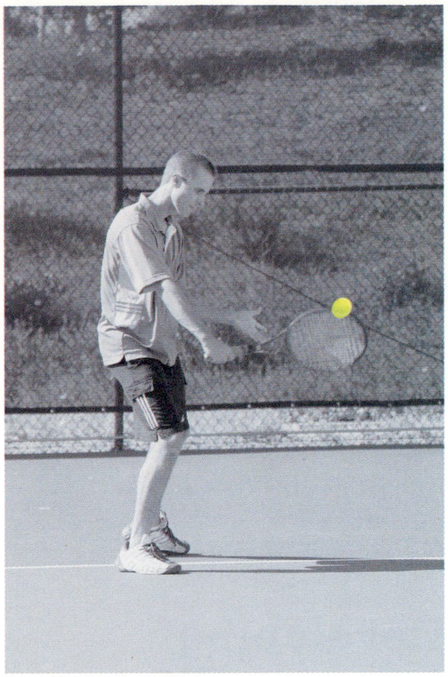

PHOTO 1.13 Backhand groundstroke.

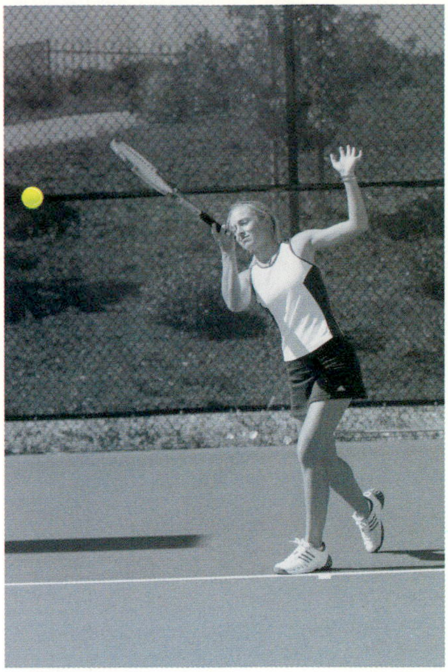

PHOTO 1.14 Lob.

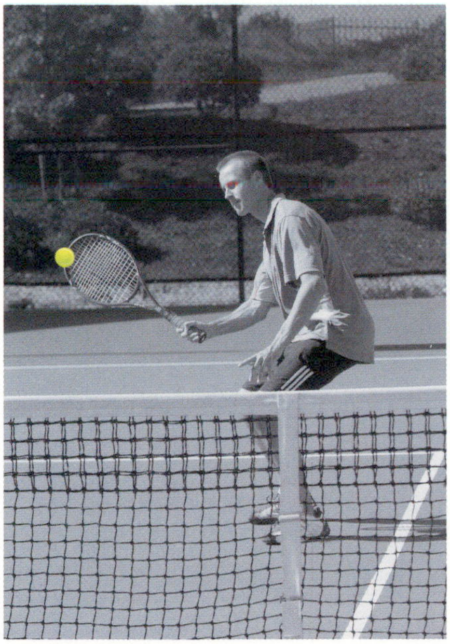

PHOTO 1.15 Volley.

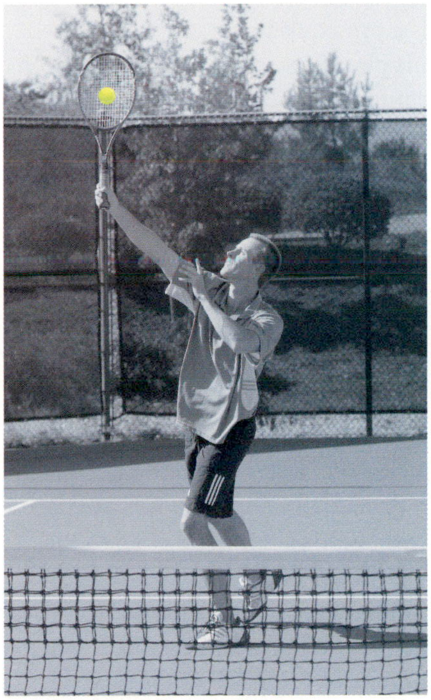

PHOTO 1.16 Overhead.

The *backhand groundstroke* (Photo 1.13) is played under the same conditions as the forehand groundstroke, with the same ball action. Both are swinging action strokes, with the forehand hit on the racket side of the body and the backhand hit on the nonracket side of the body.

Both strokes are foundations for more advanced strokes, including *topspin* and *slice (underspin) groundstrokes*. *Approach shots*, which are an extension of groundstrokes, are characterized by a player advancing from the baseline and toward the net to hit a ball.

Lobs, Volleys, Overheads

All *lobs* (Photo 1.14) are also an extension of groundstrokes. In terms of the swinging action, there is a lifting action designed to hit the ball deep to the baseline and with a loft.

The *volley* (Photo 1.15) is a punching action characterized by playing the ball before it contacts the court surface. Both forehand and backhand volleys usually are played at the net. *Half-volleys* are an extension of a volley shot, but they are hit on a short bounce.

The *overhead* (Photo 1.16) is a continuation of the basic flat service,

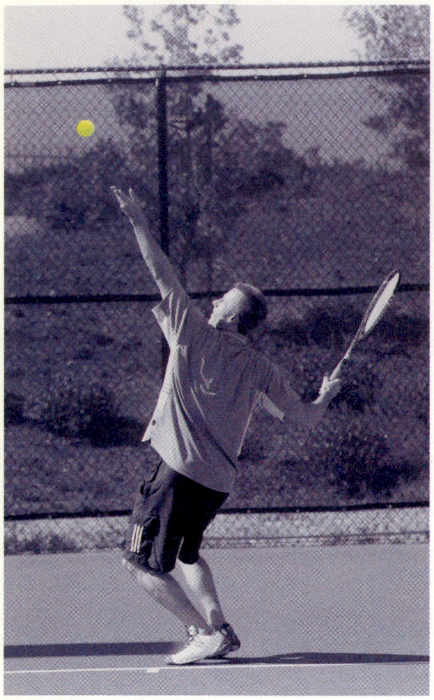

PHOTO 1.17 Flat serve.

from a skill perspective. Key parts of the serve are reflected in the overhead stroke. It differs from the serve in that the ball is hit either on the fly or after a bounce on the court surface when the offensive player is positioned near the net.

The basic *flat serve* (Photo 1.17), is described as a throwing action. Strokes that develop from the flat service are the slice service (sidespin), the topspin service, and an advnced stroke known as the American twist (another sidespin rotation).

Developing a Feel for Hitting the Ball

Developing a *feel* for the tennis ball is a prerequisite for successful tennis play. Regardless of racket control, spin of the ball, and various stroke fundamentals, execution of each stroke depends on feeling for the ball through *eye–hand coordination, timing*, and *focus*.

Eye–Hand Coordination

Eye–hand coordination is based on past experiences of throwing and catching an object similar in size to a tennis ball. The swinging, throwing, and punching actions associated with tennis are fundamental to the ball games of batting, throwing, and catching that most American children play during their childhood. If you have played softball or racquetball or have engaged in activities such as playing catch, the game of tennis will be easy for you, compared to individuals who have not had those experiences.

Timing

Timing in tennis is related to where the ball eventually will be positioned to be hit rather than to where it bounced originally. You must perceive where the ball will go after it bounces and set up behind and away from the ball so that you can step into the ball to hit it (Photo 1.18). Players tend to get too close to the ball or too far away, which either "ties them up" or causes them to lurch to hit the ball rather than step smoothly into the ball. If the ball is too far away, the player can adjust (and not lose timing) by stepping toward the ball with a weight transfer (Photo 1.19A). If the ball is too close, the player should step away, yet forward, to hit the ball (Photo 1.19B). The key factor in stepping away is to open the upper body as the racket is brought through the ball at contact.

Part of timing involves controlling the speed of the racket head. Players under pressure tend to swing too hard or too fast, particularly when returning service. You must remember to play from a relaxed position and to control the racket-head speed. The same pressure can exist when hitting an overhead or a groundstroke when the opposing player is at the net. The added pressure tends to break down timing, forcing the player to rush through the stroke. The focal points have to be *relaxation, confidence* in hitting the ball, and *concentration* on the ball. Timing is improved immeasurably by watching the ball as long as possible. This is the part of focus that is most often ignored.

Focus

The ability to *focus* is extremely important in tennis. It is critical that you "see" the ball and perceive the racket striking the ball. Being able to focus on the ball is based on the same past experiences as with eye–hand coordination. Focus requires recognizing the bounce of the ball in terms

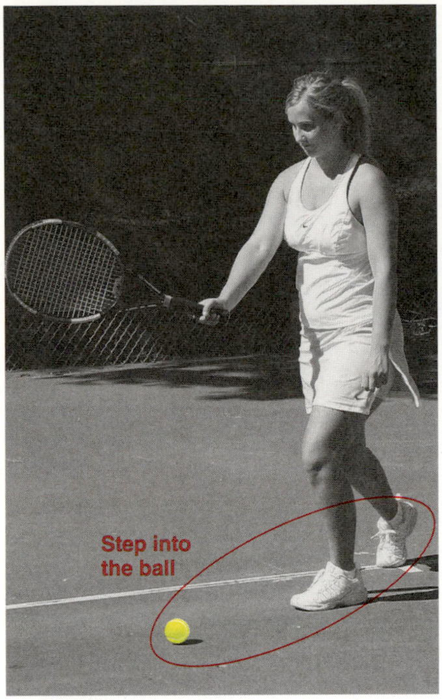

Photography by Terrell Lloyd; assisted by Anna Symonds Myers

PHOTO 1.18 Position of ball and feet away and behind the ball.

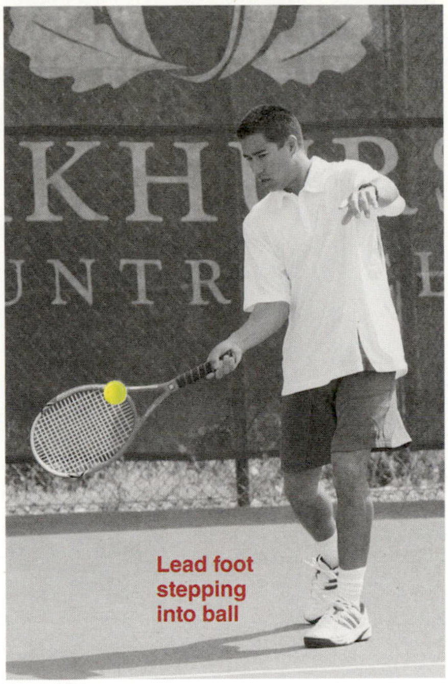

PHOTO 1.19A Stepping into the ball.

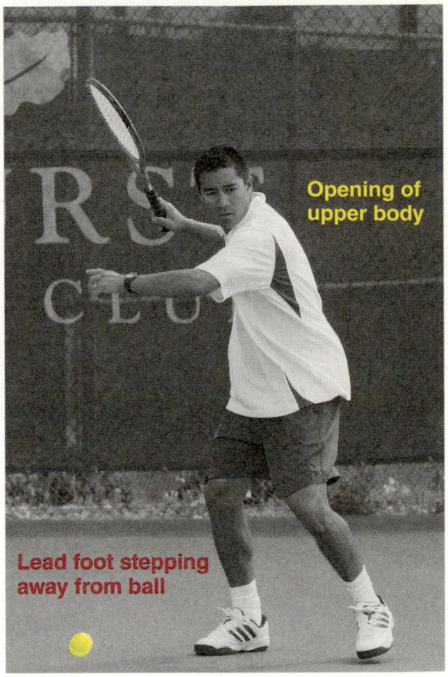

Photography by Terrell Lloyd; assisted by Anna Symonds Myers

PHOTO 1.19B Stepping away from the ball.

of height, estimating distance of the ball from the player, and judging the relationship of the ball to the body. In addition, focus entails moving to the ball, transferring the weight into the ball at contact, and being in the correct position at the correct time. A final consideration in focusing is the ability to block out all outside distractions and keep the tennis ball as the only target.

Ready Position

The foundation for timing and focus rests with establishing a *ready position* from which to hit groundstrokes and volleys (Photo 1.20A). The ready position is the primary foundation for all strokes.

The feet should be spaced slightly wider than shoulder width and parallel to each other. The knees are slightly bent, and the weight of the body is centered over the balls of the feet. The buttocks should be "down," with the upper body leaning slightly forward in a straight alignment. The head should be "up," looking toward the ball on the opposite side of the net. The racket is held "up" with a forehand grip on the handle, with the nonracket hand lightly maintaining contact with the throat of the racket. The racket head is above the hands, and the elbows are clear of the body.

The ready position gives the player the opportunity to move equally to the right or left as well as to advance forward or retreat backward. The first response from a player in the ready position is to rotate the shoulders immediately when recognizing the direction of the ball from across the net (Photos 1.20B and 1.20C). A player with good mobility will be able to move the feet quickly from the ready position. If a player can be relaxed in a ready position, keep the weight on the balls of the feet, and then react to the approaching ball with an early turn of the shoulders and quick foot movement, then the stroke will have been initiated positively.

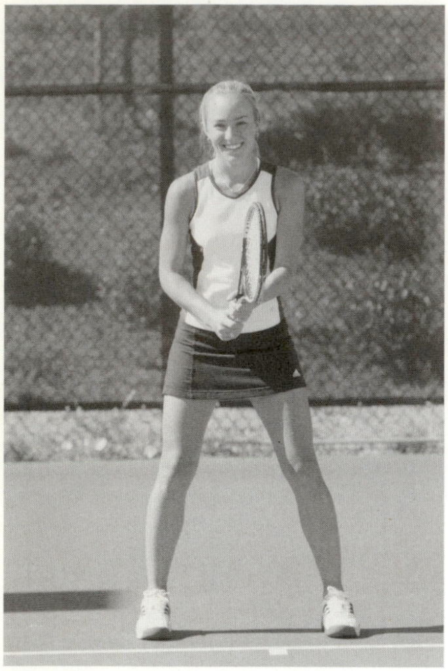

PHOTO 1.20A Ready position for a groundstroke.

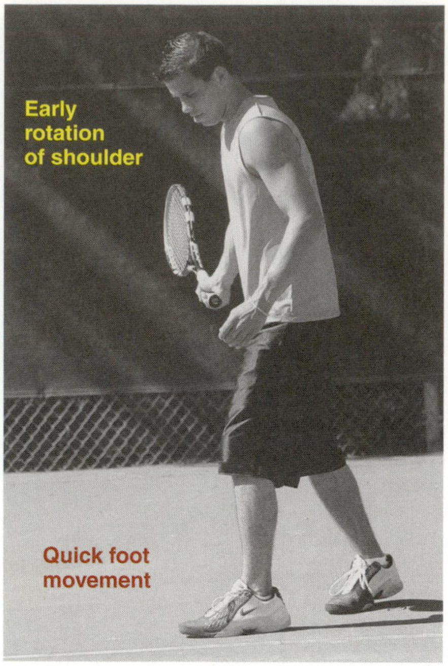

PHOTO 1.20B Ready position—turn of shoulders (forehand).

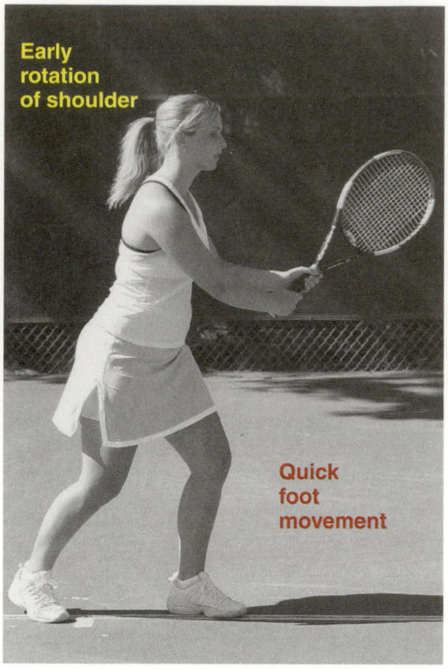

PHOTO 1.20C Ready position—turn of shoulders (backhand).

Photography by Terrell Lloyd; assisted by Anna Symonds Myers

POINTS *to* REMEMBER

READY POSITION

1. Maintain a base with the feet a shoulder width apart.
2. Focus on the ball on the other side of the net.
3. Keep the knees bent slightly and the weight on the balls of the feet.
4. Be relaxed and ready to react.
5. As the ball crosses the net, turn the shoulders and move the feet.

COMMON ERRORS & HOW TO CORRECT THEM *(Ready Position)*

The Error	What Causes the Error	To Correct the Error
Falling off balance.	Feet too close together.	Widen the base.
Incorrect timing of the ball.	Not focusing on the ball and not getting the shoulders rotated early with the feet moving.	Watch the seams of the ball and rotate your shoulders early.

Racket Control and Ball Spin

Your first concern as a beginning player is simply to hit the ball when it comes to you. As your skills improve, you will have to direct attention to racket control and ball spin to improve further.

Racket Control

Racket control is essential to good strokes and thus to successful play. When swinging a racket, three basic actions will provide racket-head control and consequently will accomplish a stroke. The basic *swinging action* is reflected in the forehand and backhand groundstrokes and the various lobs. The serve and overhead strokes are described through the *action of throwing*. The *punch action* is used with forehand and backhand volleys. By executing each of these actions or patterns, you will eliminate all extraneous motion, which will help you to simplify the action of each stroke.

Racket-Face Positions

Three basic *racket-face* positions will also affect the control and flight pattern of the ball and the bounce of the ball on the surface of the court. The effect of these three positions on the resulting action of the ball depends on the speed of the racket head while hitting through the ball and on the angle of the racket face when it contacts the ball. If contact is made with the *racket face flat* to the ball (Photo 1.21), the flight of the ball will be straight. An *open racket face* (Photo 1.22) will cause the ball to have a floating action in its flight. A *closed racket face* (Photo 1.23) will force the flight pattern of the ball downward.

Each racket-face position is important to all skill levels. Understanding what causes the drop or rise of the ball gives the beginning player greater insight into the total concept of hitting the ball and reacting to the bounce.

Comprehending spins is a direct carryover from understanding racket-head and racket-face control. A tennis shot that is hit without spin is affected by three aspects of the overall stroke.

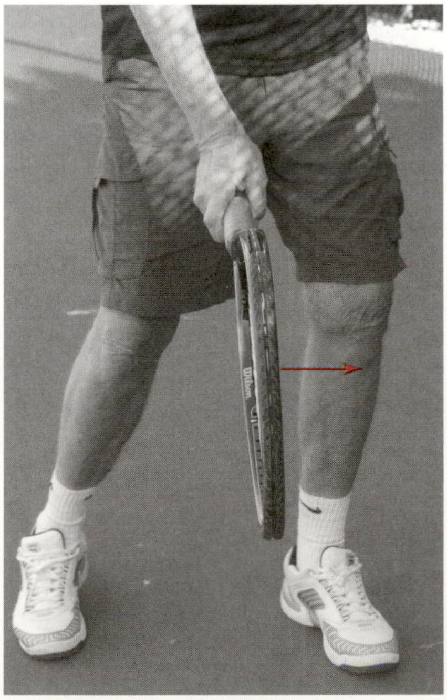

Photography by Virginia Bryant

PHOTO 1.21 Flat racket face.

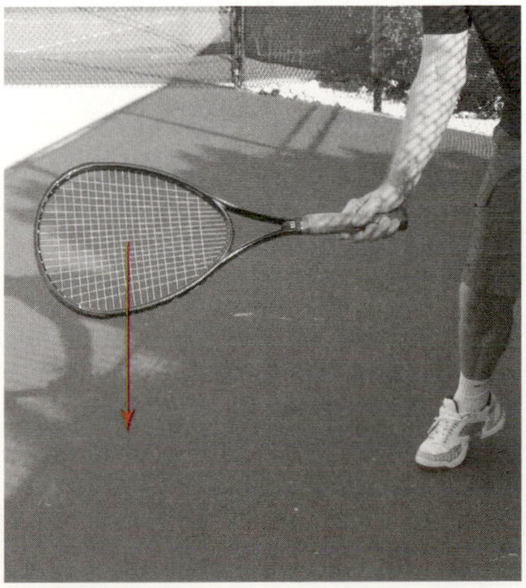

Photography by Virginia Bryant

PHOTO 1.22 Open racket face.

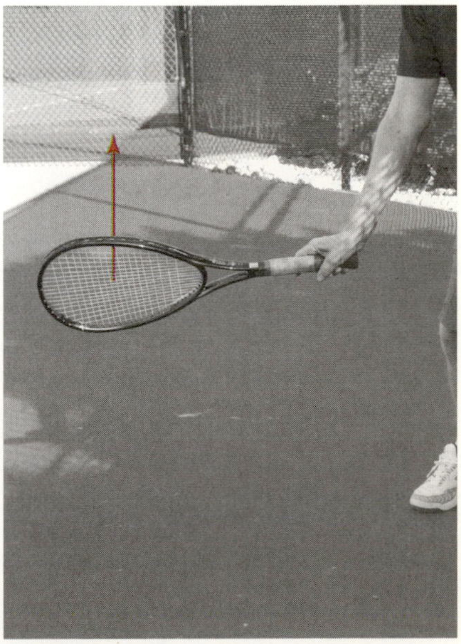

Photography by Virginia Bryant

PHOTO 1.23 Closed racket face.

1. As the ball strikes the racket face, a direct force is applied to the ball, which provides velocity.
2. That velocity is countered by air resistance and gravity; the former impedes the velocity of the tennis ball, and the latter pulls the ball down toward the court.
3. The ball will strike the tennis court surface at an angle equal to the rebound of the ball off the court surface.

Spin Action on the Ball

When a ball spins in its flight pattern due to application of spin to the ball, the tennis player must cope with the behavior of the ball as it strikes the court surface. There are three *basic spinning actions for balls in flight* (see Figure 1.2).

1. *Topspin* is caused by the action of the top surface of the ball rotating against air resistance. This creates friction on the top part of the ball, forcing the ball in a downward path.
2. *Underspin* is caused by the bottom of the ball meeting air resistance and forcing the ball to stay up longer than normally is found with a nonspinning ball.
3. *Sidespin* is created when the side of the ball meets air resistance and pressure. This causes the ball to veer in the direction of the spin.

Spin Action when Striking the Court

The *action of the ball striking the court surface* is the end result of racket control action on the ball and the spin of the flight of the ball (Figure 1.3). As the tennis ball makes contact with the tennis court, the ball will behave in a highly predictable manner. A *topspin* action will hit the court surface with a high, deep bounce because of the forward rotation of the ball. A ball hit with *underspin* usually is hit with power and at a low angle, creating a skidding action as ball meets surface. The *sidespin* strikes the court with the same action and direction as the sidespin on the ball.

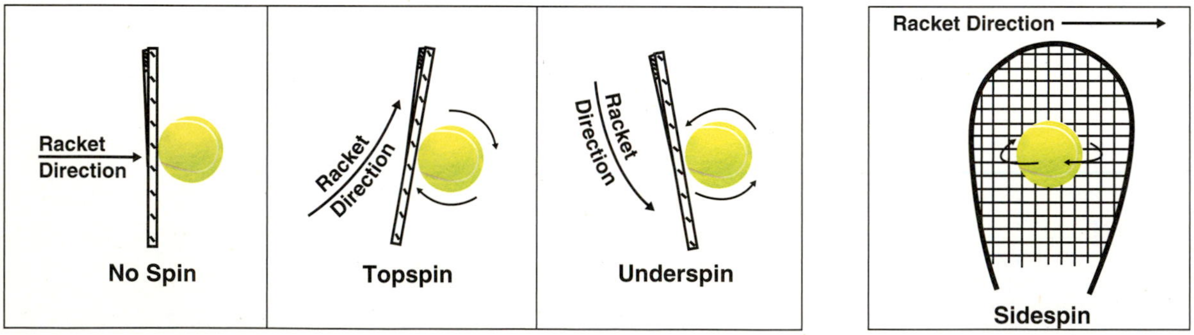

FIGURE 1.2 Basic actions for balls in flight.

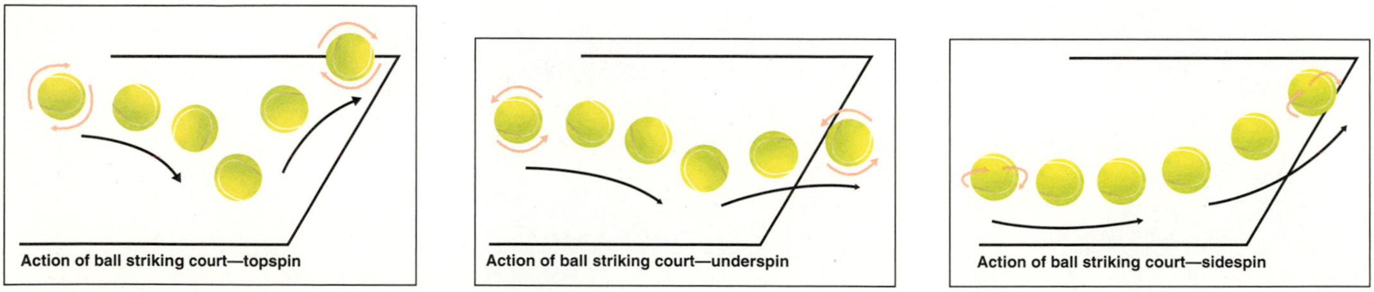

FIGURE 1.3 Basic actions for ball striking the court.

To Summarize

In summary, racket control and spin of the ball have a cause–effect relationship. A flat racket face at contact will cause a flat flight pattern and a flat equal-angle bounce off the court. An open racket face will result in underspin during the flight of the ball and a skidding action upon contact with the court surface. A closed racket face moving in a plane from low to high will provide a topspin ball action, with a resulting high and deep bounce off the court surface.

A closed racket face striking the ball on the side, as when serving, will create a sidespin action followed by a sideward bounce when the ball strikes the court. The beginning player has to understand the various spins applied to a ball in order to cope with balls hit with spin and to learn how to supply spin to various strokes.

CHECKPOINTS

1. The eastern forehand grip is described as
   a. trigger finger, "V" formed by index finger and thumb, with "V" pointed to racket shoulder.
   b. grasp of racket, "V" formed by index finger and thumb, with "V" pointed to racket shoulder.
   c. trigger finger, "V" formed by index finger and thumb, with "V" pointed to center of chest.
   d. trigger finger, "V" formed by index finger and thumb, with "V" pointed to nonracket shoulder.
2. The continental grip is described as
   a. similar to a two-handed grip.
   b. halfway between an eastern forehand and a western forehand grip.
   c. halfway between an eastern forehand and an eastern backhand grip.
   d. halfway between an eastern backhand and a western forehand grip.
3. The continental grip is used most effectively for
   a. playing the baseline.
   b. playing the baseline and the net.
   c. playing the baseline and serve.
   d. playing the net and serve.
4. The basic racket control actions are
   a. punch action, swing action, and throw action.
   b. punch action and swing action.
   c. throw action and swing action.
   d. punch action and throw action.
5. The three types of spin imparted on a ball in flight are
   a. topspin, sidespin, underspin.
   b. reverse spin, topspin, backspin.
   c. reverse spin, sidespin, topspin.
   d. sidespin, reverse spin, slice.
6. Feel for the tennis ball requires
   a. eye–hand coordination, focus, and foot coordination.
   b. eye–hand coordination, timing, and focus.
   c. focus, foot coordination, and timing.
   d. foot coordination, eye–hand coordination, and timing.
7. The first response from a ready position is to
   a. rotate the shoulders.
   b. turn the racket-side shoulder.
   c. turn the nonracket-side shoulder.
   d. rotate the shoulders with the direction of the ball seen across the net.
8. The tennis racket should be grasped
   a. tightly.
   b. loosely.
   c. firmly.
   d. in a fistlike grip.
9. The two-hand backhand grip is described as
   a. two hands separated by an inch of space.
   b. two hands snug, next to each other, with the dominant hand using a continental grip and the nondominant hand using an eastern forehand grip.
   c. two hands snug, next to each other, with both hands using an eastern back hand grip.
   d. two hands snug, next to each other, with both hands using a semi-western grip.
10. Top spin of a ball is caused by
    a. the side of the ball meeting air resistance and pressure, causing the ball to move in the direction of the spin.
    b. the bottom of the ball meeting air resistance, forcing the ball to strike the court with underspin.
    c. action of the top surface of the ball rotating against air resistance, forcing a downward path.
    d. a swing straight through the ball with air resistance directly behind the ball.

Answers to Checkpoints can be found on page 167.

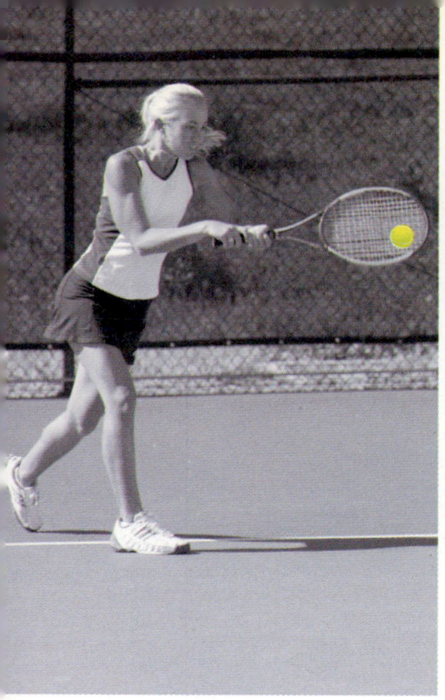

Photography by Terrell Lloyd; assisted by Anna Symonds Myers

2 Groundstrokes

Groundstrokes are crucial to success in tennis. They are executed by the player hitting the tennis ball from the baseline area following one bounce of the ball on the court. The *groundstroke* involves a swinging action designed to hit the ball deep to the opponent's baseline. Both the *forehand* and the *backhand* groundstrokes develop from the basic (little spin) flat stroke and evolve into other groundstrokes, termed *topspin* and *slice* (underspin) groundstrokes.

Groundstrokes—Basic Forehand

The *basic forehand groundstroke* is the foundation for all forehands hit with spin. It is the stroke that players use most often if they are given the choice between a backhand and a forehand.

The eastern forehand grip is used to execute the basic forehand groundstroke. Fundamentally, there are three stages to hitting a forehand: preparing to hit the ball, contacting the ball, and following through. These three stages must be performed in sequence.

Preparing to Hit the Ball

When preparing to hit the ball, the player is in the ready position. Two reactions follow:

1. Rotation of the shoulders.
2. Movement of the feet. As a result of the shoulder and foot movement, the racket, with timing, is placed in an early backswing position. To do this, the player may either bring the racket straight back or loop the racket. Either is acceptable because the goal is to get the racket back in a low position, in line with the flight of the ball. The loop is emphasized as an example in this situation.

The *loop* is divided into three parts.

1. The shoulders turn, allowing the racket to pull back in a line even with the eye (Photo 2.1).
2. The racket moves to a general position perpendicular to the fence located behind the baseline and aligned with the direction of the ball's flight (Photo 2.2).
3. The racket drops below the line of the flight of the ball at about a 12-inch position below and behind the intended contact area with the ball (Photo 2.3).

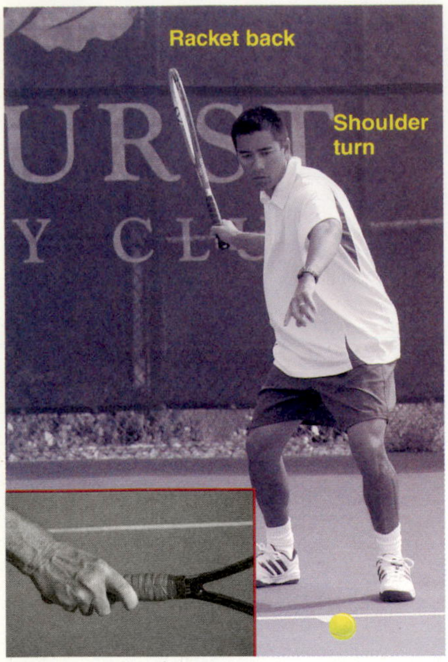

Photography by Terrell Lloyd; assisted by Anna Symonds Myers; inset photo by Virginia Bryant

PHOTO 2.1 Pull the racket back in a line even with the eye (eastern forehand grip).

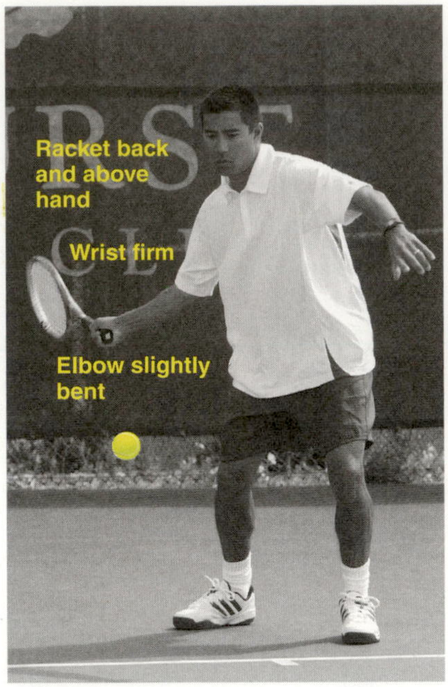

Photography by Terrell Lloyd; assisted by Anna Symonds Myers

PHOTO 2.2 Backswing—racket perpendicular and high.

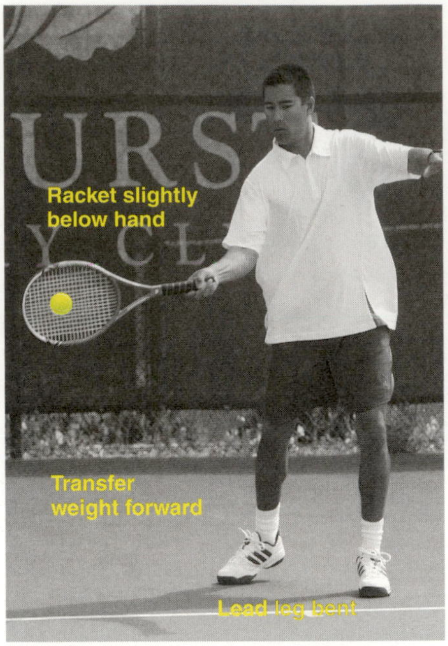

Photography by Terrell Lloyd; assisted by Anna Symonds Myers

PHOTO 2.3 Preparation for contact with the ball.

The loop will provide rhythm to the swing, add extra velocity to the ball following impact, and ensure a grooved swing.

The full pattern for this preparation is to bring the racket back in a rhythmical movement by reacting early to the ball and turning the shoulders at a 45-degree angle to begin inertia. As the racket starts back in the loop following the shoulder turn, both feet will move and pivot automatically to accommodate the upper body turn. The feet are positioned in either an open or closed stance (Photos 2.1 through 2.4 show an open stance). By the time the racket moves to a position perpendicular to the fence beyond the back court, the wrist and arm should be firm, with the elbow bent slightly and away from the body. The nonracket arm is positioned forward, enabling the player to focus on the ball as a reference point and to provide balance (Photo 2.1). The final part of the preparation is to bend the legs.

Contact with the Ball

Contact with the ball begins when the racket moves from the backswing (Photo 2.2). The weight is transferred from back foot to lead foot. The lead leg is bent at contact while the back leg is beginning to straighten. The palm of the hand grasping the racket is behind the ball at impact, with a firm wrist and with the arm extended 8 to 10 inches from the body. The nonracket arm is extended toward the ball, giving direction to the ball and balance to the body.

The ball is hit off the lead leg at slightly above midthigh to above waist level. The sequence of backswing to contact with the ball requires stepping into the ball, transferring the weight forward, and keeping the ball away from the body at a position toward the net and sideline (Photo 2.3).

Follow-Through

The final part of the sequence is the *follow-through*. The wrist remains firm and fixed, and the arm extends

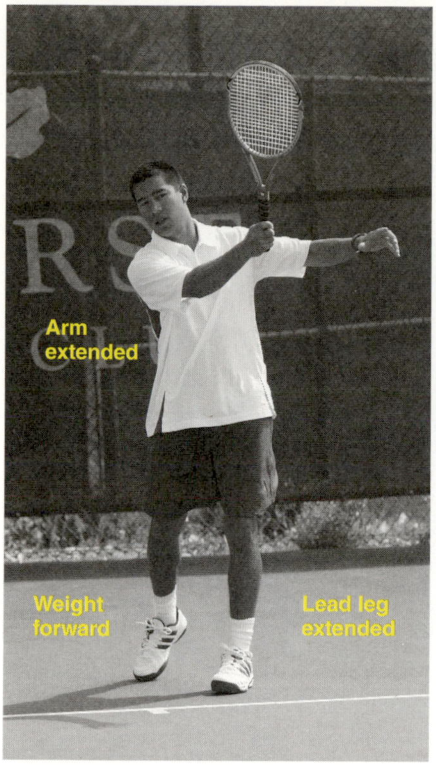

Photography by Terrell Lloyd; assisted by Anna Symonds Myers

PHOTO 2.4 Forehand groundstroke follow-through.

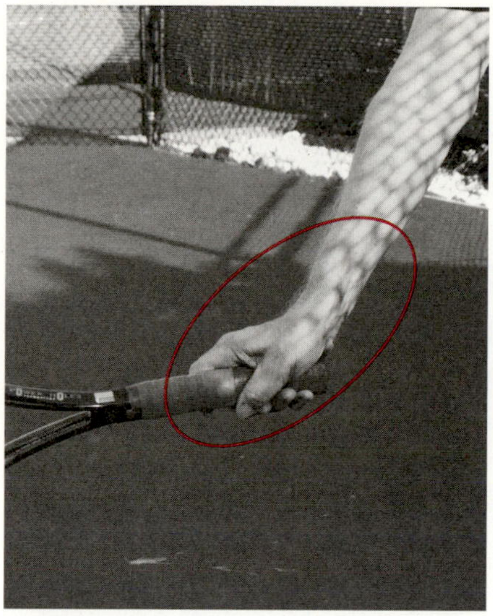

Photography by Virginia Bryant

PHOTO 2.5 Forehand groundstroke, closeup of shoulder, elbow, and wrist.

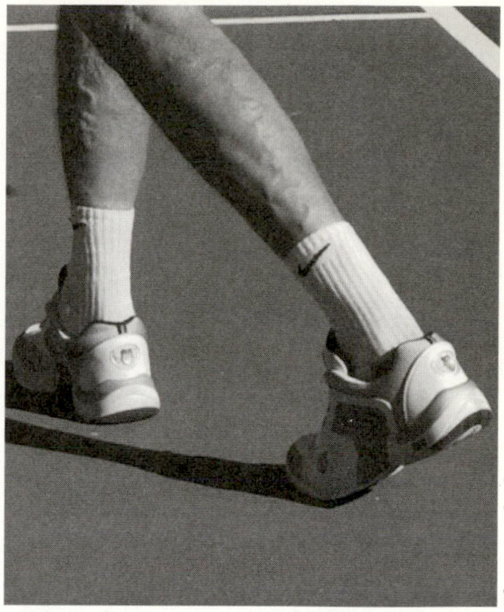

Photography by Virginia Bryant

PHOTO 2.6 Weight centered over balls of the feet.

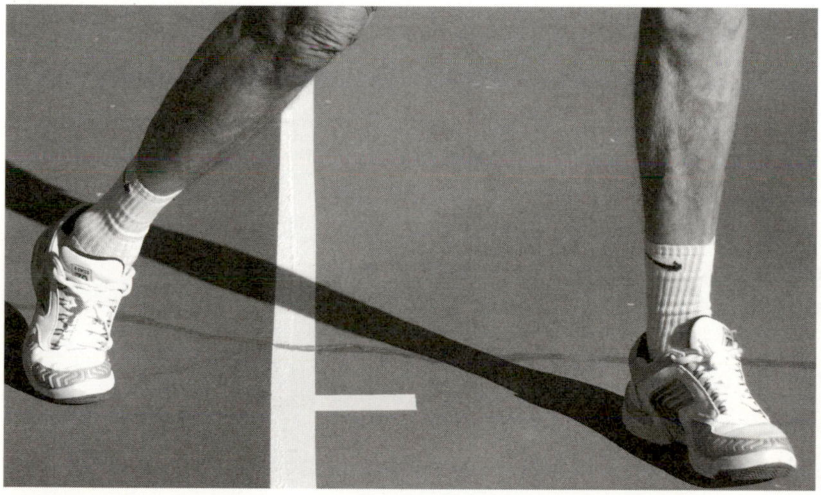

Photography by Virginia Bryant

PHOTO 2.7 Pivoting and lifting actions through the stroke.

out across the body, with the inside of the upper arm nearly touching the chin. The legs lift throughout the follow-through, with the lead leg fully extended and the back leg slightly bent. The purpose of the follow-through is to eliminate premature lifting or pulling of the ball before it leaves the racket strings at contact (Photo 2.4).

Full Sequence

Crucial to executing the stroke are the *position of the elbow and wrist* and the *transfer of weight*. The wrist and arm *must* remain firm but relaxed throughout the stroke. The tendency is to lay back the wrist and to hyper-extend the elbow. The wrist should not rotate, and the elbow should remain slightly bent. Both should remain firm (Photo 2.5).

Weight transfer provides the needed drive behind the ball, with the center of gravity directed forward through the stroke by a stepping motion into the ball. During the weight transfer, the legs must be bent, with a change in the degree of bend through the full stroke.

Footwork and *early preparation* are both critical to success with the forehand groundstroke. Footwork supplies the mobility and balance that provide the base for the stroke, and it sets the stage for weight transfer and leg power. Weight has to be centered over the balls of the feet to effect ease of movement, and the pivoting and lifting actions aid throughout the stroke in placing the body in a position to hit the ball (Photos 2.6 and 2.7). The early preparation includes good shoulder

Basic Forehand Groundstroke

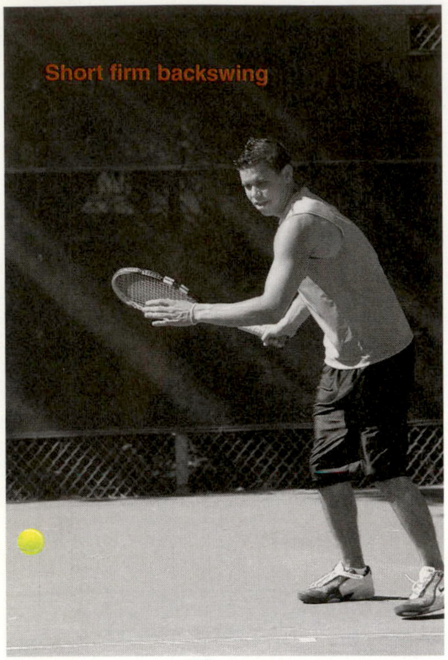

PHOTO 2.8A Backswing.

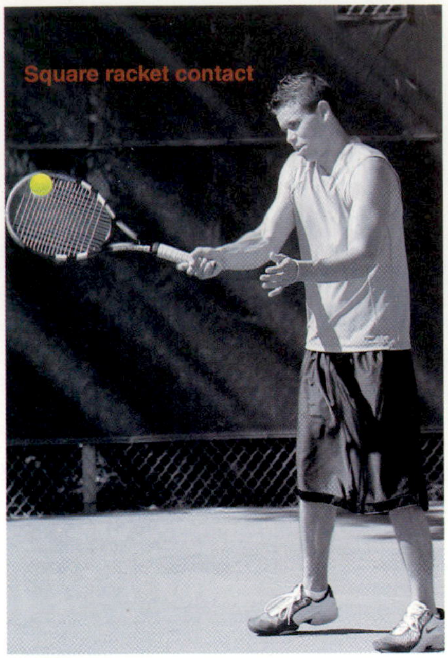

PHOTO 2.8B Contact.

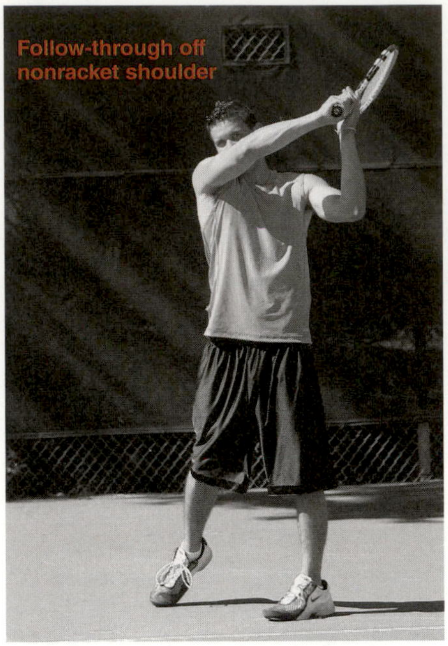

PHOTO 2.8C Follow-through.

Photography by Terrell Lloyd; assisted by Anna Symonds Myers

rotation and accompanying foot pivot with a loop backswing. That early response to the opponent's shot is the base for all that follows.

The stroke must be performed in full sequence, with a fluid movement from one part to the next. Any jerky, nongrooved action will detract from the stroke. The acceptable sequence has to include coordination of feet, legs, shoulder, arm, and wrist (Photos 2.8A–C).

POINTS *to* REMEMBER

BASIC FOREHAND GROUNDSTROKE

1. Always start from a ready position.
2. Prepare with an early shoulder rotation and pivot of the feet.
3. Activate the loop or a straight-back backswing.
4. Step into the ball at contact by transferring your weight forward, whether using an open or closed stance.
5. Contact the ball with a firm wrist.
6. Swing through the line of the ball, with the follow-through extending high and across the body.
7. Maintain a full, synchronized sequence to the timing of the stroke.

COMMON ERRORS & HOW TO CORRECT THEM *(Basic Forehand Groundstroke)*

The Error	What Causes the Error	To Correct the Error
Ball pulled to the nonracket side of the court.	Hitting too far out in front of the body or turning the racket shoulder too much through the stroke.	Step into the ball, hitting off the lead leg. Keep your nonracket shoulder consistent with transfer of weight forward. Keep your nonracket hand out in front of your body as a reference to the ball.
Ball directed to the near racket side of the court.	Being late in the backswing position, backswing beyond the perpendicular position to the fence, or laying the wrist too far back.	React early to the flight of the ball with a 45-degree turn of the shoulders, initiating an early backswing. Keep elbow and wrist firm, from backswing to contact.
Balls hit short, with little velocity.	Not stepping into the ball with weight transfer. Racket also may be too high in the backswing. Too short of a backswing and follow-through.	Transfer your weight into the ball at contact. Change the swinging pattern to be in line with the ball, and extend both backswing and follow-through.
Balls hit long or high against opponent's back fence.	Hitting the ball with poor timing, or too hard with the weight on the back foot, or in a lifting pattern at contact; also "breaking wrist" at contact.	Synchronize the timing of the stroke through backswing contact and follow-through range. Use good weight transfer. Keep your wrist firm; don't lean back at contact with the ball.

Groundstrokes—Basic Backhand

The basic backhand groundstroke is the easier of the two strokes (forehand vs. backhand) to hit mechanically, yet it is the stroke that most players fail to execute successfully in competition. Hitting a backhand is easy and fun, but first the player must develop confidence.

The *grip* used for the basic backhand is the *eastern backhand grip*, with the hand rolled onto the top of the racket grip so the "V" is pointed to the nonracket shoulder when the racket is held in front of the body. Another guide for the grip is to align the knuckles of the racket hand with the net when the racket makes contact with the ball.

As with all forehand strokes and backhands, the stroke has three phases that all mesh into a consistent, grooved feeling.

Preparation to Hit the Ball

From the ready position preparing to hit the ball is based on an early reaction to the ball, with an immediate rotation of both shoulders. The feet pivot during the shoulder rotation, and the racket starts its backswing movement with either the loop or straight-back technique. The loop is pulled back at eye level and then dropped about 8 inches below the contact point of the ball (Photo 2.9).

A change of grips also occurs in the preparation phase. The player begins the stroke from a ready position with an eastern forehand grip. As the player reacts to the ball and turns the shoulders and pivots the feet, the racket begins its backward journey. As the racket initially moves back, the player uses the nonracket hand to adjust the grip by turning the racket at the throat until the top of the hand is seen as the racket follows the

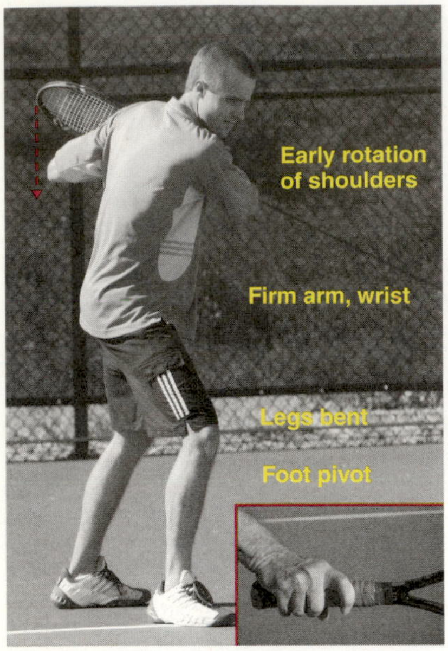

Photography by Terrell Lloyd; assisted by Anna Symonds Myers; inset photo by Virginia Bryant

PHOTO 2.9 Backhand groundstroke preparation (eastern backhand grip).

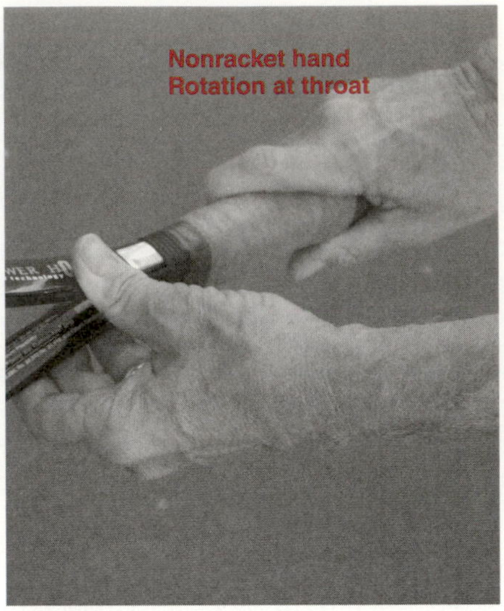

Photography by Virginia Bryant

PHOTO 2.10 Changing grips for the backhand.

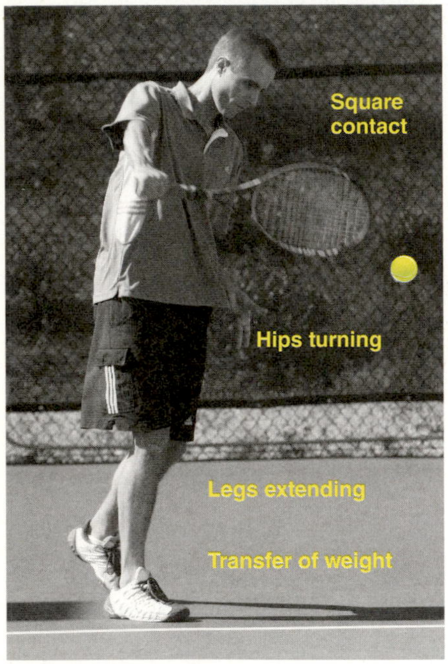

Photography by Terrell Lloyd; assisted by Anna Symonds Myers

PHOTO 2.11 Backhand groundstroke contact.

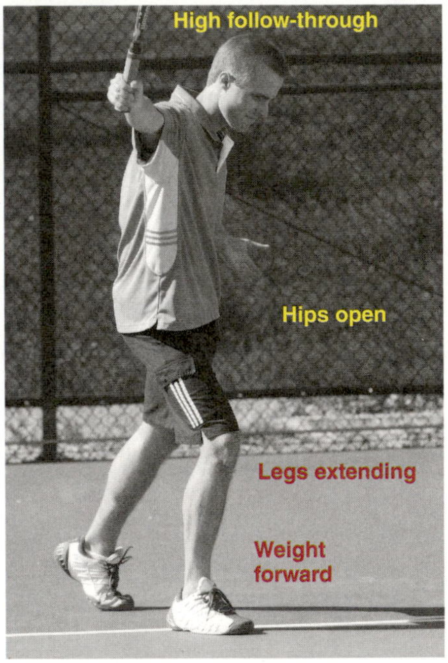

Photography by Terrell Lloyd; assisted by Anna Symonds Myers

PHOTO 2.12 Backhand groundstroke follow-through.

shoulder to the backswing position (Photo 2.10).

The nonracket hand stays in contact with the throat of the racket throughout the backswing and into the movement forward to hit the ball. During the final extension backward, the racket is perpendicular to the back fence. The weight of the body is centered over the back foot, and the legs are bent, permitting the body to be coiled for the next phase of the stroke.

Contact with the Ball

Contact with the ball occurs with a level-to-high swinging pattern that will ensure direction for the ball. The shoulder leads the elbow into the swing, and the elbow leads the wrist. This provides an accumulating effect so that at contact the racket is square to the ball and the joint alignment from shoulder to wrist is a straight line. That joint alignment provides a firm base of support as the ball strikes the racket face. The weight of the body is transferred to the lead leg just prior to contact with the ball, and the position of the racket to the lead leg at contact is midthigh to slightly above waist level (Photo 2.11).

Follow-Through

The follow-through is an extension of the level-to-high swinging action, with the weight continuing forward off the lead leg as the lead leg straightens and the back leg bends slightly (Photo 2.12). This provides a degree of balance to the base of the stroke. The wrist remains firm as the racket finishes high, facing the racket side of the sideline.

Key elements in the basic backhand groundstroke are the *wrist, elbow*, and *shoulder positions*. The initial shoulder turn followed by the shoulder leading into the stroke are essential movements in completing the action. The elbow and the wrist never should be physically ahead of the racket (Photo 2.13). The racket should rotate around the wrist, and the wrist should rotate around the elbow from backswing to contact with the ball.

At follow-through the racket should lead the wrist and elbow.

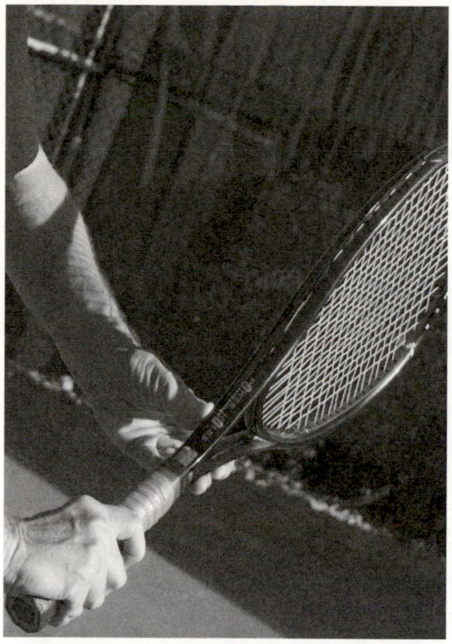

Photography by Virginia Bryant

PHOTO 2.13 Backhand groundstroke, closeup of shoulder, elbow, and wrist.

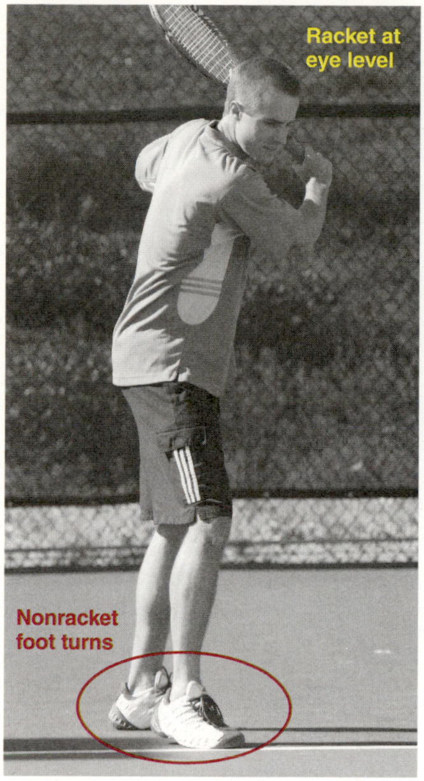

Photography by Terrell Lloyd; assisted by Anna Symonds Myers

PHOTO 2.14 Backhand groundstroke loop—pull the racket back at eye level.

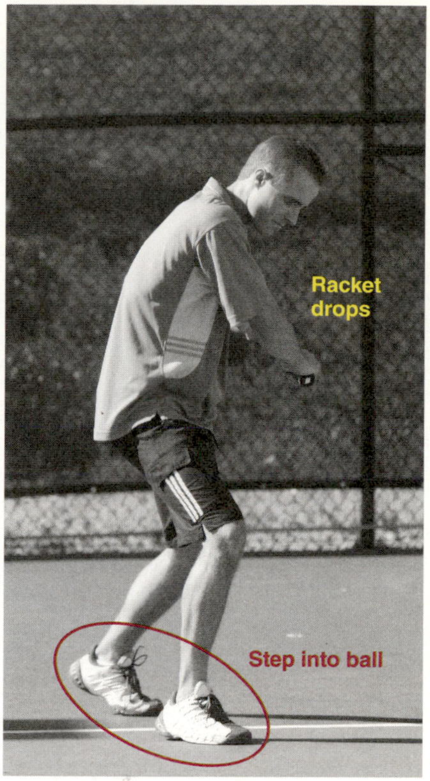

Photography by Terrell Lloyd; assisted by Anna Symonds Myers

PHOTO 2.15 Backhand groundstroke loop—drop the racket below the projected contact point of the ball.

If the elbow or wrist leads the racket at contact, a pushing action will result, decreasing the velocity of the ball. In addition, if you lead with the elbow, that incorrect mechanical position can eventually lead to tennis elbow, an injury discussed in Chapter 10. A final aspect of the follow-through requires that the racket arm stay closer to the body—at a distance of perhaps 6 to 8 inches—than with the forehand.

Full Sequence

Racket control, weight transfer, footwork, and *leg power* all contribute to the success or failure of the backhand groundstroke. Racket control is characterized by the loop—pulling the racket back at eye level (Photo 2.14) and then dropping the racket below or even with the projected contact point of the ball (Photo 2.15).

Balance and weight transfer occur when the player uses proper footwork from the ready position to the final follow-through. The critical part of the footwork involves the singular turn of the nonracket foot when the shoulder rotates (Photo 2.14—see circle) and the subsequent stepping into the ball with the racket-side foot just prior to contact with the ball (Photo 2.15—see circle). The weight transfer is a total exchange of weight, from the back foot during preparation to the lead leg at contact and then on through follow-through.

The full sequence of actions involved in the basic backhand groundstroke will determine the outcome of the stroke. Movement must be a fluid sequence void of all jerky or shaky movement. That sequence should include coordination of shoulders, feet, legs, elbow, and wrist into a mechanically

Basic Backhand Groundstroke

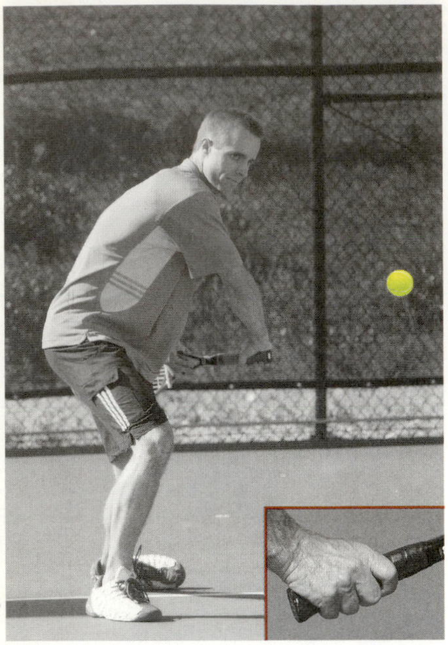
Virginia Bryant

PHOTO 2.16A Backswing.

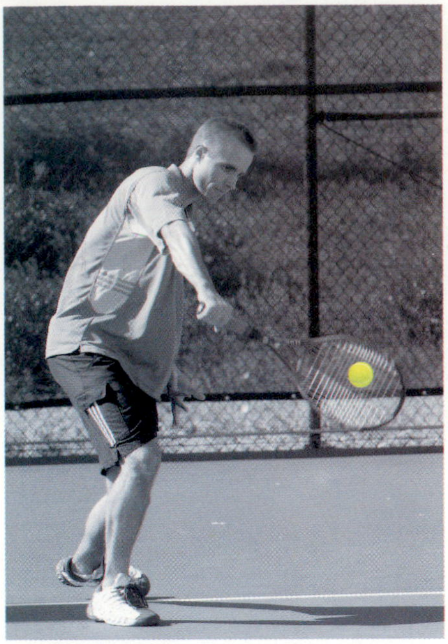

PHOTO 2.16B Contact.

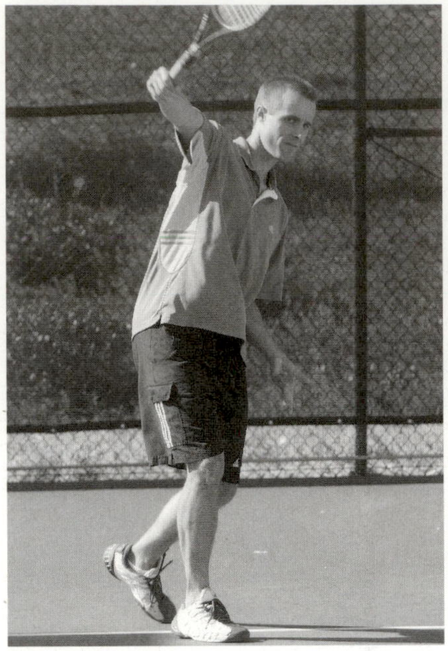

PHOTO 2.16C Follow-through.

Photography by Terrell Lloyd; assisted by Anna Symonds Myers; inset photo by Virginia Bryant

smooth, grooved stroke that causes the racket to contact the ball in a nearly square position and that flows to an ultimate follow-through (Photos 2.16A–C). As a final thought, the mechanics of the stroke have to be combined with the belief that the backhand is easier to execute and mechanically more sound than the forehand.

POINTS *to* REMEMBER

BASIC FOREHAND GROUNDSTROKE

1. Always start from the ready position.
2. Prepare with an early shoulder rotation and pivot of the feet.
3. Activate the loop or a straight-back motion backswing.
4. Change the grip, using your nonracket hand to turn the racket, from an eastern forehand to an eastern backhand as the racket is brought to the backswing position.
5. Keep a firm wrist, and keep the elbow and wrist behind the racket to contact.
6. Transfer the weight from the back to the front foot as the racket moves from backswing to contact to follow-through.
7. Swing low to high, with the racket finishing high and parallel to the racket-side sideline.
8. Keep a full synchronized sequence to the timing of the stroke.

COMMON ERRORS & HOW TO CORRECT THEM (Basic Backhand Groundstroke)

The Error	What Causes the Error	To Correct the Error
Ball pulled to the nonracket side of the court.	Hitting too far out in front of the body or turning the racket shoulder too early.	Stay sideways as long as you can during the swing. Avoid pulling your racket shoulder at contact.
Ball directed to the nonracket side of the court.	Too late in shoulder turn to initiate a backswing.	Anticipate early, and turn your shoulder to set up the backswing. Keep elbow and wrist firm from backswing to contact.
Ball hit short or into the net with little velocity.	Not stepping into the ball at contact, with minimal weight transfer. Too short of a backswing and follow-through.	Step into the ball and transfer your weight forward. Hit with the flat racket face and follow a racket pattern from semilow to high. Hit with an extended and fixed racket arm.
Ball hit long or high against opponent's fence.	Hitting with poor timing or weight on back foot. Also, opening racket face too much and not following through and/or "breaking" wrist at contact.	Synchronize the timing, and transfer your weight to the lead foot at contact and follow-through. Step into the ball at contact, with racket face square. Make sure to follow through. Also, check your grip and make sure it is an eastern backhand grip.

Groundstrokes—Two-Hand Backhand

The two-hand backhand is immensely popular today with people who need the added strength for force and velocity as well as more control, particularly the beginner who has trouble hitting the *sweet spot* of the racket face. The player using the two-hand backhand will gain confidence in the backhand but at the same time sacrifice the reach related to the conventional backhand stroke. The two-hand backhand provides a natural topspin application to the ball, eliminating the basic flat backhand stroke.

In the *two-hand backhand*, the dominant hand grips the racket with a continental or eastern backhand grip at the butt end of the racket handle. The nondominant hand rests on top of the racket-side hand in an eastern forehand grip. The heel of the support hand is nestled snugly between the thumb and index finger of the racket-side hand.

Preparation to Hit the Ball

Preparation for hitting the ball involves basic rotation of the shoulders, except that the rotation will be limited because of the two-hand position. Rather than a loop backswing, the racket is brought straight back and then dropped low toward the feet. The same foot pivot and weight transfer occur with the two-hand backhand as with the conventional eastern forehand and backhand (Photo 2.17A).

Basic Two-Hand Backhand Groundstroke

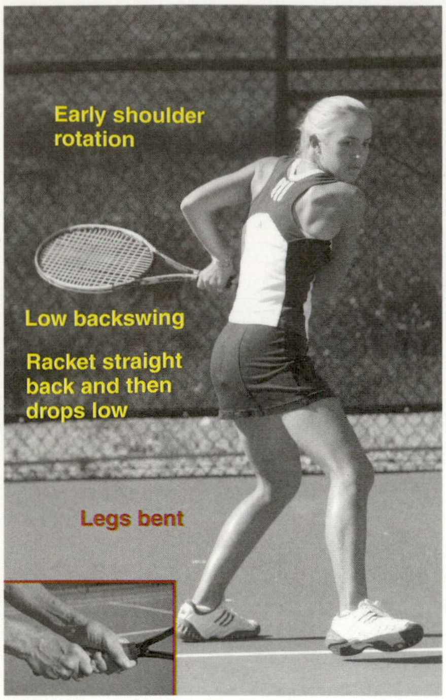

PHOTO 2.17A Backswing (two-hand backhand grip).

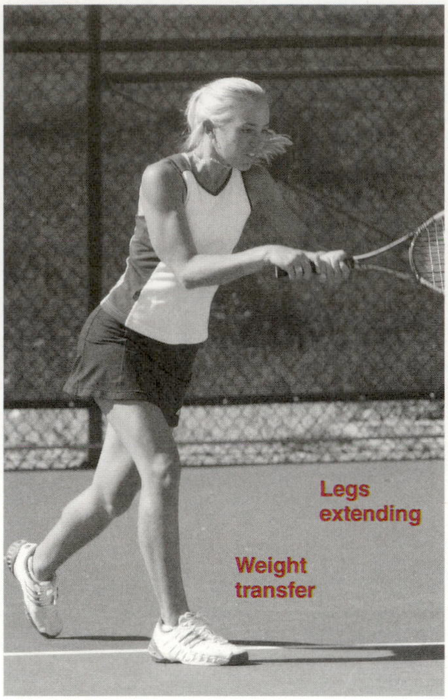

PHOTO 2.17B Contact.

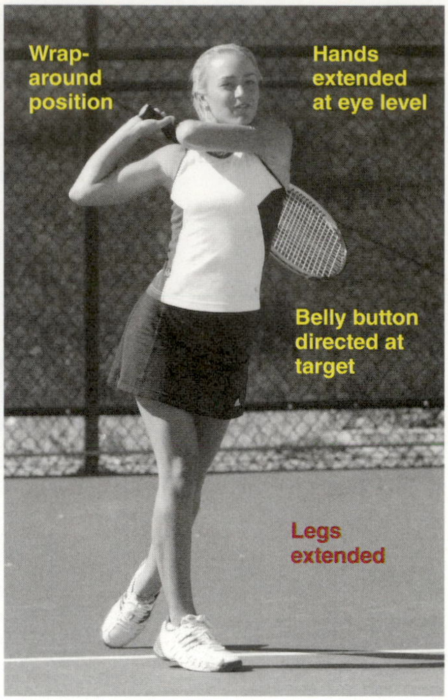

PHOTO 2.17C Follow-through.

Photography by Terrell Lloyd; assisted by Anna Symonds Myers; inset photo by Virginia Bryant

Contact with the Ball

Contact with the ball involves continuation of the low-to-high pattern, with the arms close to the body and the wrists firm. As with all strokes, the weight is transferred forward to the lead foot as the player steps into the ball to make contact off that lead foot. As the weight is transferred, the contact of the ball occurs between midthigh and waist level (Photo 2.17B).

Follow-Through

The follow-through is a simple continuation of the stroke, with the legs extended and with the hands extended and at eye level, your belly button turned to your target. The full wraparound swing comes from your shoulders and requires a solid, compact swing action. The hands work together throughout the swing (Photo 2.17C).

POINTS *to* REMEMBER

TWO-HAND BACKHAND GROUNDSTROKE

1. Keep your arms close to your body throughout the stroke, and keep your wrists firm.
2. Make sure that the two hands are snug to each other on the grip.
3. Use a low backswing to a high follow-through.
4. Make contact with the ball at midthigh-to-waist level.
5 Incorporate a compact, full wraparound swing.

COMMON ERRORS & HOW TO CORRECT THEM *(Two-Hand Backhand Groundstroke)*

The Error	What Causes the Error	To Correct the Error
Stroking the ball into the net.	Hitting too far in front of the lead leg or not following the low-to-high pattern.	Start with a low backswing, moving through the ball in an upward movement at contact, and then follow through to a high wraparound position.
Hitting the ball long or high against the fence.	Dropping the racket to a low position and bending the knees in an exaggerated low-to-high follow-through and leg extension. Opening the racket face through backswing, contact, and follow-through.	Swing low to high, and use a low leg bend followed by an extension of the legs, but eliminate the exaggerated movement. Make sure your grip is a combination of continental or eastern backhand next to the nondominant eastern forehand grip.
Hitting the ball off the end of the racket or not getting to the ball in time.	Poor reaction time and little anticipation of where the ball will be hit. Reaching when you should be moving your feet.	Concentrate on the ball when it is in on the far side of the net. Remember that the radius of the reach is shorter with a two-hand backhand than with a one-hand backhand.

Synopsis of the Groundstroke

Groundstrokes are the basis of all play in tennis. The developing player has to grow with the game and progress from a stationary position of hitting groundstrokes to a moving situation that will allow setting up to hit a ball. To balance the skill aspect of hitting groundstrokes, the player has to work on both sides of the body equally to develop both forehand and backhand. The beginning player has to be skilled at simple tasks ranging from dropping a ball and hitting a groundstroke to knowing where homebase is and moving from homebase to retrieve and stroke the ball.

Self-Drop

Learning how to *drop and hit the ball* to begin a rally is necessary if a player is going to practice, warm up, or actually play the game. With a forehand groundstroke, the drop should be toward the sideline and toward the net so that the player has to extend the arm to reach the ball and step, transferring weight to the lead leg to hit the ball. Dropping the ball anywhere else would confuse the player, eliminate form development for each stroke, and provide a difficult setup to begin a rally. One of the reasons for a forehand developing more quickly is that a player tends to practice more on the forehand side. Typically this is because it is more convenient to drop the ball on that side to begin a rally (Photos 2.18A and B).

The drop for the backhand should be attempted as often as the forehand drop to encourage development of the backhand stroke. The backhand differs from the forehand drop only in that the drop is completed under the racket on the backhand side and the racket is not yet in a complete backswing position. The ball is dropped in a palm-up position, and a lifting action allows the ball to bounce and come straight back up off the rebound to midthigh level to be hit. During the drop and swing, the body is turned to

Self-Drop for Forehand

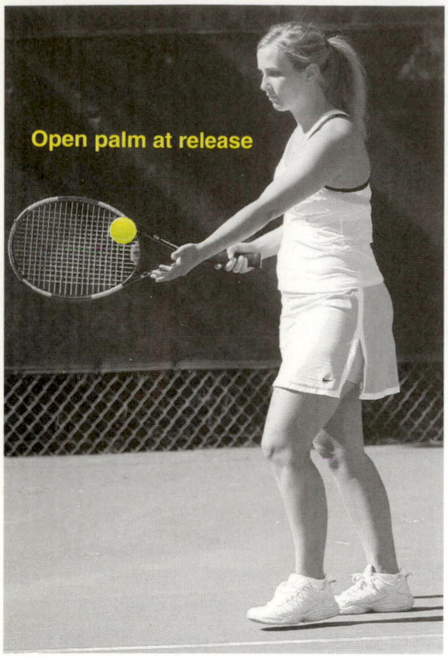

PHOTO 2.18A Drop the ball toward the sideline and toward the net.

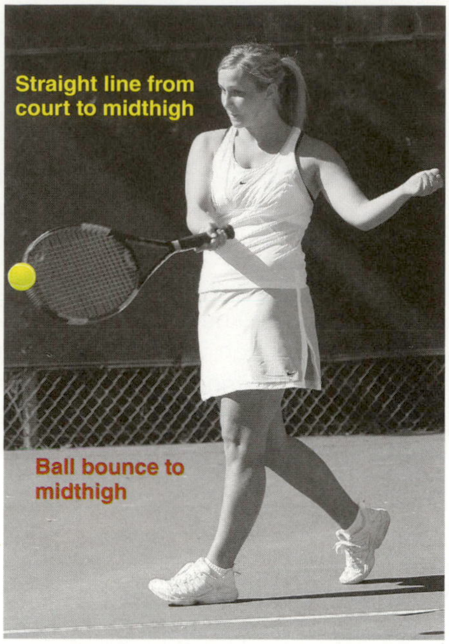

PHOTO 2.18B Ball should bounce and come straight back up to midthigh.

Photography by Terrell Lloyd; assisted by Anna Symonds Myers

Self-Drop for Backhand

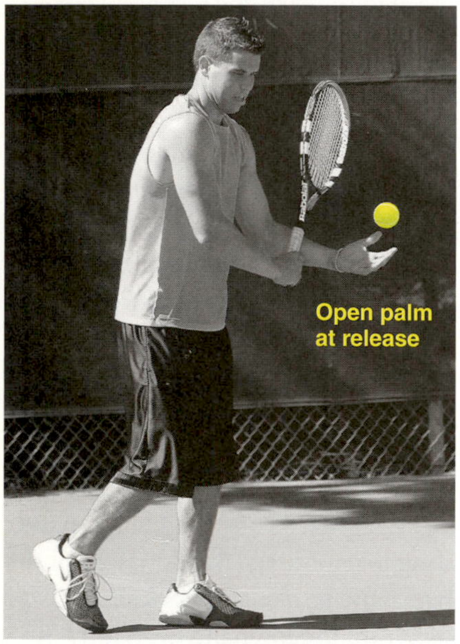

PHOTO 2.19A Drop the ball toward the sideline and toward the net.

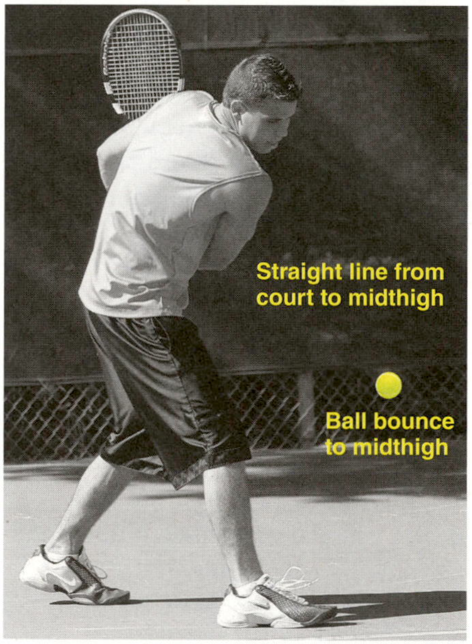

PHOTO 2.19B Ball should bounce and come straight back up to midthigh.

Photography by Terrell Lloyd; assisted by Anna Symonds Myers

the side, facing the appropriate sideline (Photos 2.19A and B). The drop for the two-hand backhand is the same as for the basic backhand, except you need to regrasp with your two-hand grip after dropping the ball.

Homebase

Practice with groundstrokes usually begins from a stationary position. The area behind the baseline is known as *Homebase* (Figure 2.1). It is a great learning experience for the player just beginning to develop the mechanics of a sound groundstroke to have all balls hit deep to that position. The rationale for having balls thrown to students in the early stages of skill development or having a ball machine direct balls to a player is to ensure that homebase is identified and that practice is as consistent as possible. There comes a time, however, when the player has to leave homebase and move after a ball hit a distance away. The player must leave the homebase area, move toward the ball, and hit a groundstroke—then return to homebase.

Moving to the Ball

Moving to the ball, which involves proper footwork, is a major problem for the beginning tennis player. If the ball is hit deep, with a high and deep bounce, the player must retreat behind the baseline to get to the ball, set up, and then step back into the ball with weight transfer. To respond to a deeply hit ball, the player first must turn the shoulder (remember—the player always starts from a ready position) and take a sideward step with the foot that is on the same side as the turning shoulder. From that point, the movement is either a sideward response or a total turn and run to at least a step beh... from the ball. The turning move... away must occur as soon as possible, preferably before the ball crosses the net (Photo 2.20).

Moving to the ball when it is in front of the player is a little easier, but it requires early anticipation of where the ball is going. The player moves in a direct line forward, with timing that will provide opportunity to set up behind the ball and away from the line of the ball's flight. The last part of the movement involves slowing down and gathering the body in a controlled manner and then stepping in a direct line to the ball with the racket-side foot first, thereby aligning the body to the path of the ball and establishing the next sequential step.

The next step involves stepping into the ball with the nonracket-side leg in a timed movement to synchronize with the contact part of the full stroke. As the racket-side leg steps first, the racket is in a backswing position; then it comes through into the ball at contact (Photo 2.21). There is no difference between hitting a forehand and a backhand groundstroke. The point is to set up behind and to the side of the ball as described when hitting the ball to start a rally.

Moving to the ball or hitting from the baseline will be enjoyable if a foundation is built from the baseline that is consistent for all groundstrokes. The foundation of hitting with a stepping movement, having good weight transfer, and developing a sound stroke pattern is basic. The foundation must be repeated so often that each stroke becomes an instinctive reaction that requires no thought and assures fluidity of movement.

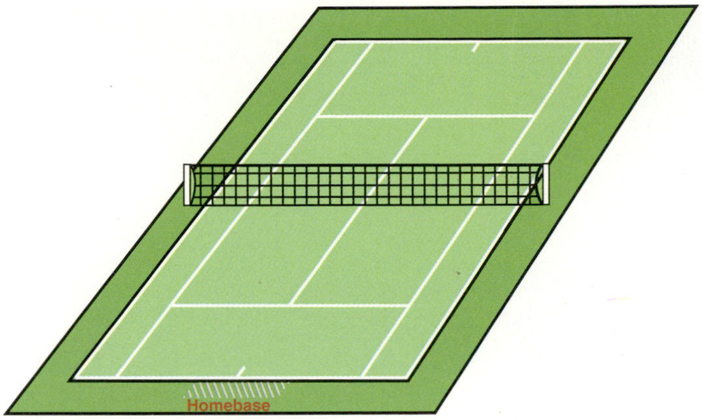

FIGURE 2.1 Homebase.

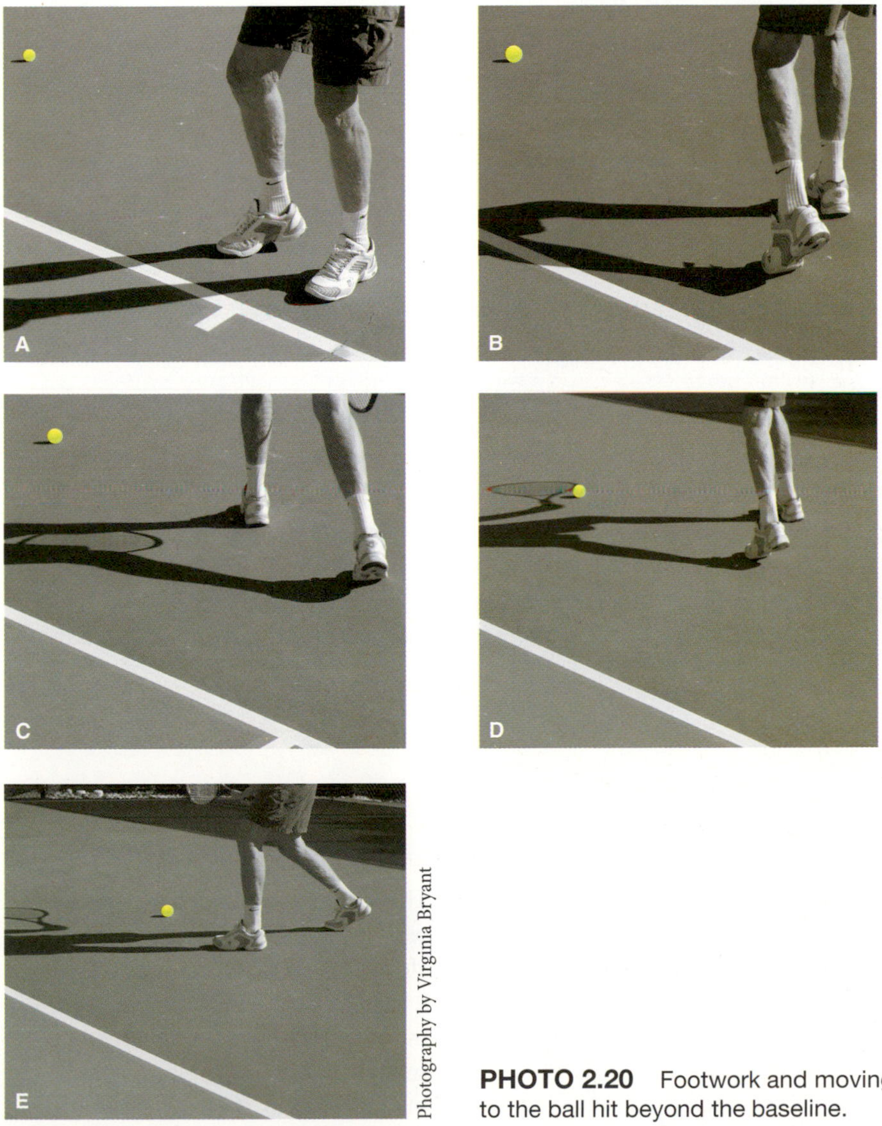

Photography by Virginia Bryant

PHOTO 2.20 Footwork and moving to the ball hit beyond the baseline.

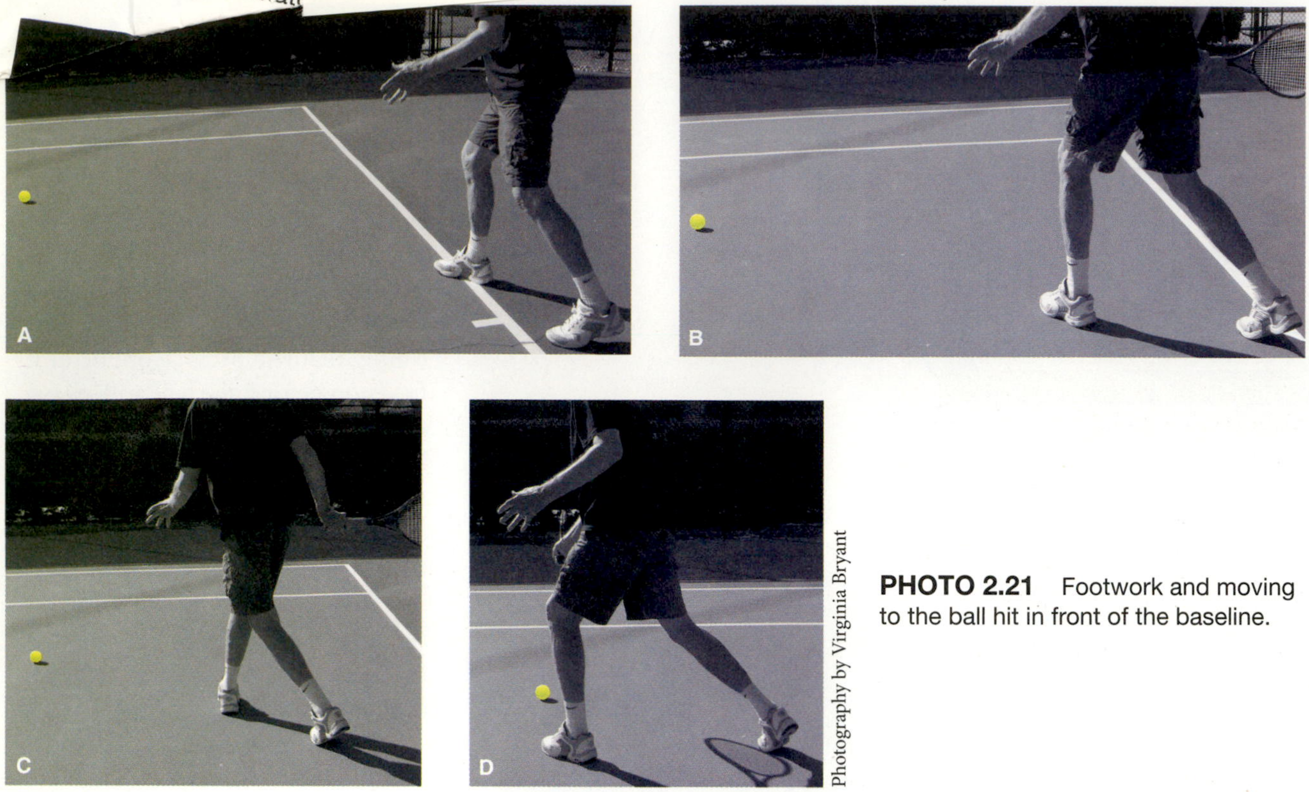

Photography by Virginia Bryant

PHOTO 2.21 Footwork and moving to the ball hit in front of the baseline.

POINTS *to* REMEMBER

SYNOPSIS OF THE GROUNDSTOKE

1. Learn to self-drop the ball to begin a groundstroke, keeping the ball a step in front and to the side of you.
2. Hit from homebase when practicing groundstrokes; when forced to move to hit a ball, make sure you return to homebase.
3. When moving to hit a ball beyond you or in front of you, remember to pivot first and then set up away from the ball, allowing yourself to step into the ball at contact.

Increasing Beginner Skills: Forehand Groundstroke—Slice and Topspin

The basic forehand groundstroke is the stroke that beginners start with. But if they are to increase their skills, they have to identify and eventually hit a *forehand slice groundstroke* and a *forehand topspin groundstroke*.

Forehand Topspin Groundstroke

The topspin stroke begins with a very low backswing, a slightly closed racket face at contact, and a high follow-through. At contact the forearm rotates somewhat. In addition, the legs play a part in this stroke, with a low bend of the knees during the backswing followed by an extension of the legs in the follow-through position (Photos 2.22A–C). The spin

Forehand Topspin Groundstroke

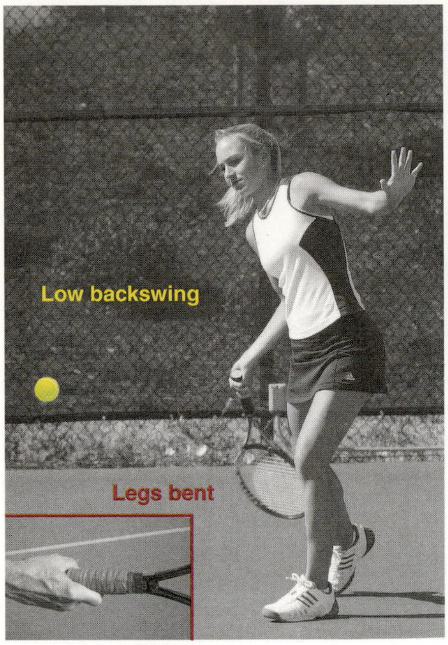

PHOTO 2.22A Backswing (Semi-Western Forehand Grip).

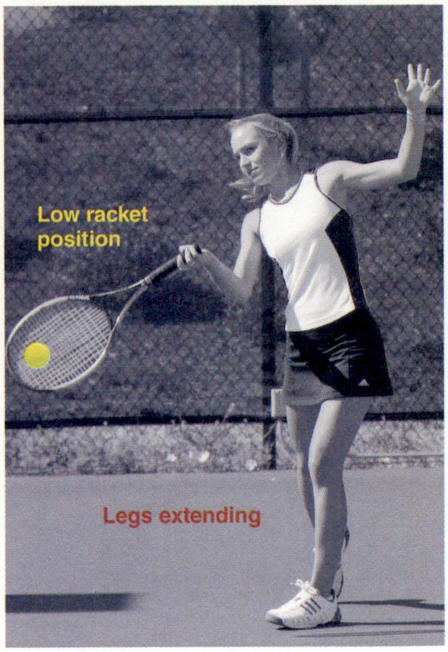

PHOTO 2.22B Contact.

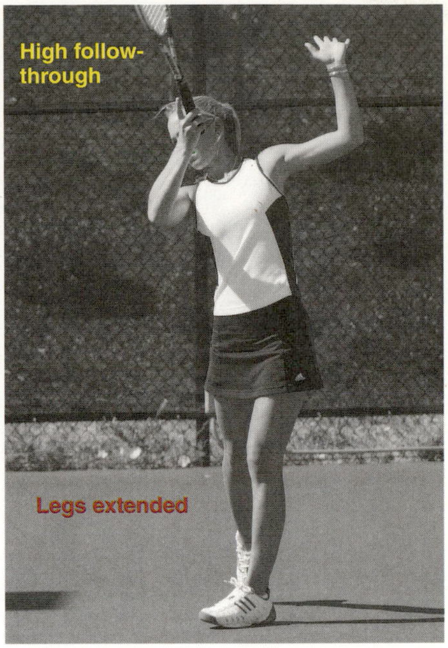

PHOTO 2.22C Follow-through.

Photography by Terrell Lloyd; assisted by Anna Symonds Myers; inset photo by Virginia Bryant

of the ball is an overspin, or topspin, and the ball action upon striking the court surface is a high bounce. The grip used for a slice is still the eastern forehand grip; but to gain additional spin, the grip for the topspin changes to a semi-western grip.

Forehand Slice Groundstroke

The slice requires a high backswing and a slightly open-face contact point, followed by a high follow-through (Photos 2.23A–C). The spin imparted to the ball is underspin, with the ball staying low to the net, followed by a skidding action or a low bounce when rebounding off the court.

Forehand Groundstroke Progression

The beginner first has to develop the basic stroke and then move to the slice and topspin in a progression. For most beginners, the slice is more difficult to develop. In contrast, the forehand topspin groundstroke comes naturally to many players, and often it is typically the first forehand groundstroke that young players learn.

Increasing Beginner Skills: Backhand Groundstroke—Slice and Topspin

As with the forehand slice and topspin groundstroke, the basic backhand is the starting point for a beginner. But two strokes add to the groundstroke development: the *backhand slice groundstroke* and the *backhand topspin groundstroke*.

Forehand Slice Groundstroke

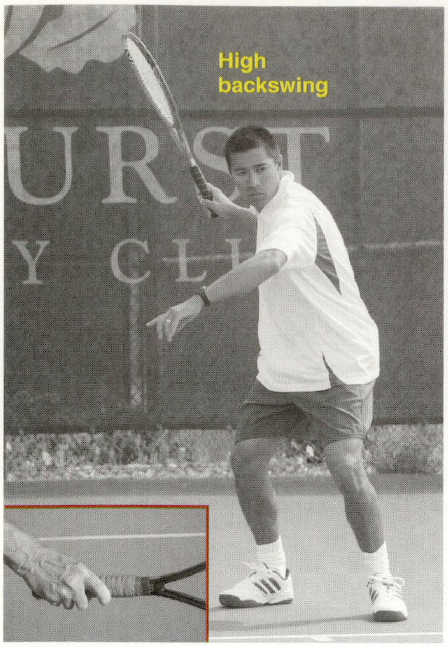

PHOTO 2.23A Backswing (eastern forehand grip).

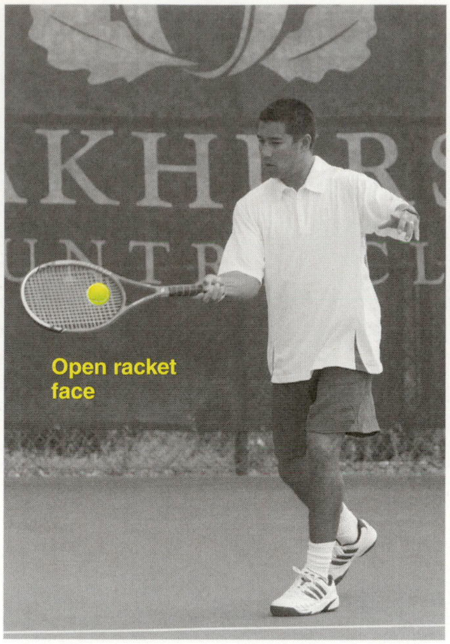

PHOTO 2.23B Contact.

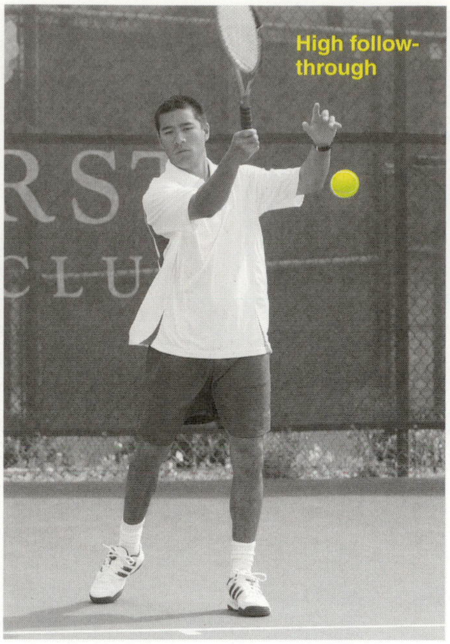

PHOTO 2.23C Follow-through.

Photography by Terrell Lloyd; assisted by Anna Symonds Myers; inset photo by Virginia Bryant

Backhand Topspin Groundstroke

The topspin groundstroke starts with a low backswing, a slightly closed face at contact, and a high follow-through (Photos 2.24A–C). The forearm does rotate slightly from contact to follow-through, and the legs bend and extend from backswing to follow-through. The eastern backhand grip is used for both the slice and the topspin.

Backhand Slice Groundstroke

The slice is executed with a slightly high backswing, an open racket face at contact, and a high follow-through (Photos 2.25A–C). The ball action is the same underspin with a skidding action as it rebounds from the court. The eastern grip is used with this stroke.

Two-Hand Backhand Topspin Groundstroke

A two-hand backhand topspin stroke is particularly successful because the stroke is compact and already programmed to begin low in the backswing and continue on through to an extensive high follow-through. It becomes particularly successful when hitting a topspin backhand because the stroke is compact and already programmed to begin low in the backswing and continue on through to an extensive follow-through (see Photos 2.17A–C).

Two-Hand Backhand Slice Ground Stroke

A two-hand backhand slice groundstroke requires minor adjustments from the topspin stroke. First, the backswing needs to be adjusted to a higher position. Second, the contact

Backhand Topspin Groundstroke

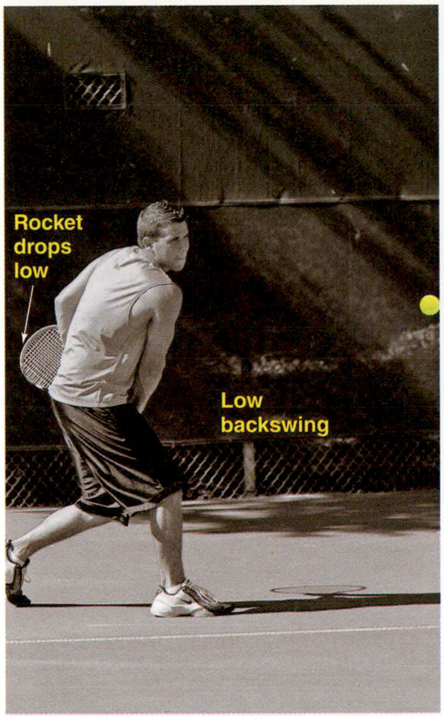

PHOTO 2.24A Backswing.

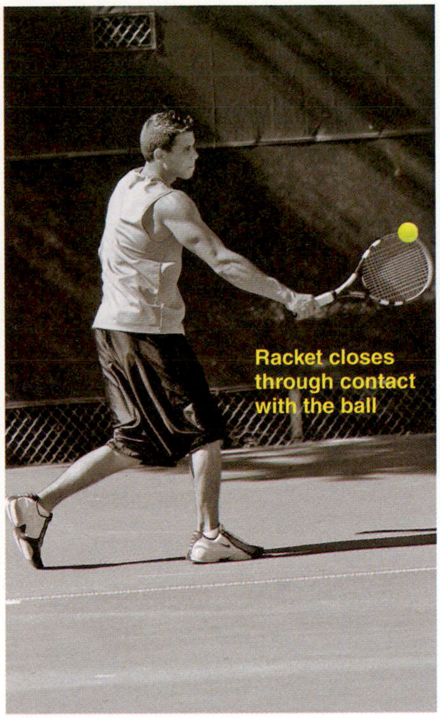

PHOTO 2.24B Contact.

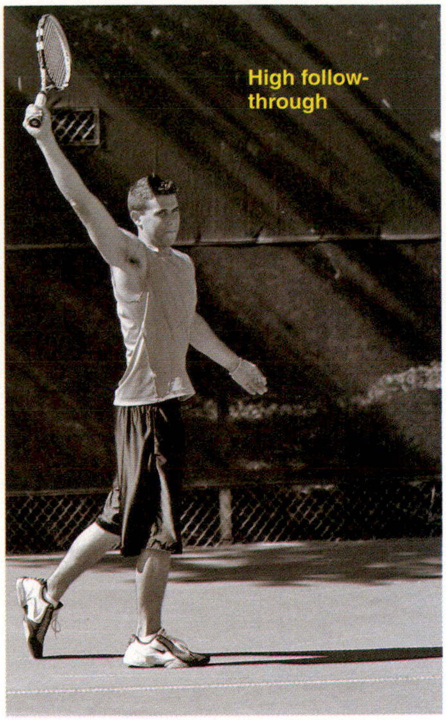

PHOTO 2.24C Follow-through.

Photography by Terrell Lloyd; assisted by Anna Symonds Myers

Backhand Slice Groundstroke

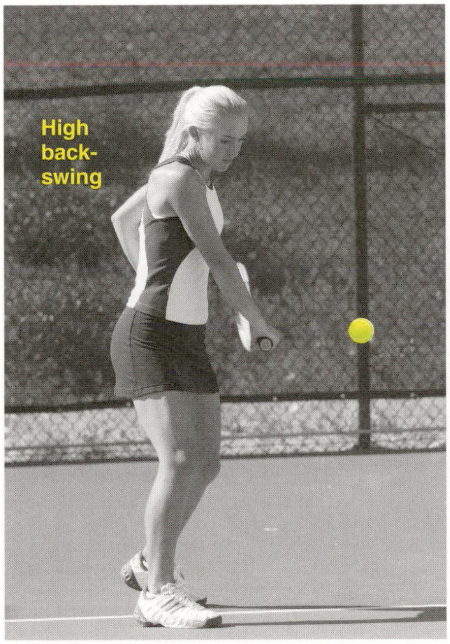

PHOTO 2.25A Backswing.

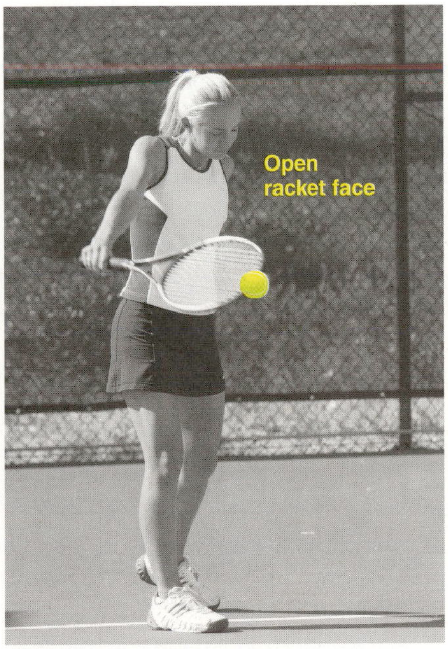

PHOTO 2.25B Contact.

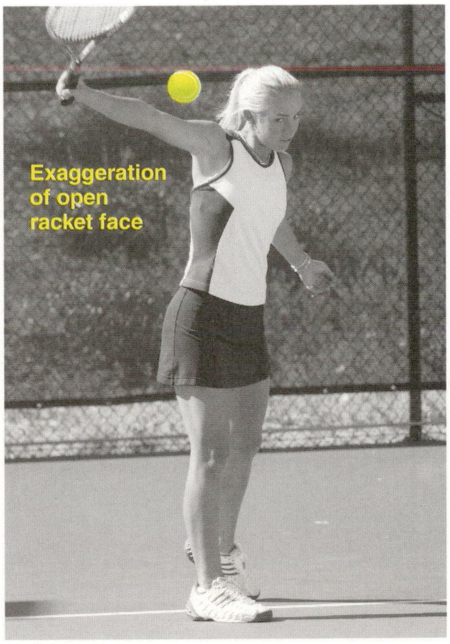

PHOTO 2.25C Follow-through.

Photography by Terrell Lloyd; assisted by Anna Symonds Myers

Two-Hand Backhand Slice Groundstroke

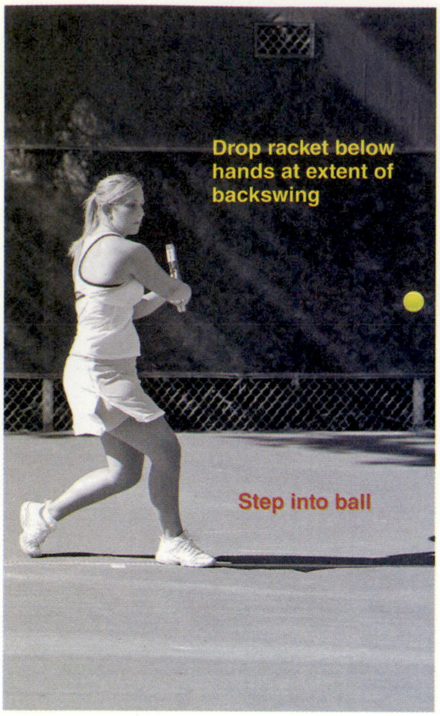

PHOTO 2.26A Backswing.

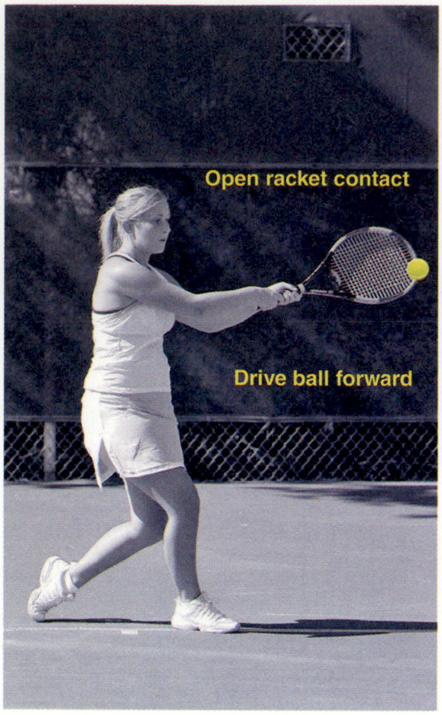

PHOTO 2.26B Contact.

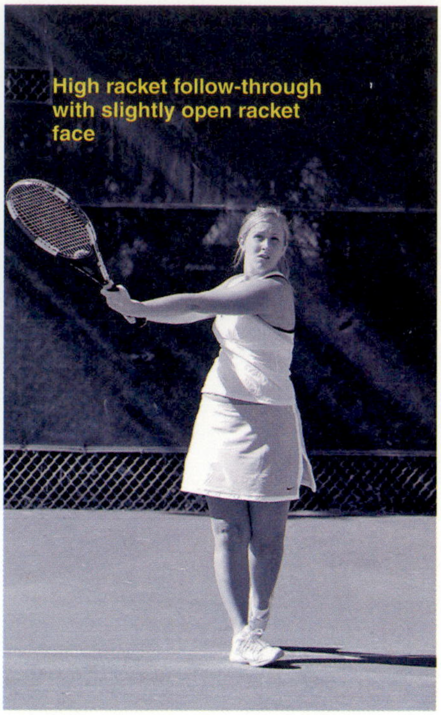

PHOTO 2.26C Follow-through.

Photography by Terrell Lloyd; assisted by Anna Symonds Myers

with the ball requires an open racket face, and third, the follow-through finishes high, in line with the direction that you hit the ball (Photos 2.26A–C).

Just as with the comments regarding the forehand groundstroke, beginners have to start with the basic backhand and progress to spin strokes. Often the slice becomes an extremely reliable stroke for the developing player, and the topspin can become quite lethal, particularly for a player who develops a two-hand backhand.

POINTS to REMEMBER

INCREASING BEGINNER GROUNDSTROKE SKILLS—SLICE AND TOPSPIN

1. A slice backswing is high, and contact is with an open-face racket. Follow-through is high and in line with the flight of the ball.
2. A topspin backswing is low, and contact is an upward brushing motion. There is a slight forearm roll as the racket continues to a follow-through off the nonracket shoulder.
3. A two-hand backhand topspin is a basic backhand alternative to a one-handed backhand executed with a natural low backswing and high follow-through.
4. The two-hand backhand slice requires a high backswing, an open racket face, and a high follow-through (no wraparound), in line with the flight of the ball.

Increasing Beginner Skills: Using the Groundstroke to Hit an Approach Shot

Moving to hit a ball situated between the baseline and the net is related to foot movement and also to decision making. It now is important to recognize which shots require the player to step into the ball, stroke the ball, and then return to homebase or to move up to the ball and hit it and then advance to the net. Shots that are hit at the service court line require the decision to continue to advance to the net to play a potential volley or to retreat to homebase. Balls that are hit between the service court line and the net require no decision: The player is advised to move forward to play at the net (Figure 2.2). When a decision must be made either to attack the net or to retreat to the baseline, or when the player must go to the net, a modification of the groundstroke called an *approach shot* is called for.

When it is determined that a player is going to hit an approach shot, that player must develop certain perceptions. First, a player must realize that the approach shot is simply a groundstroke that he or she must move toward in order to hit the ball. Second, the approach must be viewed as a gift given as a reward for excellent play on the baseline that forced the opponent to hit the ball short rather than deep. Third, a player must recognize that approach shots often allow for too much time to decide what to do with the ball, resulting in a shabby attempt at hitting the ball. Fourth, the approach shot must be considered a modified version of the full groundstroke swing. Fifth, as the beginning player improves, there is a transition from the use of a basic stroke to using spin.

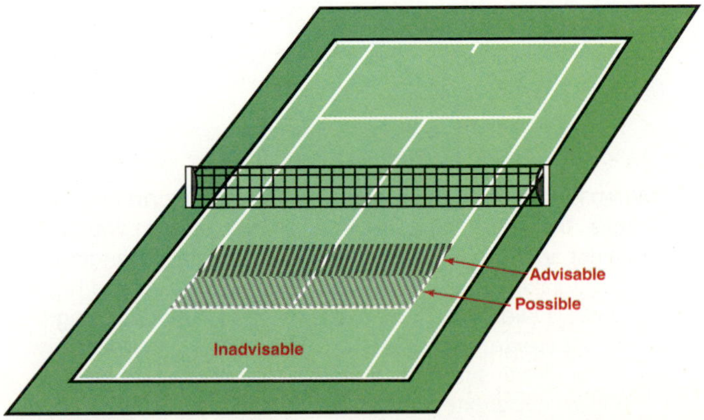

FIGURE 2.2 Foundation—when to go to the net, when to stay at homebase.

The third and fourth concepts have to be discussed in more detail. Having time to hit a shot allows the player to decide how and where to hit the ball. There is a problem, however, when the player changes the decision once it has been made. The player must make one decision on *how* to hit the ball and another on *where* to hit the ball (deep or at an angle). Both judgments are difficult for beginning players, and as a result they simply bang away at the ball, usually missing everything but the back fence. A player must be aware of the choices and continue to learn from mistakes, gaining confidence from each opportunity to hit an approach shot. The target areas are based on zones. An approach shot positioned down the line should be hit across the net to the down-the-line zone; a shot positioned in the center zone should be hit deep to the center of the court or deep to either corner zone (Figure 2.3).

Modifying the approach shot to cope with the target area is the skill adaptation to the groundstroke. Here are three adaptations to the approach shot from the groundstroke:

1. Shorten your backswing.
2. Visualize the target.
3. Select the appropriate shot sequence.

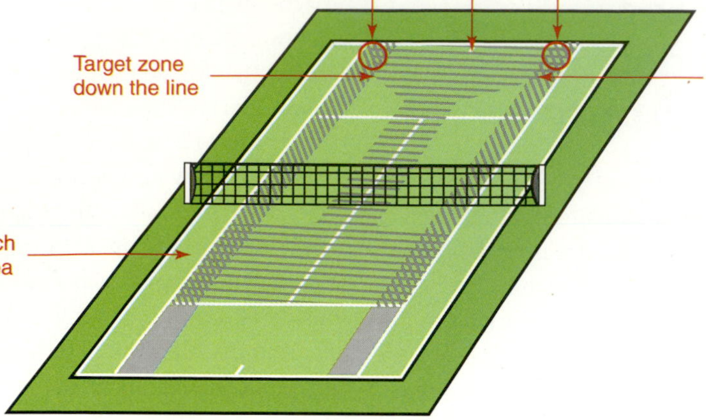

FIGURE 2.3 Approach shots down the line and in the center zone.

An approach shot doesn't require extensive force behind it, as does a shot from the baseline. Instead of bringing the racket back in a full backswing motion, it should be brought back perhaps two-thirds of that distance. If, when preparing to hit an approach shot, a player develops mental imagery of the target as being located at the opponent's service court line, the ensuing distance the ball travels probably will increase by a third of the distance. As a result, the ball will really travel to the opponent's baseline. The baseline is the spot desired for a deep hit, but the mental imagery has to give a shortened target distance to allow for the shortened distance the ball actually must travel.

The player continues the sequence once an approach shot is hit by moving to the net to play a potential volley return of the opponent's reaction to the approach shot, or the player can return to the baseline and home-base. (Discussion of the volley sequence is found in Chapter 4).

POINTS to REMEMBER

APPROACH SHOT

1. An approach shot is a groundstroke with a short backswing.
2. The establishment of an image of hitting the ball short of the opponent's baseline will enable you to keep the ball in play by not allowing for over-hitting the ball beyond the baseline.
3. A decision has to be made regarding whether to return to the baseline or to go to the net after hitting an approach shot. You just can't stay at the spot where you hit the ball.
4. If you are at least halfway to the net, your choice is usually to continue to the net. Less than halfway may suggest that you return to the baseline.

CHECKPOINTS

1. The three parts to a basic forehand groundstroke are
   a. preparation, loop backswing, and follow-through.
   b. preparation, contact, and follow-through.
   c. loop backswing, contact, and follow-through.
   d. preparation, loop backswing, and contact.
2. When hitting a forehand groundstroke, the
   a. wrist and forearm remain firm but relaxed.
   b. wrist is laid back and the elbow is hyperextended.
   c. wrist remains firm, with the elbow hyperextended.
   d. wrist is laid back and the elbow is firm but relaxed.
3. Correcting the error of shots hit short with little velocity requires
   a. changing the swing from slightly low to high.
   b. changing the swing from slightly high to low.
   c. transferring weight into the ball at contact.
   d. stepping away from the ball at contact.

4. To hit a forehand topspin groundstroke requires an adjustment from the basic stroke, which includes
   a. eastern grip, low-to-high swing, and leg flexion and extension.
   b. semi-western grip, low-to-high swing, and leg flexion and extension.
   c. semi-western grip, flat backswing to high follow-through, and leg flexion and extension.
   d. eastern grip (changing to a semi-western grip as skill improves), low-to-high swing, and leg flexion and extension.
5. A characteristic of hitting a basic backhand groundstroke is
   a. shoulder leading into contact, with racket rotating around the wrist and elbow leading the racket.
   b. shoulder leading into contact, with the wrist and elbow leading the racket.
   c. shoulder held back, with the wrist and elbow leading the racket.
   d. shoulder leading into contact, with the racket rotating around the wrist and elbow.
6. A backhand groundstroke hit long is caused by
   a. hitting with poor timing and/or weight on the back foot.
   b. too much of an open racket face with no follow-through.
   c. hitting with an open racket face, poor timing, and not following through.
   d. all three of the above causes.
7. The two-hand backhand groundstroke requires that the follow-through is a
   a. racket finish in a wraparound of shoulders and head, and the belly button turned toward the hitting target.
   b. racket finish high, with the belly button turned toward the hitting target.
   c. racket finish in a wraparound of shoulders and head, and the belly button turned to the racket side of the body.
   d. combination of *a, b,* and *c*.
8. Hitting the ball off the end of the racket when hitting a two-hand backhand is caused by
   a. not dropping the racket to a low position.
   b. poor reaction timing and limited anticipation.
   c. hitting too far out in front of the lead leg.
   d. not swinging low to high.
9. When attempting to hit a moving ball that is short or deep, the player must
   a. set up even with the ball and step up even with the ball to hit it.
   b. set up in front of the ball and step into the ball to hit it.
   c. move at an angle to set up behind the ball and step into the ball to hit it.
   d. move straight to the ball and step into the ball to hit it.
10. Approach shots should be hit
    a. with a visual image target to the opponent's service court line.
    b. with a reduced backswing.
    c. with a target of down the line to the corners and to the center.
    d. using *b* in combination with *a* and *c*.

Answers to Checkpoints can be found on page 167.

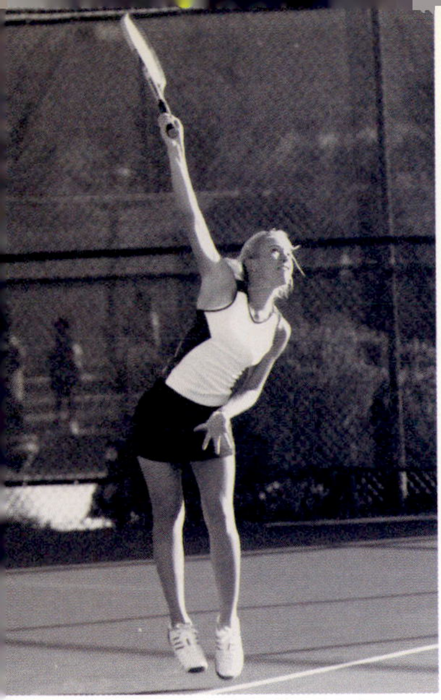

Photography by Terrell Lloyd; assisted by Anna Symonds Myers

3

Service and Service Return

The service and service return are critical to success in tennis. Groundstroke skill enables the developing player to rally from the *baseline*. Without the skills of service and service return, the beginning player is not able to place the ball into play or to return a service. The three services that are used widely in tennis are: (1) the basic flat service, (2) the slice service, and (3) the topspin service. Discussion in this chapter will be limited to the flat serve as the basic beginner serve and the slice serve as a serve to increase the beginner's skill.

Basic Flat Service

The *basic flat service* is a model for the service. A *service stance* is used in all serves. The feet are positioned approximately shoulder-width apart, with the lead foot approximately the length of a tennis ball from the baseline and the center mark of the baseline. The shoulder is pointed toward the service court target, the knees are slightly flexed, and the body from the waist up is upright (Photo 3.1).

The *grip* for the *flat service* (and for the two other services) is the continental, with some possible slight variations. The continental grip provides a flat surface for a square contact point. When learning to

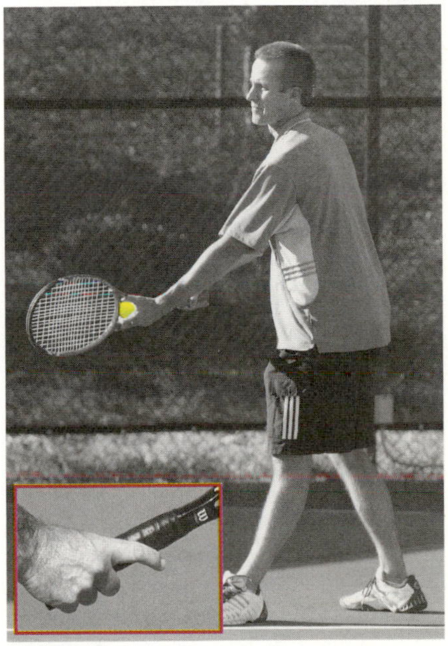

Photography by Terrell Lloyd; assisted by Anna Simmons Myers; inset photo by Virginia Bryant

PHOTO 3.1 Service stance (continental grip).

serve, you may begin by using an eastern forehand grip, but you should change to a continental grip as soon as possible.

The Ball Toss

Skill is involved in *holding the ball for the toss* that initiates the serve action and also in *actually tossing the ball*. To begin any service, you must have two tennis balls in your possession. Keep one ball in the pocket of your tennis shorts so that you have to deal with only one ball during any one serve.

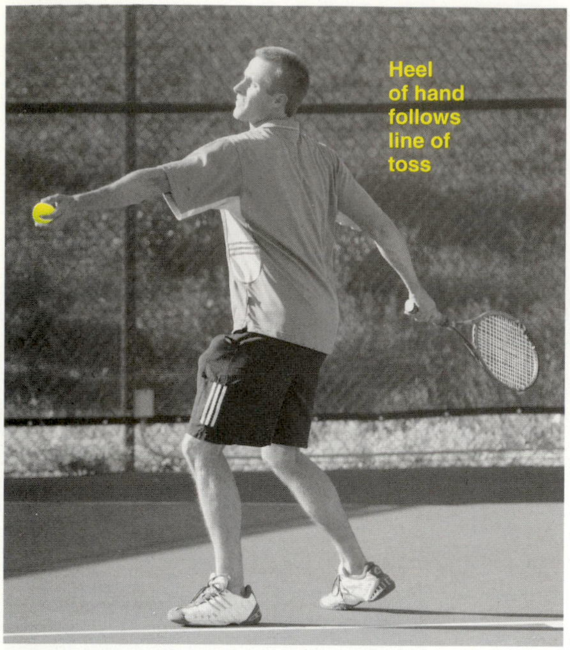

Photography by Terrell Lloyd; assisted by Anna Symonds Myers

PHOTO 3.2 Beginning of toss.

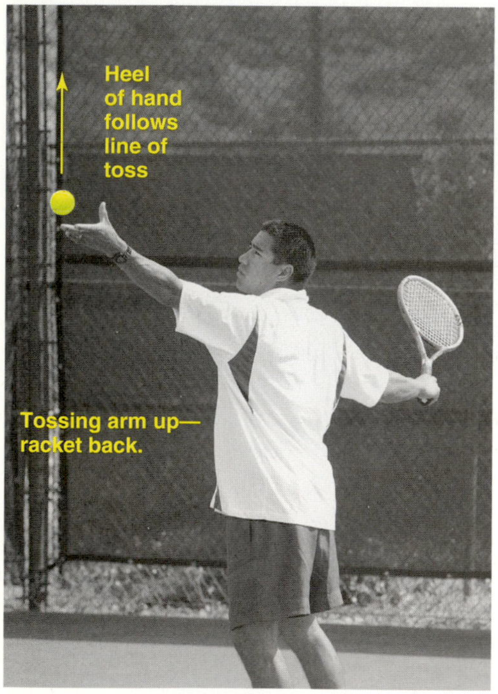

PHOTO 3.3A Release.

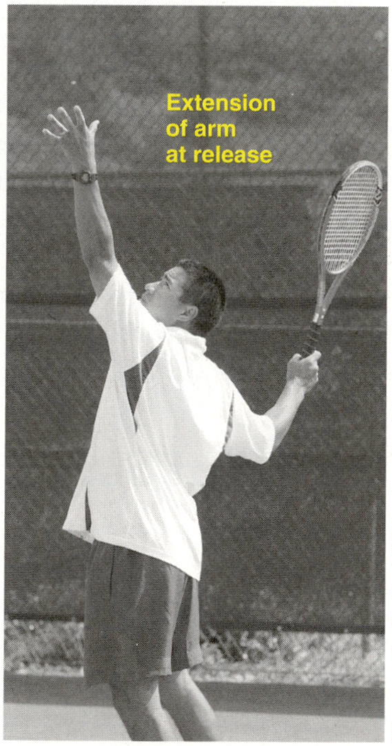

Photography by Terrell Lloyd; assisted by Anna Symonds Myers

PHOTO 3.3B Height of toss.

Grasp the ball to be tossed with the fingertips and the thumb, with the heel of the hand pointing in the direction of the toss (Photo 3.2). From this support base, the ball is placed into a position off the lead shoulder between the player and the sideline and higher than the reach of the racket. A straight arm lifts the ball from the waist to above the head. The heel of the hand is raised during the full arm movement. As the tossing arm begins the upward movement, the racket arm brings the racket back in synchronization with the toss. At the extension of the arm reach, the ball is released, culminating the lifting action. The toss must be executed the same way again and again so that you can become consistent (Photos 3.3A and B).

The Feet

When first learning the service, keep the feet a shoulder width apart throughout the serve. Initially, stability is more important than extra rhythm. Although the feet will not come together in the early stages of learning, the back foot will come forward automatically as the weight transfers toward the target on the follow-through What you should never do is step forward with your lead foot as you contact the ball (Photos 3.4A–C).

Service Backswing

The first timing aspect of the service is the *toss synchronization as preparation for the service*. As the tossing hand begins the upward lift of the ball, the racket begins a backward movement, with the arm straight. The two arms move in opposition. The racket continues back, with the elbow bending as the racket approaches the shoulder-blade area. The back of the elbow is at a right angle, and the arm is in an overhand throwing position. As the ball reaches the top of the placement and begins to fall, the tossing hand will drop away and the hitting elbow will stay in a right-angle position (see Photos 3.5A–C).

Service Contact of Ball

Following the backswing, the initiation of contact occurs. The legs straighten from a bent position in preparation for bringing the racket through in a striking position, with the wrist and forearm breaking and, along with the shoulders, rotating through the contact of the ball.

Footwork for Service

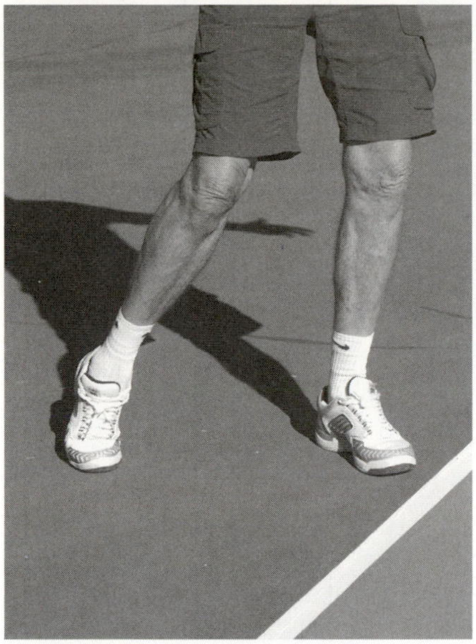

PHOTO 3.4A Backswing.

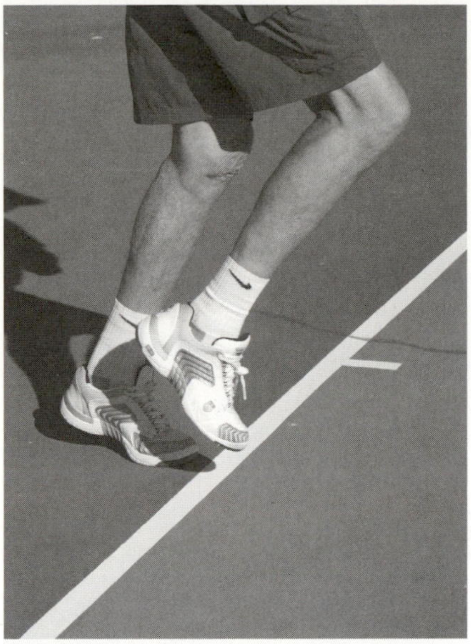

PHOTO 3.4B Contact.

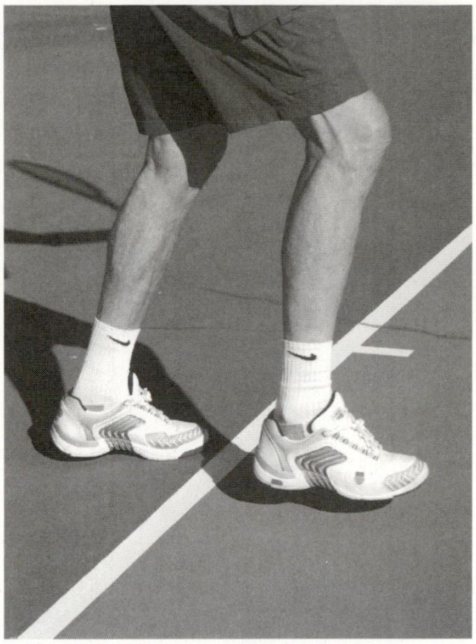

PHOTO 3.4C Follow-through.

Photography by Virginia Bryant

The arm and body are stretched fully. The back and top of the ball are hit with the racket face at approximately 4 inches down from the height of the toss. The toss is to be positioned approximately 1–2 feet off the lead foot, allowing forward movement of the racket from backswing to contact. The body, led by the shoulder, opens up to the position of the ball at contact (Photo 3.5D).

Service Follow-Through

The follow-through continues as momentum carries the racket through the ball and on down to the far nonracket-side leg. A definite weight transfer occurs during follow-through, with the momentum of the racket side pulling the body down and forward. This forces the back foot at the last moment to step forward for a balanced finish (Photo 3.5E).

Rhythmical Service

The basic flat service is designed mechanically to hit through and down on the ball. The ball cannot be hit directly down in a straight line unless the server is at least 697" tall. The racket makes an upward movement at contact, followed by a breaking of the wrist and forearm through the ball. Most beginning players have a great desire to hit the flat serve as hard as they can, assuming that the idea is to hit the service with blazing speed. The problem is that few balls are placed accurately into the appropriate *service court*, which, in turn, means that the ball isn't placed in play to begin a point. This takes away from the fun of playing the game and minimizes the possibility for success. The idea is to hit a firm, controlled, rhythmical service that is placed in the service court effectively. Rhythm and ball placement are far more effective than a sometimes-accurate, high-velocity serve.

Full Service versus Half-Service

Executing a full service versus a half-service requires discussion. Some beginning instruction actually starts with the racket already positioned between the server's shoulder blades to eliminate the initial take-back portion of the stroke preparation (Photo 3.6). The purpose is to keep the stroke as simple as possible and not to complicate coordination of the stroke by including a full swing.

Flat Service

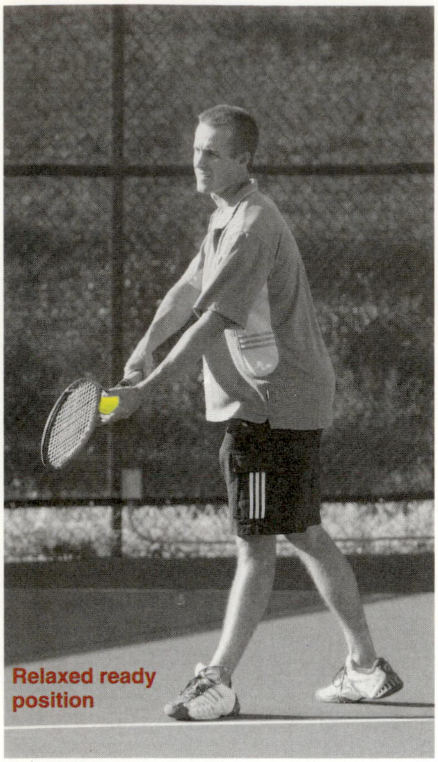

PHOTO 3.5A Ready position.

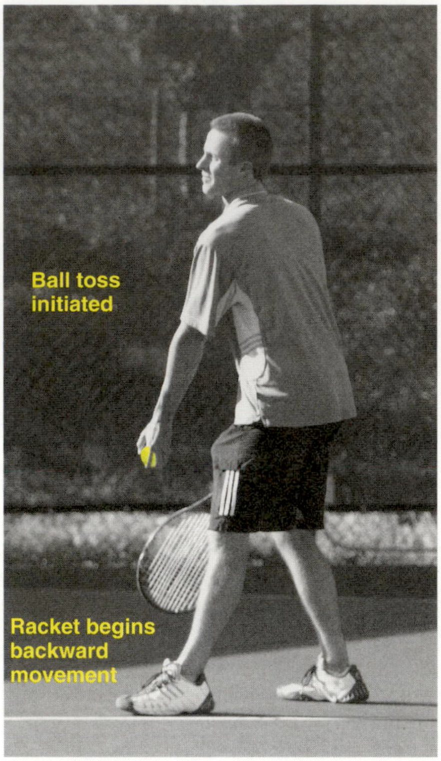

PHOTO 3.5B Initiation of release of ball and take-back of racket.

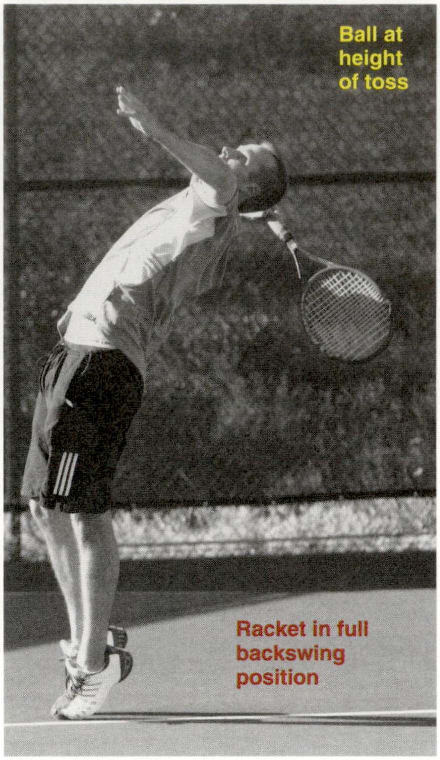

PHOTO 3.5C Backswing continuation in preparation sequence.

Flat Service

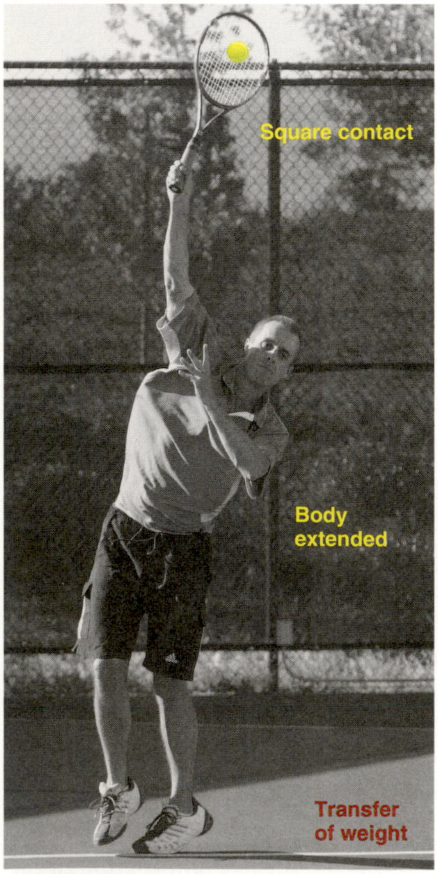

PHOTO 3.5D At contact.

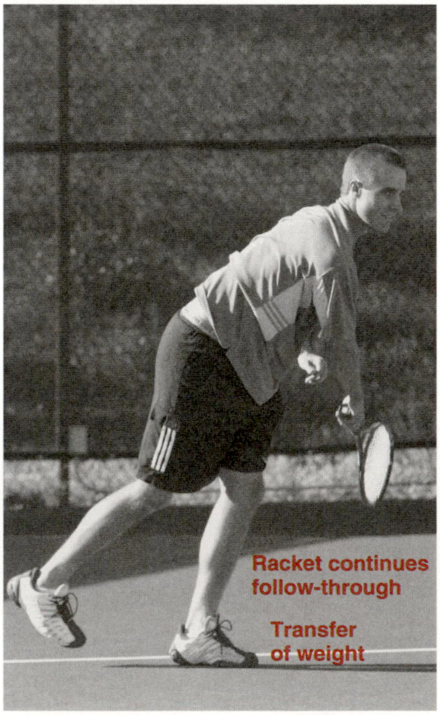

PHOTO 3.5E Follow-through sequence.

Photography by Terrell Lloyd; assisted by Anna Symonds Myers

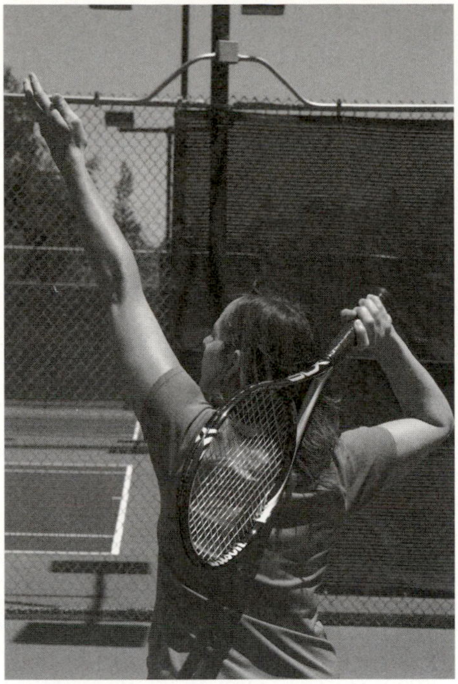

Photography by James E. Bryant

PHOTO 3.6 Half serve position.

The choice of a full serve versus a half-serve is simply one of efficiency. Some highly skilled players use a half-service position, and many less skilled players use a full service. Some players are more comfortable initially with a full-service sequence, but all players need to see the half-service position to understand the upward position of the elbow and the location of the racket during the backswing to permit accurate timing of the stroke.

POINTS *to* REMEMBER

BASIC FLAT SERVE

1. Use the continental grip as soon as possible.
2. Time the toss with the take-back of the racket.
3. Keep your tossing arm straight, with the heel of the hand lifting in the direction of the toss and releasing the ball at the extension of the arm.
4. Make the toss higher than the racket can reach.
5. The toss should be projected inside the baseline 1–2 feet away for forward movement of the racket from backswing to contact.
6. Coil the body by arching your back and bending your knees during preparation.
7. Bring the racket through the ball with a slight upward wrist, followed by a downward wrist and forearm break and shoulder turn.
8. Let your weight transfer carry your body and racket forward in the direction of the ball, with your back foot coming forward to regain balance.
9. Make sure the racket follows on through to the nonracket-side hip.

COMMON ERRORS & HOW TO CORRECT THEM *(Basic Flat Serve)*

The Error	What Causes the Error	To Correct the Error
Erratic placement of the serve.	Inconsistent toss.	Toss the ball by placing it in front of the lead shoulder and opposite the sideline, at a height above the reach of the racket.
Balls served short.	Ball hit too far out in front of the server toward the net; or server attempting to hit over ball; or ball too low at contact.	Toss the ball off the lead shoulder, at a height above the reach of the racket. Focus on brushing through the back and top of the ball.
Ball toss goes behind the head.	Not lifting in a straight line with the tossing arm.	Use the heel of the hand as the lifting agent, along with a straight arm, thereby giving direction to the ball.
Ball served long.	Racket under the ball at contact, pushing the ball up; trying to hit the ball too hard.	Toss the ball off the lead shoulder, at a height above the reach of the racket and in front of the lead shoulder. Focus on brushing through the back, top of the ball at contact.
Stepping on the baseline during the serve.	Toss is too far over baseline toward net, or player steps with foot as if throwing a ball.	Toss the ball by placing it off the lead shoulder no more than 1 to 2 feet from the lead shoulder. Make sure the toss is above the reach of the racket. Keep the lead foot firmly on the court.

Return of Service

Because serves have different velocities, trajectories, and spins, the beginning player may be confronted with a series of decisions on how to cope with each type of serve.

Positioning for Return of Serve

Return of serve positioning is a matter of mathematics. The receiver must split the court in half in a line from the server to the receiver (Figure 3.1). The receiver cannot overplay to the side, attempting to return all serves with a forehand, because a server with a wide serve or an adequate slice serve can place a ball that will kick off the court and out of reach of the player. It is much better for the receiver to position with the potential to hit either a forehand or a backhand equally.

The depth of the receiver's position depends on the velocity of the ball. If a player pushes the ball when serving and simply gets the ball in play, the receiver can move up and stand inside the baseline about halfway between the baseline and the service court line. If the server has a strong serve with high velocity, the receiver should stand at or slightly behind the baseline.

Returning the served ball effectively requires a special set of skills. First, the receiver should develop a relaxed attitude and appropriate ready position. The ready position (Photo 3.7) should be high to permit quick lateral movement and enable the receiver to hit through the ball with minimal adjustment. As the serve is hit, the receiver has to rotate the shoulders to a hitting position at the earliest possible moment. The receiver then must transfer weight into the stroke by stepping into the ball at contact.

When receiving a serve hit at a high velocity, the backswing and follow-through have to be shortened. This shortened backswing enables the receiver to control the racket and bring it through in time to contact the ball. The action of the racket is more of a blocking or punching movement that pushes the ball back across the net, reversing the velocity of the serve. If there is limited velocity applied to the ball by the server, a regular groundstroke execution will

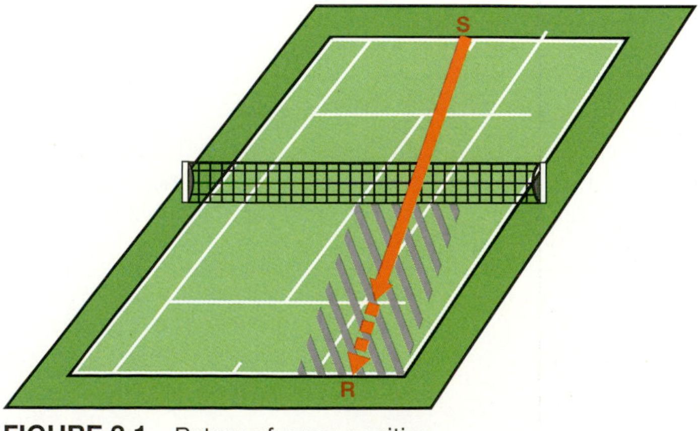

FIGURE 3.1 Return of serve position.

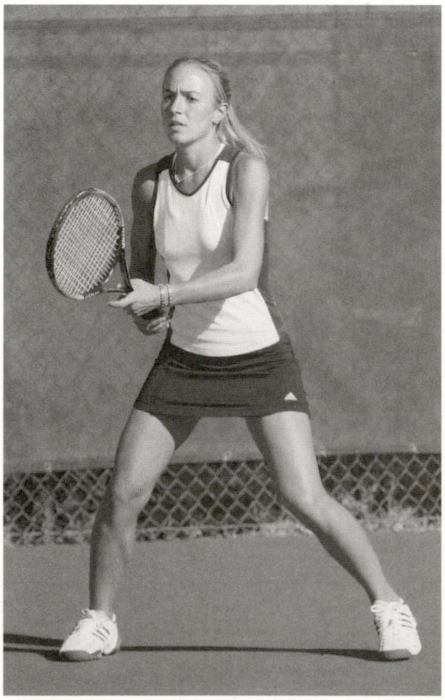

Photography by Terrell Lloyd; assisted by Anna Symonds Myers

PHOTO 3.7 Ready position for return of serve.

be more effective, as opposed to a punching action.

The racket should be square to the ball and a little out in front of the lead leg, with a short follow-through to add direction to the ball. The racket should be held firmly throughout the stroke, particularly at contact. Finally, the receiver must watch the ball as long as possible up to the point of contact. Return of serve follows the same process and skill pattern whether hitting a forehand (Photos 3.8A–C) or a backhand (Photos 3.9A–C). Selecting which side to hit from depends on the spin and direction of the ball and a responsive early rotation of the shoulders based on anticipating the position of the ball.

Where to Hit the Ball

Target for return of serve is a moot point if the return player is just trying to get the racket on the ball. But with a degree of skill at returning a serve, the receiver can return the ball to spots on the court. The first consideration is where *not* to place the ball. Balls hit short to the server reward that server, so short returns should be eliminated. Serves that pull a return player off the court should be returned down the sideline rather than cross-court, and most returns hit soft and "up" should be avoided. If the receiver can remember to return deep with pace and velocity on the ball, subsequent play should enable the receiver to gain equal footing in a baseline rally.

Anticipating the Serve

Anticipation of the serve is both a physical and a mental exercise in the return of service. The receiver must look at the server's body language and concentrate on the ball. The

Return of Serve: Forehand

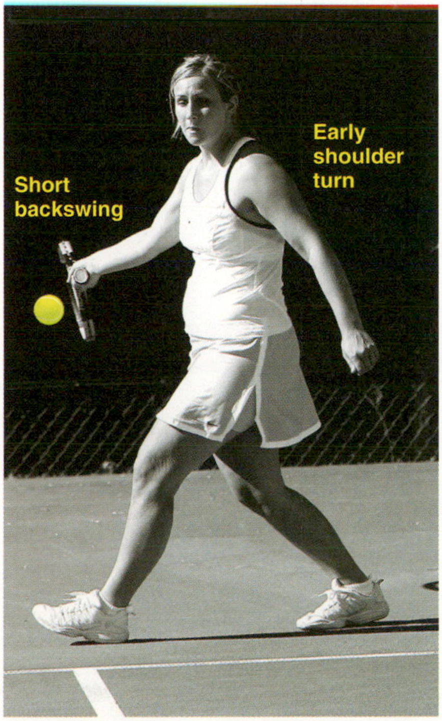

PHOTO 3.8A Backswing.

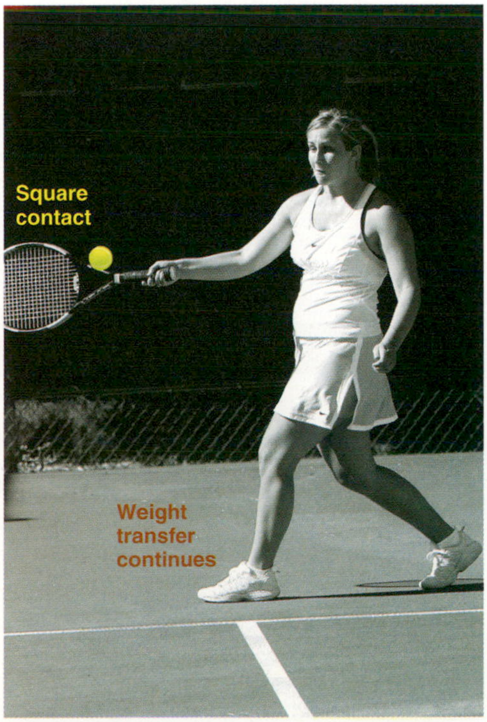

PHOTO 3.8B Contact.

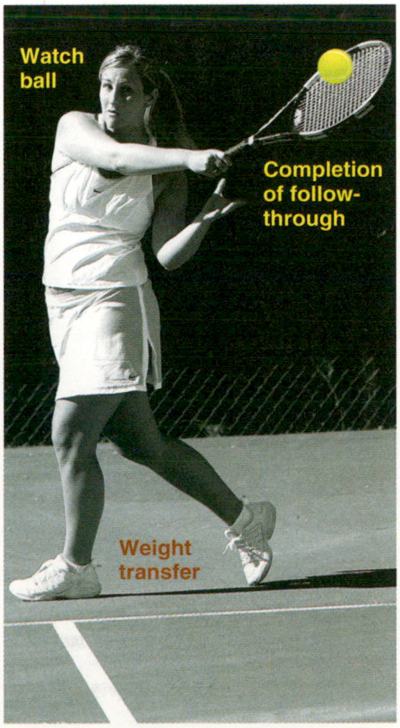

PHOTO 3.8C Completion of follow-through.

Photography by Terrell Lloyd; assisted by Anna Symonds Myers

Return of Serve: Backhand

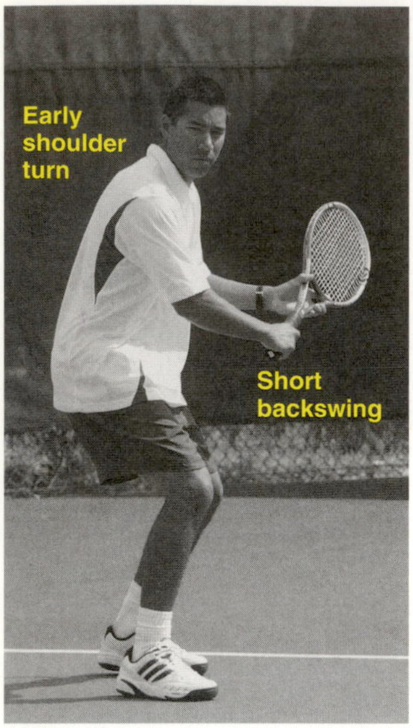

PHOTO 3.9A Backswing.

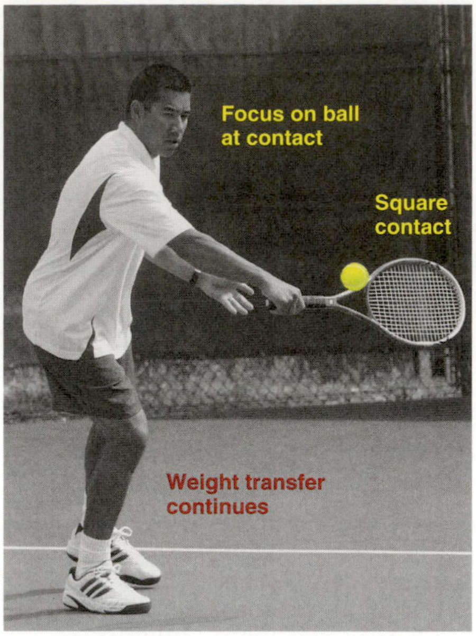

PHOTO 3.9B Focus on ball at contact

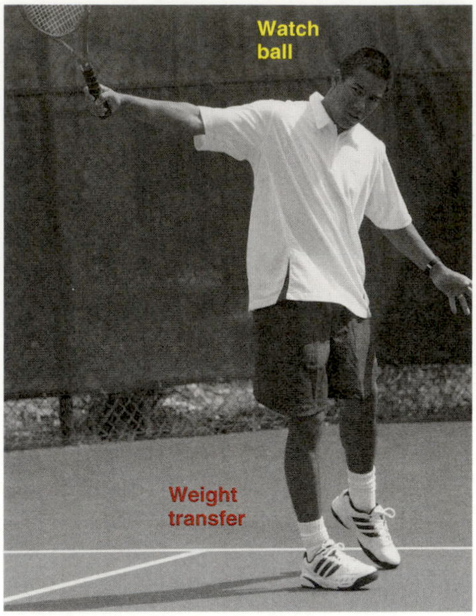

PHOTO 3.9C Follow-through.

Photography by Terrell Lloyd; assisted by Anna Symonds Myers

body language will provide clues to the spin and velocity of the ball. If the server's racket-face pattern is to the outside of the ball and the toss is short and back toward the racket shoulder, the serve will be a slice. If the toss is off the lead shoulder and toward the net, the ball will be a flat serve. A topspin serve will be interpreted by a toss above the head with more back arch than usual.

Velocity of the ball can be observed to some extent by the server's effort. Concentrating on the seams of the ball will permit the receiver to react physically to the direction of the ball. The mental efforts all combine to allow the receiver to make an early shoulder turn and pivot of the feet, thereby placing the racket in a backswing position.

POINTS *to* REMEMBER

RETURN OF SERVE

1. Throughout the serve, concentrate on the server's body language and on the ball.
2. Get the racket back early.
3. Be aggressive and step into the ball at contact.
4. Use a compact swing with a short backswing and follow-through against high-velocity serves.
5. Maintain a firm grip on the racket at contact.
6. Hit deep on all returns of serve.

COMMON ERRORS & HOW TO CORRECT THEM (Return of Serve)

The Error	What Causes the Error	To Correct the Error
Hitting the ball out beyond the server's baseline.	Swinging with a full groundstroke swing.	Use a compact swing; block high-velocity serves.
Pulling the ball across the court to the sidelines.	Racket contact with the ball too far out in front of the projected contact point.	Judge the velocity of the ball, and time your swing.
Ball coming off the racket late, with direction toward the near sideline.	Not anticipating early and, as a result, not getting the shoulders turned and the racket back early.	Watch the ball, and react by turning the shoulders and pivoting the feet early.
Cannot control direction of the ball.	Wrist isn't firm and grip isn't tight. Timing is inconsistent.	Keep a firm wrist and grip at contact. Judge speed of ball for timing.

Increasing Beginner Skills: Slice Service

A slice serve is often considered an intermediate skill, but in reality it can be taught as a beginning serve. Actually, it may be an easier serve for a beginner to learn.

The slice service puts a sidespin action on the ball. It can be used as a first or second serve, although it usually is used as a second serve in singles and a first and second serve in doubles. The spin permits the server to hit with greater accuracy and still place the serve deeply. A sidespin is imparted by contacting the back and side of the ball in sequence. The racket grip is a continental grip; as more spin is needed, the grip can be adjusted to an eastern backhand grip. The result is that the ball lands in the court and kicks away from the server's position.

Comparison of Flat and Slice Serves

The slice service differs from the flat service in the toss position and in the racket's movement pattern. The toss is the same distance from the body, but with less height (one of the advantages when the wind is blowing is that a lower toss with a slice service is less affected). The ball is tossed between the lead shoulder and the middle of the body. More spin and less velocity can be achieved the closer the toss is to the back of the racket shoulder.

The difference between the slice and the flat serve toss is that the flat serve toss is above the reach of the racket, as compared to the shorter toss for a slice service, and the toss is in front of the lead shoulder instead of between the lead shoulder and the middle of the body (Photos 3.10A–B and 3.11A–B for comparison).

During a slice service, contact is made on the side and back of the ball just below center. The wrist and forearm move through a controlled motion with forceful action at contact. The shoulders are turned more with a slice service, leaving the body even more open at contact than with the flat service (Photos 3.12 and 3.13 for a comparison of flat serve versus slice serve).

Toss for Flat Serve

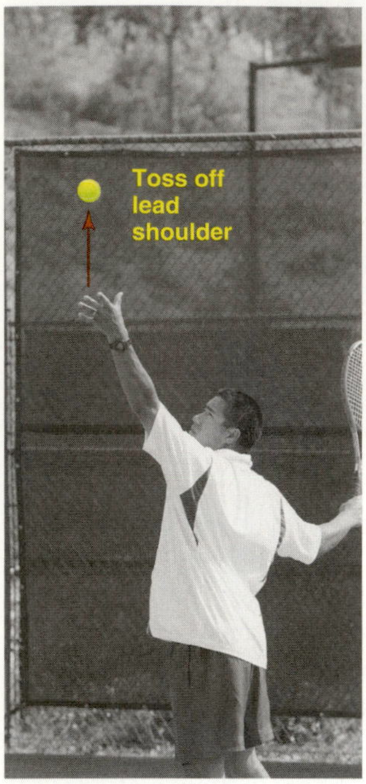

PHOTO 3.10A Toss off lead shoulder.

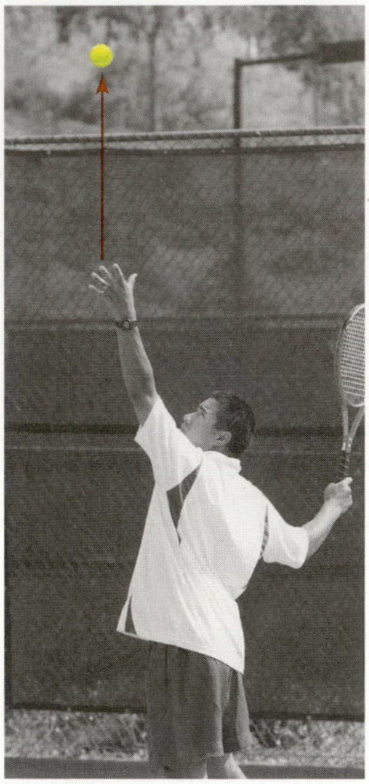

PHOTO 3.10B Toss above the reach of racket.

Photography by Terrell Lloyd; assisted by Anna Symonds Myers

Toss for Slice Serve

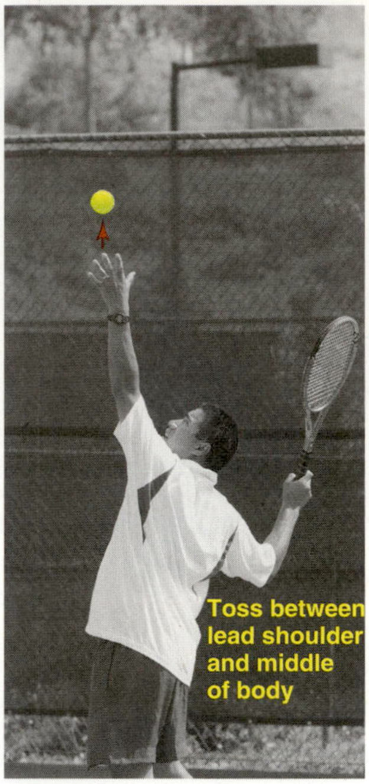

PHOTO 3.11A Toss between lead shoulder and middle of body.

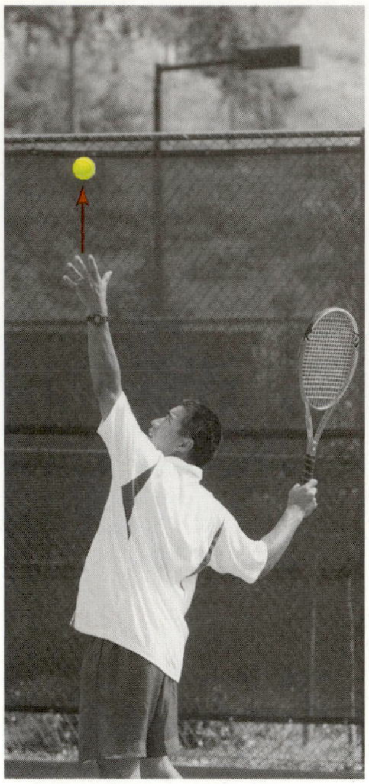

PHOTO 3.11B Short toss.

Photography by Terrell Lloyd; assisted by Anna Symonds Myers

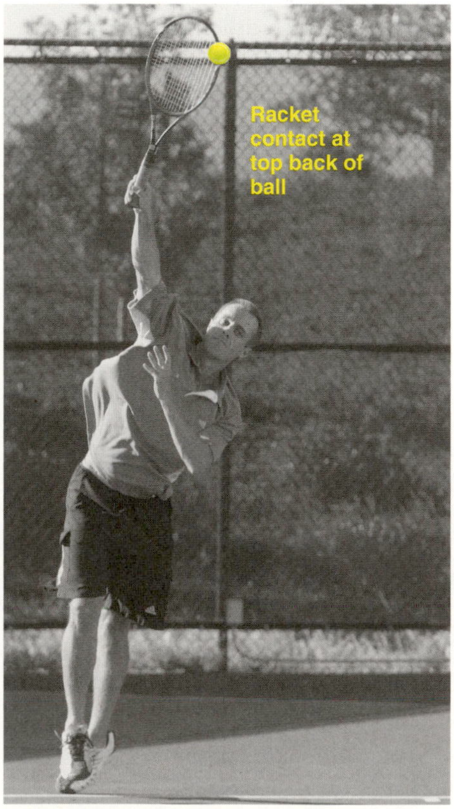

Photography by Terrell Lloyd; assisted by Anna Symonds Myers

PHOTO 3.12 Flat service contact.

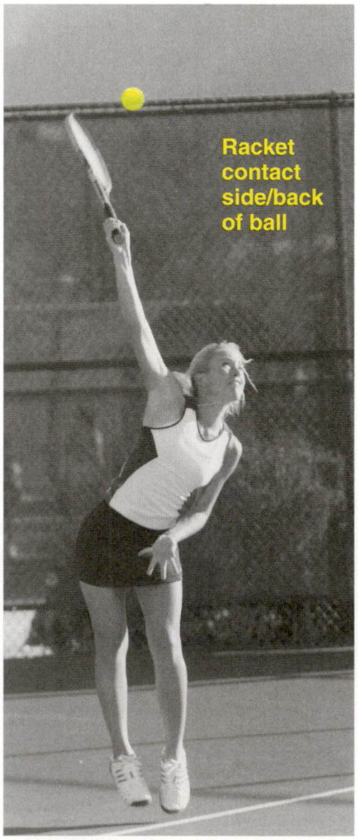

Photography by Terrell Lloyd; assisted by Anna Symonds Myers

PHOTO 3.13 Slice service contact.

Slice Serve

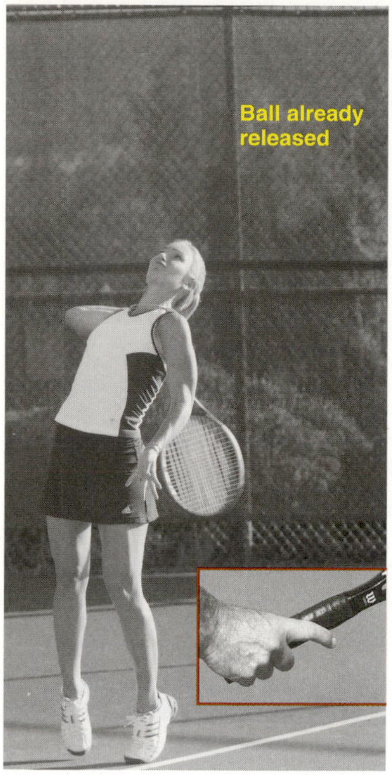

PHOTO 3.14A Backswing (continental grip).

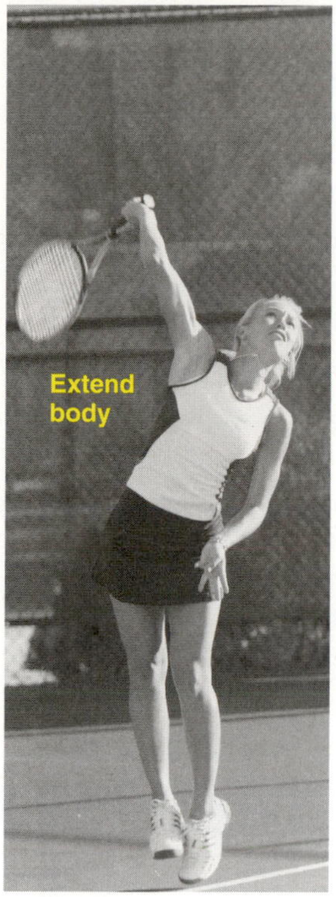

PHOTO 3.14B Continuation of backswing.

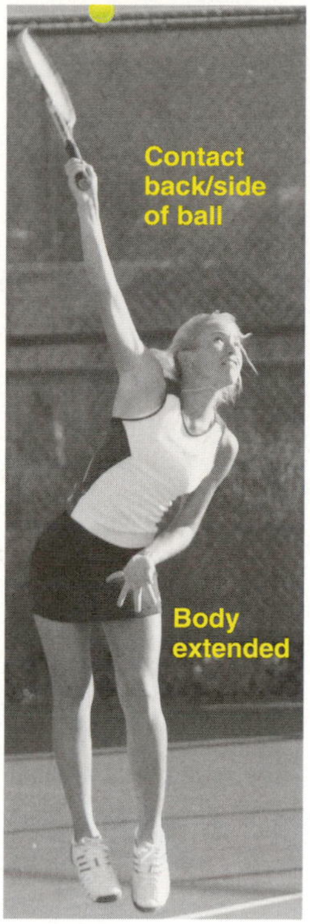

PHOTO 3.14C Contact.

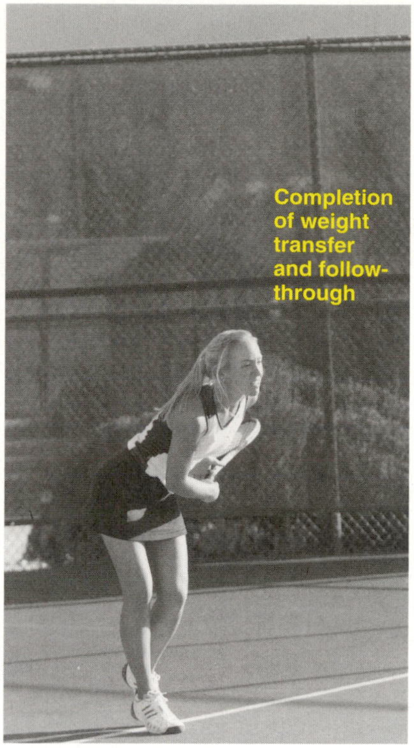

PHOTO 3.14D Completion of follow-through.

Photography by Virginia Bryant

Photography by Terrell Lloyd; assisted by Anna Symonds Myers

Sequence of Slice Serve

The full sequence of the slice service, including the exceptions identified, is a rhythmical one, with the take-away, followed by contact with the ball, and culminating with a follow-through down off the hip of the nonracket side. The weight transfer is an aid to that sequence, as is the leg bend followed by extension of the leg at contact (Photos 3.14A–D).

Summary of Differences and Commonalities of Two Serves

A summary of the differences and commonalities of the two services may be helpful to the developing player. The differences, related to ball-toss position, racket-pattern movement, and foot position on the baseline, are outlined in Table 3.1. The commonalities involve weight transfer, elbow position on the backswing, and follow-through off the nonracket-side hip.

TABLE 3.1
Differences between the Two Major Services

Type of Service	Ball-Toss Placement	Foot Position on Baseline	Racket-Pattern Movement	Contact Position on Ball
Flat	In front of lead shoulder, above racket reach	Even	Straight through	Back-top
Slice	Between lead shoulder and racket shoulder, lower than racket reach	Back foot slightly back	Curving line	Back-side just below center

POINTS to REMEMBER

SLICE SERVE

1. Use a continental grip.
2. Open the serving stance more than with the flat service.
3. Toss the ball lower than with the flat service, and toss more toward the back shoulder to obtain more spin.
4. Contact the ball sequentially on the back and side below center.
5. Pull the shoulder through the ball at contact.
6. Use a forceful action with the wrist and forearm at contact to increase velocity and spin.
7. Transfer your weight forward through the sequence of the service, allowing the back foot to move forward to regain balance after contact.

COMMON ERRORS & HOW TO CORRECT THEM *(Slice Serve)*

The Error	What Causes the Error	To Correct the Error
Lack of spin on the ball.	Toss not far enough back to the racket shoulder or no continental grip; body doesn't open to the ball.	Toss between the two shoulders; check to make sure the grip is continental. Turn the lead shoulder more through the stroke.
Pulling the ball out of the serving court.	Turning the nonracket shoulder into the ball too early, and pulling the shoulder too far through the ball.	Point the nonracket shoulder to the service court target area from contact through follow-through, thereby reducing excessive shoulder turn.
A great amount of spin, but little velocity or distance.	Hitting the ball too far back on back shoulder, or racket pattern too far to the outside of the ball at contact. Also, using eastern backhand grip.	Move toss more toward the lead shoulder and/or control racket pattern through a sequential brushing action of the back and side of the ball.
Hitting the ball off the racket edge.	Too much of an eastern forehand grip.	Use a continental grip.

CHECKPOINTS

1. The toss for serve is a key to success. It should be executed
   a. by grasping the ball with the fingertips and thumb.
   b. with the heel of the hand pointed in the direction of the toss.
   c. by a straight lifting action of the arm.
   d. by using all three of the above skills.
2. The toss synchronization requires
   a. the racket beginning a backward movement as the tossing hand lifts.
   b. the racket placed in the middle of the shoulder blades as the tossing hand lifts.
   c. the racket beginning backward movement as the toss reaches its top height.
   d. use of all three of the above techniques.
3. The racket follow-through
   a. continues on a downward pattern, finishing off the nonracket leg.
   b. continues on a downward pattern, finishing off the racket leg.
   c. stops at waist level.
   d. can be any of the above three, depending on the type of serve used.
4. Weight of the body should
   a. be transferred forward by stepping with the lead foot.
   b. be centered at contact with the ball.
   c. rest on the back foot at contact with the ball.
   d. be transferred forward at contact with the ball.
5. The cause of the ball being consistently served into the net is
   a. that the toss is too high.
   b. that the server is attempting to hit over the ball.
   c. that the ball toss is too far out in front of the server.
   d. any of the three causes listed above.
6. The contact position on the ball for a slice serve is
   a. top-back.
   b. side-back.
   c. top.
   d. side.
7. The position of the ball on the toss for a slice serve is
   a. off the lead shoulder.
   b. off the racket shoulder.
   c. between the lead shoulder and the racket shoulder.
   d. any of the above three positions.
8. A lack of spin applied to the ball when hitting a slice serve is caused by
   a. the toss being placed not far enough back toward the racket shoulder.
   b. turning the racket shoulder into the ball too soon.
   c. too extreme a continental grip.
   d. contact on the side of the ball.
9. The return of serve ready positioning should be
   a. with the receiver standing to the forehand side of the line of the serve.
   b. with the receiver standing 2–4 feet inside the baseline.
   c. with the receiver standing 2–4 feet behind the baseline.
   d. with the receiver splitting the court in half in a line from the server to the receiver.
10. The correction for hitting a return of serve long is
    a. to use a compact swing and swing through the ball.
    b. to use a compact swing and block all serves.
    c. to use a compact swing and block all high-velocity serves.
    d. to use a full swing.

Answers to Checkpoints can be found on page 167.

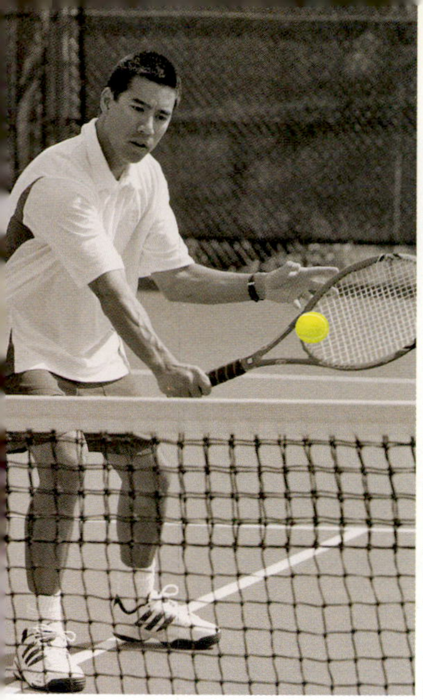

Photography by Terrell Lloyd; assisted by Anna Symonds Myers

4
Net Play

The *volley* is one of two strokes hit when the ball is in midair prior to striking the court on the bounce. It is an uncomplicated punching action stroke, also described as a "blocking-the-ball action." The volley is used in singles play following an approach shot or in a serve-and-volley combination. In doubles, the volley also is used following an approach shot and as a serve-and-volley combination, and it is used with a player positioned at the net during a serve.

Early in their development all players must learn the skills involved in the volley. A singles player may avoid most situations involving the volley, but in doubles play there is no choice but to be located at the net on most shots played.

The volley shot begins from the *ready position*, as described when preparing to hit a groundstroke, except that the racket is held higher, at chin level (Photo 4.1). From this position the player who is at the net may respond with either a forehand or a backhand volley. Part of the preparation in the ready position is to assume a grip that is both comfortable and functional.

The *continental grip* usually is recommended for the volley, because no adjustment has to be made for a forehand or a backhand volley (Photo 4.1). Often there is not enough time to change grips when at the net because of the high velocity of a ball and the short distance from the opposing player. The strength of the continental grip is that the backhand is firm and solid when hitting the volley. The weakness is that the grip for a forehand provides a weaker base for balls

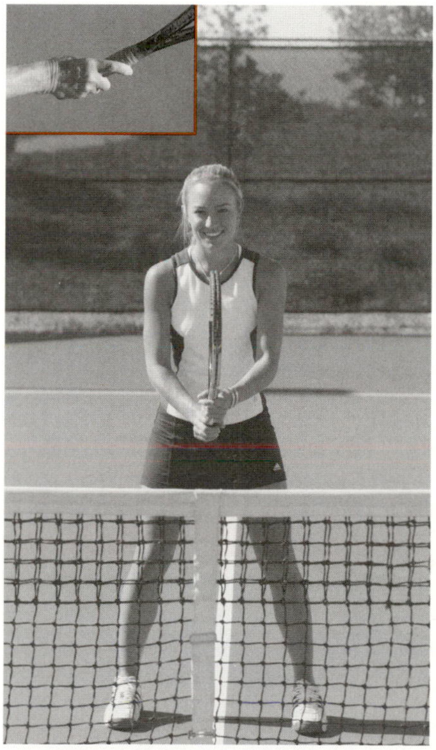

Photography by Terrell Lloyd; assisted by Anna Symonds Myers; inset photo by Virginia Bryant

PHOTO 4.1 Volley ready position (continental grip).

hit above the net, forcing the player to adjust at the net by changing to an eastern forehand when time permits. Most successful players do "cheat" and move the hand on the grip for most high volley shots, provided they have the time to change and also to change back following the stroke.

Forehand Volley

Forehand Volley Backswing

The *forehand volley* begins with a "short" backswing created by a shoulder turn. The racket head is located above the hand as the racket is taken back even with the racket shoulder (Photo 4.2A). The *preparation* is completed with the weight centered on the racket-side foot.

Forehand Volley Contact

The racket comes forward at *contact* with the ball, with the face of the racket striking the back of the ball squarely at the front of the lead leg (Photo 4.2B). A slight downward path of the stroke with a slightly open racket face at the point of contact imparts some underspin to the ball.

At contact the racket head is positioned above the hand, the wrist remains firm, and the grip also is firm to prevent the racket from turning in the hand at impact. A step is taken with the opposing leg, and the weight is transferred to that leg. The knees are bent from backswing to contact. It should be repeated that the racket must be in front of the lead leg at contact.

Forehand Volley Follow-Through

The *follow-through* (Photo 4.2C) is the final part of the punching action. A short downward motion, with the bottom edge of the racket leading and a continuation of a slightly open racket face, completes the stroke. The lead leg is still bent during follow-through, with the weight centered over that leg. Upon completing the follow-through, the player

Backhand Slice Groundstroke

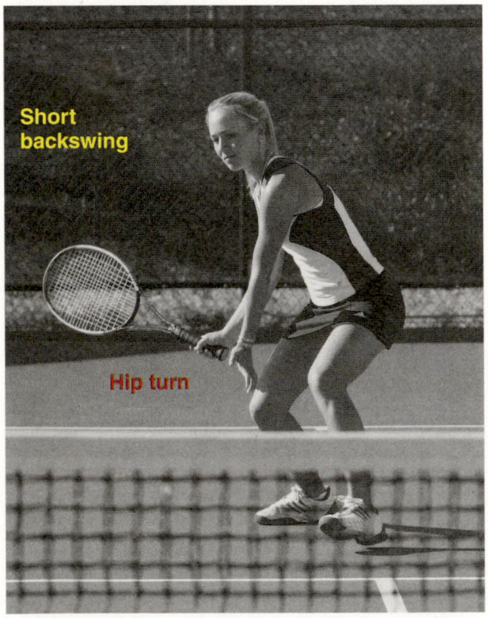

PHOTO 4.2A Preparation.

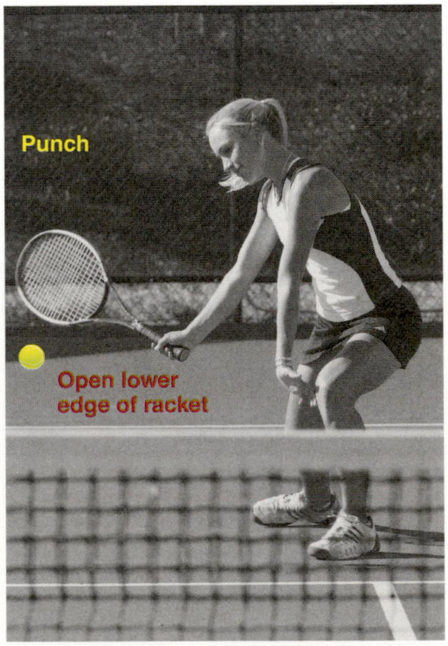

PHOTO 4.2B Contact with the ball.

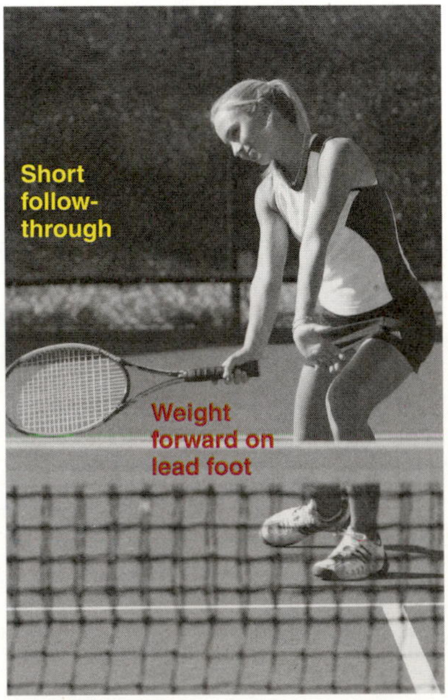

PHOTO 4.2C Follow-through.

Photography by Terrell Lloyd; assisted by Anna Symonds Myers

Backhand Volley Sequence

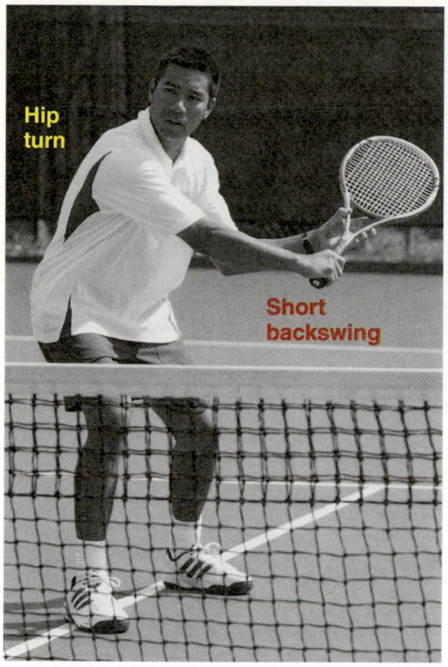

PHOTO 4.3A Preparation.

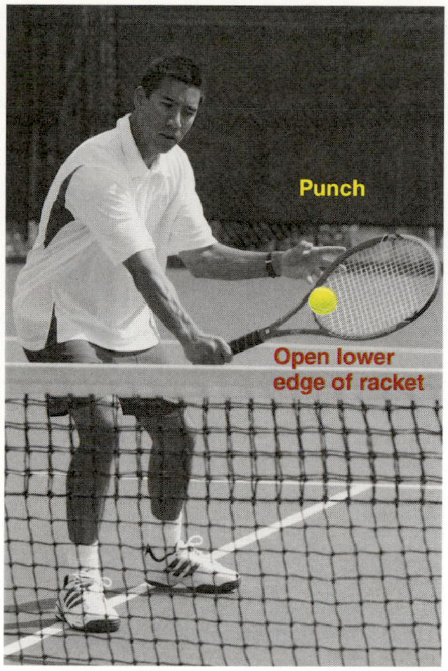

PHOTO 4.3B Contact with the ball.

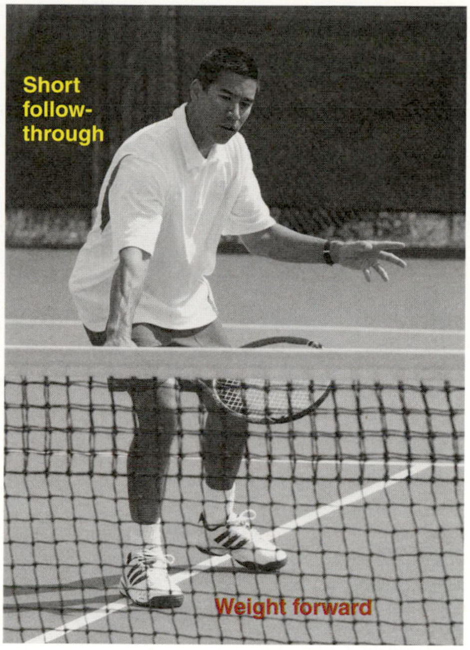

PHOTO 4.3C Follow-through.

Photography by Terrell Lloyd; assisted by Anna Symonds Myers

must return to a ready position in preparation for the next volley.

Backhand Volley

The *backhand volley* is executed in a manner similar to the forehand volley, but it is easier to complete mechanically.

Backhand Volley Backswing

The backswing is aided, since the shoulder turn is already to the backhand side and the elbow and shoulder work as a firm backboard when striking the ball. In *preparation*, the nonracket hand grips the throat of the racket to provide stabilization of the racket position when in a ready position. The racket head is then brought back to the nonracket side and is positioned above the hand. The weight of the body is centered over the nonracket-side foot, and the backswing is short, with a firm wrist (Photo 4.3A).

Backhand Volley at Contact

At *contact*, the weight shifts forward to the racket leg as that leg steps into the ball. The racket-face strings make full square contact with the back of the ball with a punching action that includes a firm wrist and arm and a firm grip on the racket. Contact is made slightly in front of the lead leg, with the racket above the hand (Photo 4.3B). The knees are bent from preparation through contact and into the follow-through.

Backhand Volley Follow-Through

The *follow-through* is a continuation of the punch action, with the bottom edge of the racket continuing to lead in order to apply a slight backspin to the ball (Photo 4.3C). At the end of the follow-through, the weight is

Two-hand Backhand Volley Sequence

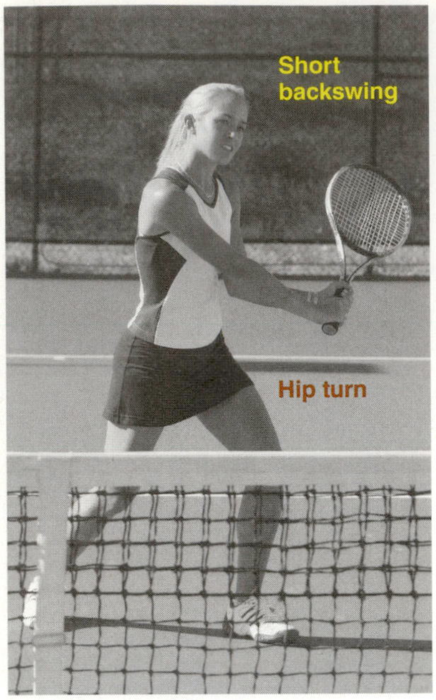

PHOTO 4.4A Preparation.

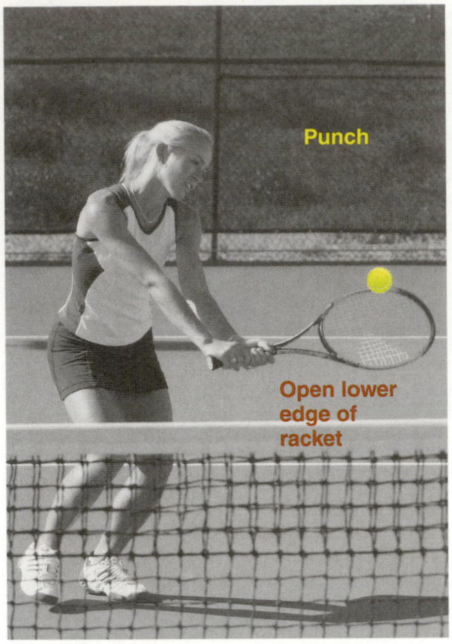

PHOTO 4.4B Contact with the ball.

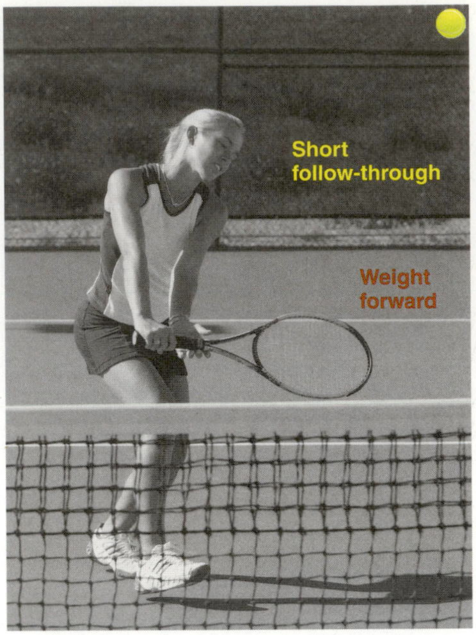

PHOTO 4.4C Follow-through.

Photography by Terrell Lloyd; assisted by Anna Symonds Myers

centered on the leading leg and the racket is extended a short distance forward. The recovery must be quick as the player returns to the ready position at the net.

Two-Hand Backhand Volley

A *two-hand backhand volley* also can be used at the net. The stroke is the same as the basic *backhand volley*, but you are limited in terms of arm and leg extension. This is a relatively severe limitation; but with good footwork and the reminder to keep your arms into your body, it is an effective volley stroke (Photos 4.4A–C). As you develop confidence and skill at the net, you need to move away from two hands to a more effective one-hand backhand volley stroke.

POINTS *to* REMEMBER

VOLLEY

1. Punch the ball—don't swing at it.
2. Keep the backswing and follow-through brief.
3. Keep the racket above the hand throughout the stroke.
4. Step into the ball if time allows.
5. Stay low on the ball.
6. Hit behind the ball at contact, and then follow through with the bottom edge of the racket leading in order to impart backspin to the ball.
7. Make contact in front of the lead leg.
8. Maintain control of the racket with a firm grip and firm wrist throughout the stroke.

COMMON ERRORS & HOW TO CORRECT THEM (Volley)

The Error	What Causes the Error	To Correct the Error
Balls that have no pace or just drop off the racket strings.	Not hitting in front of the lead leg; not transferring weight into the ball at contact.	Hit slightly in front of the lead leg between the body and the net. Step into and punch through the ball.
Racket turns in the hand, causing lack of control of the ball.	Lack of a firm grip, or grip size is too small.	Tighten the grip or increase the size of the grip for better control.
Ball strikes the net following contact.	Player not getting "down on the ball" and bending the knees. Or racket face is not open enough at contact.	Bend the knees all the way through the shot. Open the racket face and punch through the ball, allowing the racket face to open from contact to follow-through.
Ball is hit long.	Elbow usually not firm and/or swinging at the ball as if hitting a groundstroke.	Maintain a short backswing and follow-through.

Increasing Beginner Skills: Insight When Hitting a Volley Shot

Hitting a volley shot requires anticipation, footwork, set up, body elevation, and knowing how to incorporate the volley into your total game.

Volley Anticipation

Anticipation is a key to playing well at the net. If the player at the net is afraid of the ball, he or she cannot anticipate. If the player "sees" the ball early, reacting as the ball comes off the opposing player's racket rather than waiting until the ball arrives at the net, the volleying player will be effective at the net. Once the reaction time has been established, the next important phase is to attack by stepping into the ball rather than waiting for the ball to arrive. Even guessing, as part of anticipation, is better than standing at the net and waiting.

Volley Footwork

Footwork for the volley is important to the stroke so that form can be added to the total maneuver. Footwork enables the player to step into the ball with body weight behind the punch and to move efficiently to get to the ball. The first part of the footwork involves a shoulder turn and hip pivot. From a ready position, the player should pivot the hips toward the anticipated position of the ball. With the hip turn, the shoulders will turn also, and the racket-side foot will react by pivoting until the body weight centers over that foot.

Three basic ball positions are presented to you when hitting a volley shot:

1. The setup volley with the shoulder and hip turn, involving a small cross-step.
2. The wide-ball volley that forces the player to take a lengthened cross-step.
3. The ball hit at the player, which requires a defensive reaction volley.

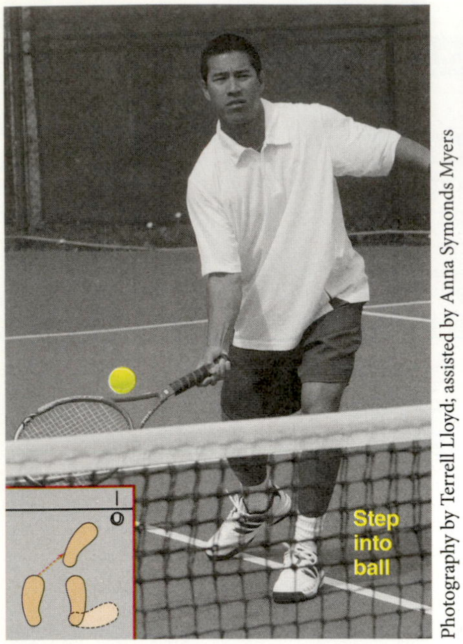

PHOTO 4.5 Footwork for the setup volley (forehand).

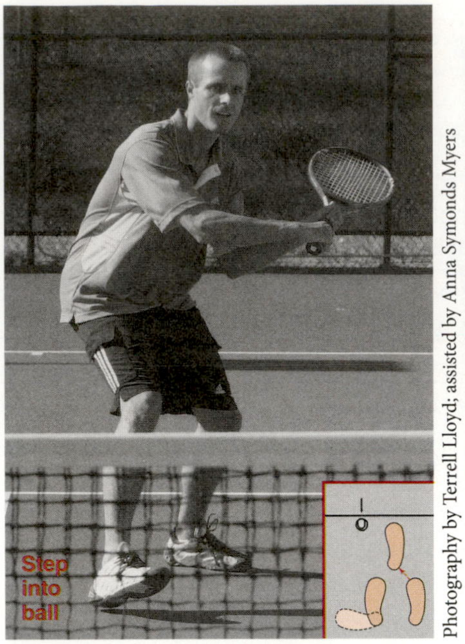

PHOTO 4.6 Footwork for the setup volley (backhand).

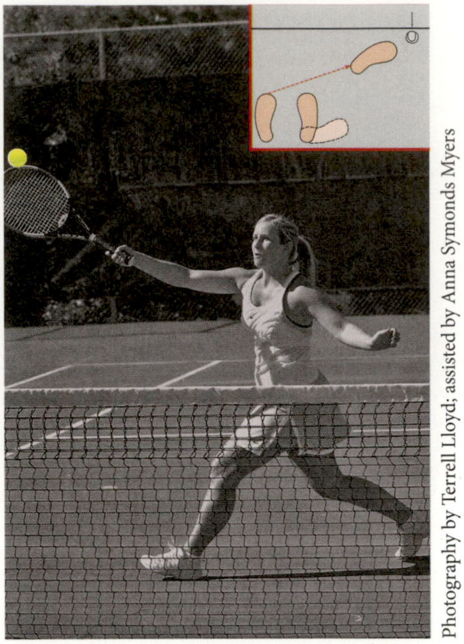

PHOTO 4.7 Footwork for the wide-ball volley (forehand).

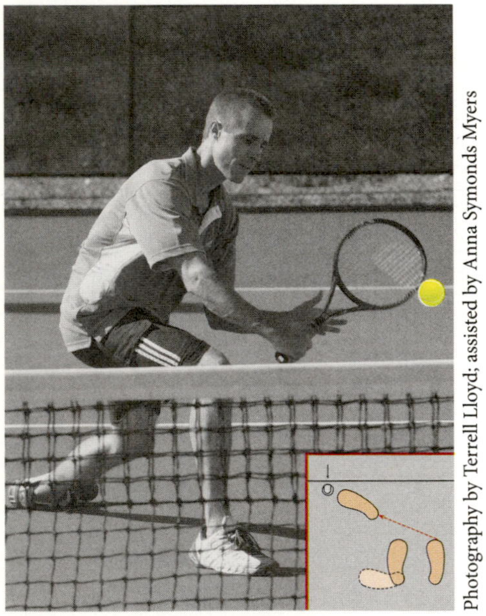

PHOTO 4.8 Footwork for the wide-ball volley (backhand).

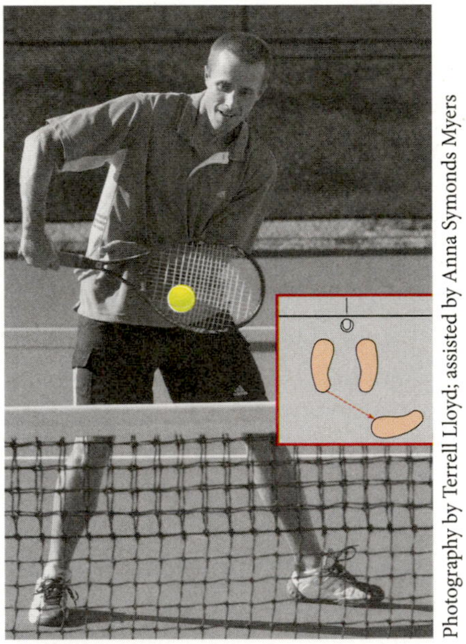

PHOTO 4.9 Footwork for the ball hit at the net player (backhand).

Volley Setup

The *setup volley* is initiated with the shoulder and hip turn, followed by the turn of the inside of the foot and a step forward and a little across the body with the opposite leg (Photos 4.5 and 4.6). The *wide ball volley* is reached by the same movement used for the setup, but the step across the body with the opposite leg requires an elongated, direct movement (Photos 4.7 and 4.8).

The *ball hit at the player* requires that the player hit with a backhand volley, if at all possible. The player must pivot off the racket foot and, if there is time, step with the non-racket foot behind the opposite foot to turn the shoulder sideways to the ball (Photo 4.9 diagram insert). The player then must lean back into the path of the ball (Photo 4.9).

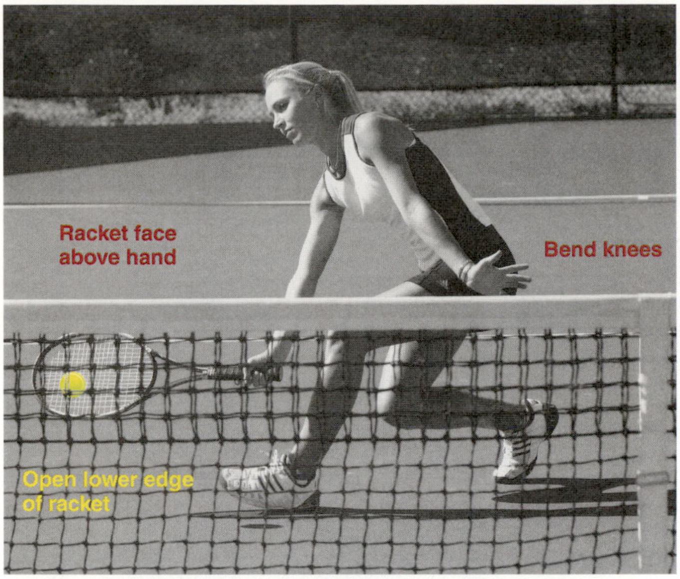

PHOTO 4.10 Low forehand volley.

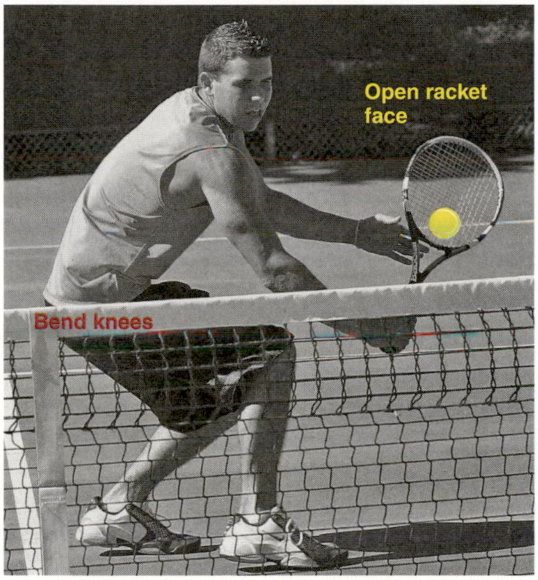

PHOTO 4.11 Low backhand volley.

Elevating to Hit the Volley

Body elevation also is important to successfully complete the volley, as balls are not going to be returned at shoulder level in all situations. The legs must be either bent or extended for many of the volley stroke situations.

A *low volley* forces the player to bend the knees and get low to the ball (Photos 4.10 and 4.11). The hip and shoulder turn must occur to position the shoulder to the ball, and the legs must bend as low as possible. The volleyer steps into the ball with the opposite foot and punches under and through the ball, using underspin to lift the ball over the net. The underspin is achieved by opening the racket face. The closer the ball is to the court at contact, the more open the racket face should be. The follow-through of the low shot continues with an upward, short movement of the racket, with the knees remaining bent. Throughout the stroke, the racket should stay at least even with the hand, if possible, to ensure proper technique and stroking action.

The *high volley* forces you to extend the body and the legs to reach the ball. The shoulder turn must occur early to permit the racket to be taken back a little farther and higher than for the basic volley. The player then steps into the ball with the opposite leg and punches down and through the ball. The follow-through moves in the direction of the ball just hit and ends at waist level. The punching pattern is a high-to-low closing stroke. The wrist is locked, and the stroke is firm (see Photos 4.12 and 4.13).

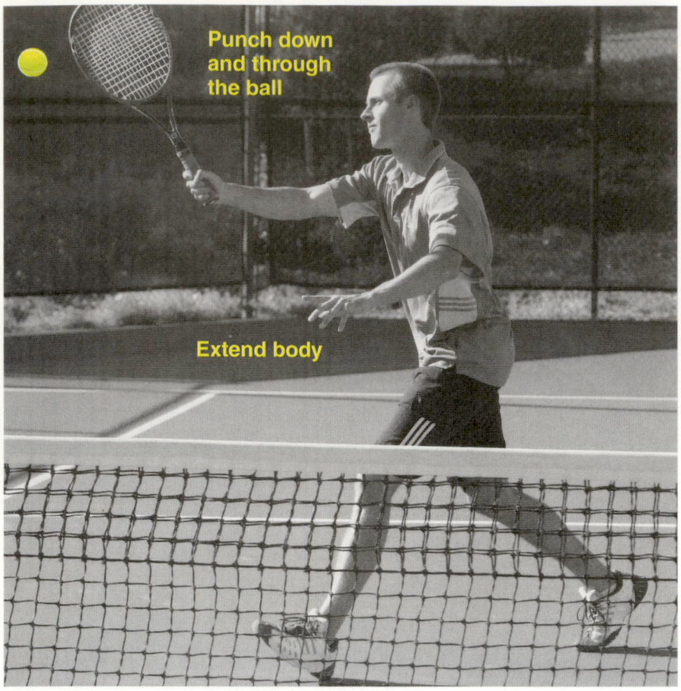

Photography by Terrell Lloyd; assisted by Anna Symonds Myers

PHOTO 4.12 High forehand volley.

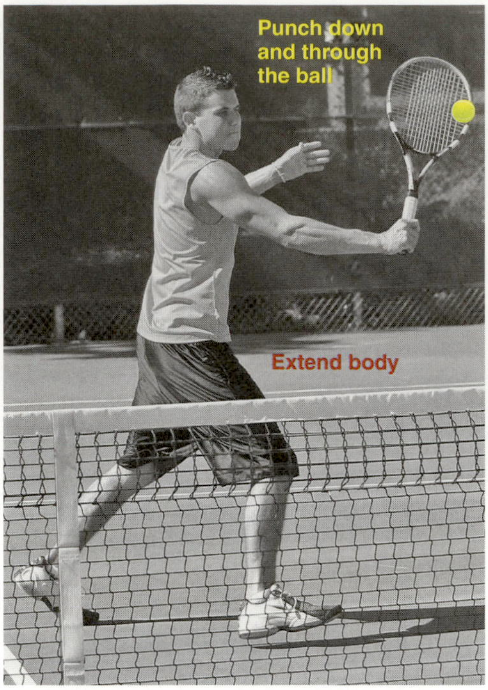

Photography by Terrell Lloyd; assisted by Anna Symonds Myers

PHOTO 4.13 High backhand volley.

Incorporating the Volley into Your Total Game

The volley has to be *incorporated into the total game* of the beginning player. At this point, the volley is an extension of the player hitting a groundstroke and advancing to the net, or hitting an approach shot and moving to the net, or hitting at the net in doubles play. The volley is a reward for forcing the opponent into a mistake, and it is executed best between the service court line and the net.

Beginning players will play most volleys off the net at a range of one to one and one-half racket lengths away from the net. More advanced players have a wider range back to the service court line, but the same players have the goal of moving closer to the net to be less vulnerable to a well-placed low shot at the feet.

Increasing Beginner Skills: Half-Volley

Half-volleys are necessary when the player is positioned in the midcourt area and is confronted with a return shot placed just in front of the feet. The player uses an eastern forehand or backhand grip, or a continental grip, and strokes the ball as a combination groundstroke and volley. The player must bend both legs to the extreme, with the lead leg bent at a right angle and the back leg nearly scraping the court surface.

The ball must be contacted on the "short" bounce. The wrist is firm at contact, and the angle of the racket face is open just enough to permit the ball to clear the net. The backswing is short, as with an approach shot, and the follow-through

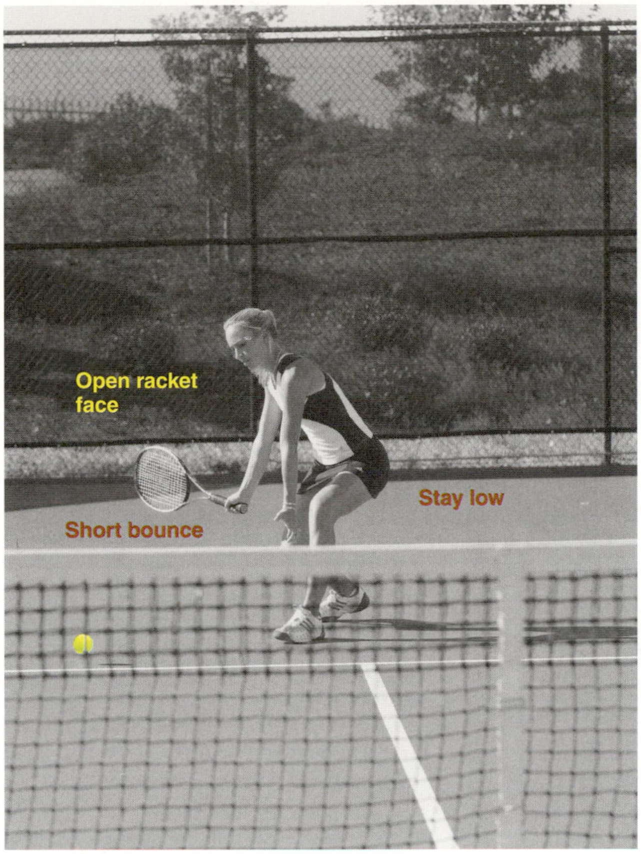

Photography by Terrell Lloyd; assisted by Anna Symonds Myers

PHOTO 4.14 Forehand half-volley.

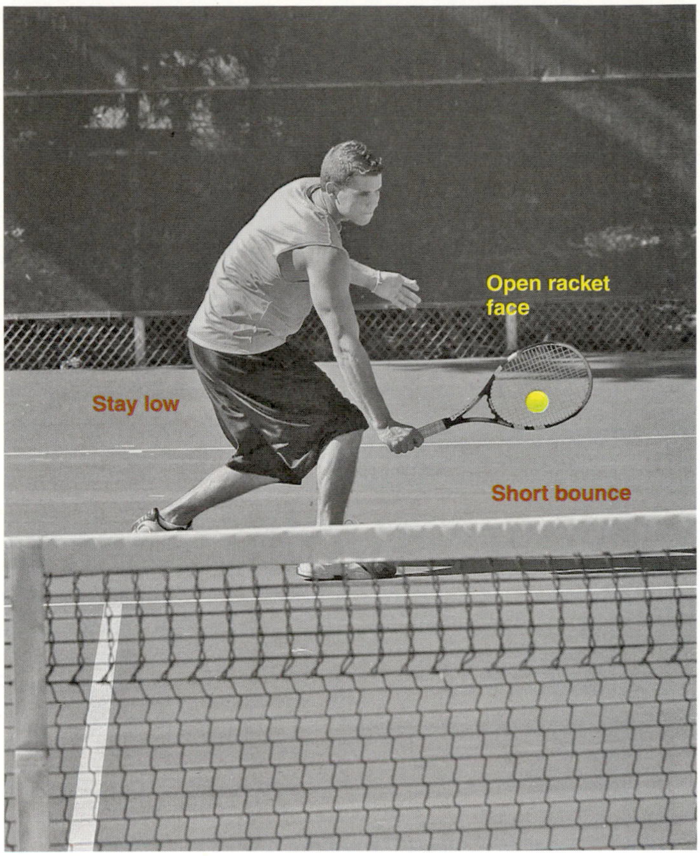

Photography by Terrell Lloyd; assisted by Anna Symonds Myers

PHOTO 4.15 Backhand half-volley.

lifts the body up from the low position. Throughout the shot, the head should stay down to ensure that the body does not lift early. The forehand half-volley contact point is at the lead leg, and the backhand point is in front of the lead leg (see Photos 4.14 and 4.15).

POINTS *to* REMEMBER

INSIGHT WHEN HITTING A VOLLEY SHOT

1. See the ball early in order to react.
2. Attack by stepping into the ball at contact.
3. A wide ball is reached by stepping across the nonracket leg and toward the net.
4. Bend, and get down on the ball, when hitting a low volley (ball below the net).
5. A high volley return requires an extension of the legs, a longer backswing and follow-through, and stepping into the ball, with the elbow closing on the stroke.
6. A ball hit into the body requires using your backhand. Remember to pivot off the racket-side foot, bringing the nonracket leg back, forcing you to turn your racket-side shoulder sideways.

POINTS to REMEMBER

HALF-VOLLEY

1. Contact ball on short bounce.
2. Get low, with leg bent.
3. Open front edge of racket face at contact.

CHECKPOINTS

1. The type of grip used for the volley is the
   a. eastern forehand.
   b. eastern backhand.
   c. western forehand.
   d. continental.
2. The backswing for a volley shot is
   a. shortened.
   b. lengthened.
   c. the same as a regular groundstroke.
   d. any of the above three, depending on the situation.
3. Contact with the ball is made
   a. in front of the lead leg.
   b. behind the lead leg.
   c. even with the lead leg.
   d. with all three, depending on the situation.
4. To correct the shot that hits the net following contact,
   a. tighten the grip.
   b. align the wrist, arms, and shoulders in a firm position.
   c. bend the knees through the shot.
   d. close the racket face.
5. The body position for a ball hit directly at the body of the volleying player is to
   a. use a backhand volley.
   b. drop step to hit the ball.
   c. use a forehand stroke.
   d. use *a* and *b* in combination with each other.
6. A low volley position requires
   a. opening the racket face at contact.
   b. closing the racket face at contact.
   c. hitting with a square face at contact.
   d. hitting off the back foot.
7. The beginning player has a comfort zone range at the net
   a. of 1 to 1½ racket lengths from the net.
   b. from the service court to the net.
   c. of 2 to 2½ racket lengths from the net.
   d. of anywhere on the court.
8. A half-volley is hit with
   a. an open racket face at the top of the ball bounce.
   b. a closed racket face off a short bounce.
   c. a square face off a short bounce.
   d. an open face off a short bounce.
9. The leg movement for volleying a wide-ball is
   a. stepping with the inside leg closest to the ball.
   b. stepping back with the inside leg closest to the ball.
   c. cross-stepping with the outside leg to hit the ball.
   d. reaching with the arm and racket, keeping the feet and legs stable.
10. The follow-through of the racket when volleying is
    a. a punch action with the lower edge of the racket open.
    b. a punch action with the lower edge of the racket closed.
    c. a semi-swing with the lower edge of the racket open.
    d. a semi-swing with the lower edge of the racket closed.

Answers to Checkpoints can be found on page 167.

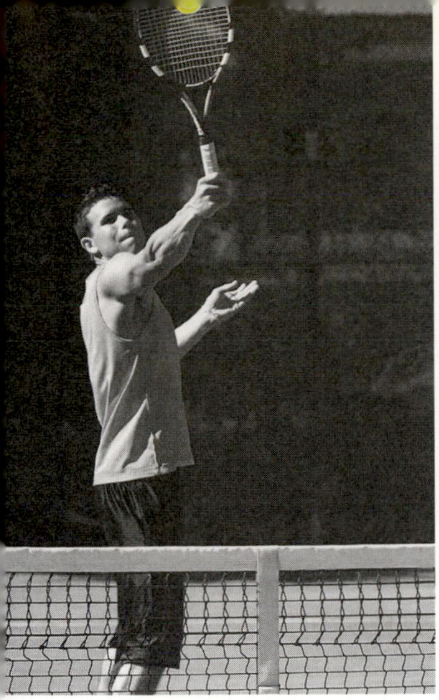

5 Aerial Game

The lob and overhead combinations are basic strokes for the beginning player, although they are usually presented last when learning various tennis skills. Each skill complements the other in tennis. The lob is an extension of the groundstroke, discussed in Chapter 2, and the overhead is an elaboration of the service, discussed in Chapter 3. Overheads are attacking weapons. Lobs are typically used to react to an opponent playing at the net.

Overheads

The basic overhead is executed as a flat serve from the half-swing position. The overhead also can be executed from the forehand or the backhand side, but typically players run around the backhand to play a forehand overhead. The two forehand overheads in tennis are the orthodox overhead, with little foot movement and a simple swing, and the more complex overhead (also termed "overhead with scissors kick"), characterized by additional agility and timing (Photo 5.1). The orthodox overhead is the only overhead to be emphasized in this chapter. The eastern forehand or continental grip is used for all forehand overheads.

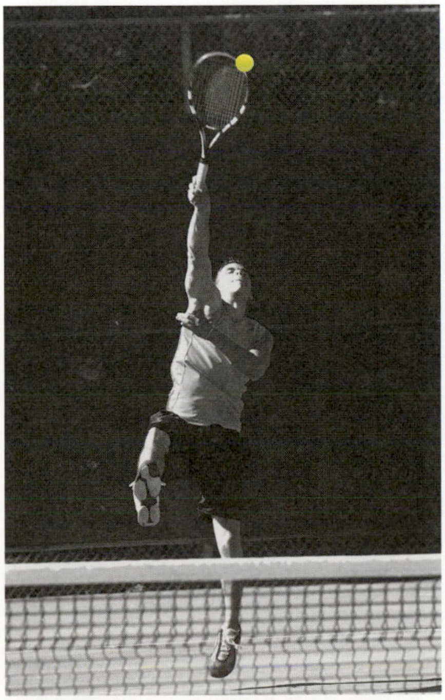

PHOTO 5.1 Complex overhead.

Overhead Transition from the Flat Service

The *orthodox forehand overhead* is a simple transition from the flat service. The player must maneuver underneath the ball that is hit as a lob, and from that position bring the racket back to the middle of the shoulder blades, with the racket elbow at a right angle. The position of the racket physically touching between the shoulder blades provides a reference point for the player hitting the overhead. When the racket moves to this position, the simultaneous reaction is for the player to point to the ball with the nonracket arm and hand as a second reference point. The line of flight of the lob is similar to the ball toss, but in this case the ball falls more rapidly and at a slightly different angle. The feet are a shoulder width apart, and the nonracket shoulder has turned to face the net and the intended target area (Photo 5.2).

Executing the Overhead

In executing the overhead, the player's body is coiled and gathered, ready to time the stroke. The ball is hit off the lead shoulder, with the legs extending and the body uncoiling. Contact of racket to ball involves an up-and-over motion, with your

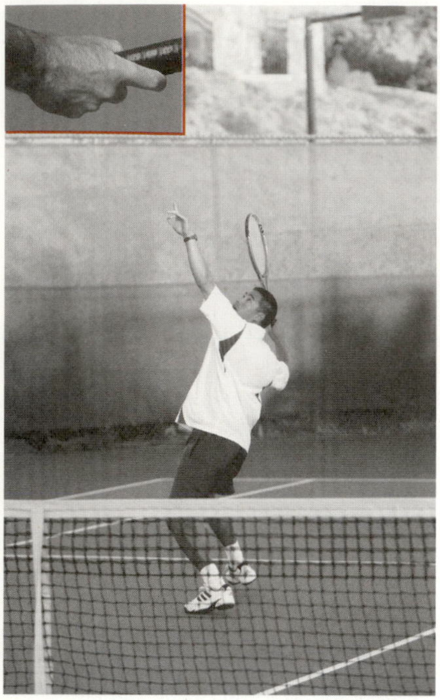

Photography by Terrell Lloyd; assisted by Anna Symonds Myers; inset photo by Virginia Bryant

PHOTO 5.2 Orthodox overhead (eastern forehand or continental grip).

forearm pronating, providing a little topspin for greater net clearance and depth. At contact, the racket arm is extended and the racket comes through the ball with a wrist break; while the nonracket hand that is used as a reference point is pulled down and back. The follow-through then continues to the far hip, but the follow-through action is shortened to accommodate the return of a ready position for the next shot (Photos 5.3A–D).

The full stroke is simple, eliminating wasted motion and extraneous actions. The feet remain stable until the follow-through pulls the back foot forward to catch the balance of the player at completion of the follow-through. The player is encouraged to hit out on the ball with smooth, rhythmical timing and control.

Increasing Agility

Advancing to more agility with the forehand overhead requires adding a few parts to the stroke. First, the player has to set up to hit the overhead. That movement consists of long, running strides to get to the general area as fast as possible and thereby allow time to set up the stroke. Once in the general area, the player will be situated behind the anticipated drop of the ball. At this point, the player takes small steps to adjust to the position of the ball. Balls that are hit over the player's head are handled in the same manner: taking long strides to get behind the ball and then short crossover steps to adjust to the falling pattern of the ball. One additional thought regarding retreating back is *never* to backpedal to the setup position. Back pedaling is not efficient and can also lead to injury caused by tripping.

Bouncing the Overhead

Bouncing the overhead means permitting the ball to bounce before executing an overhead. In two situations the lob is allowed to bounce prior to

Orthodox Forehand Overhead Sequence

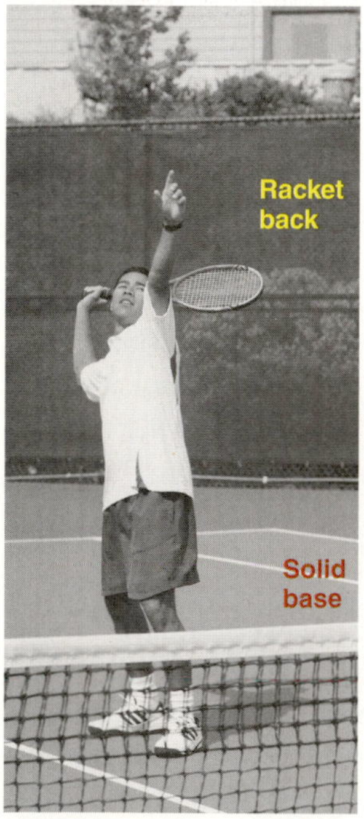

PHOTO 5.3A Preparation.

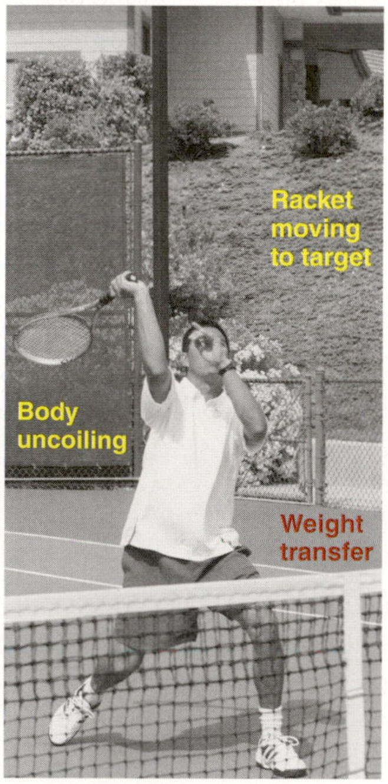

PHOTO 5.3B Initiation of swing.

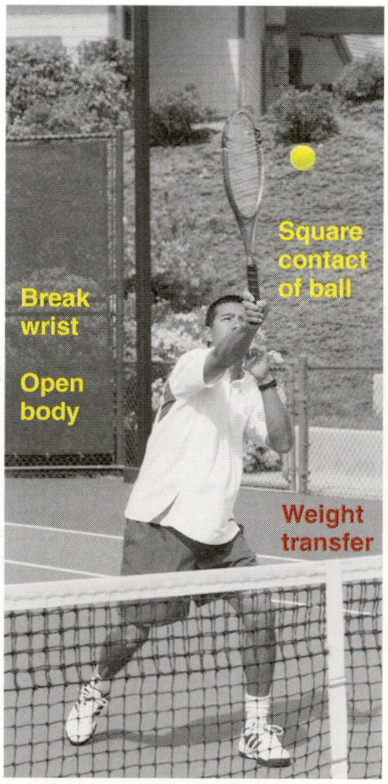

PHOTO 5.3C Contact.

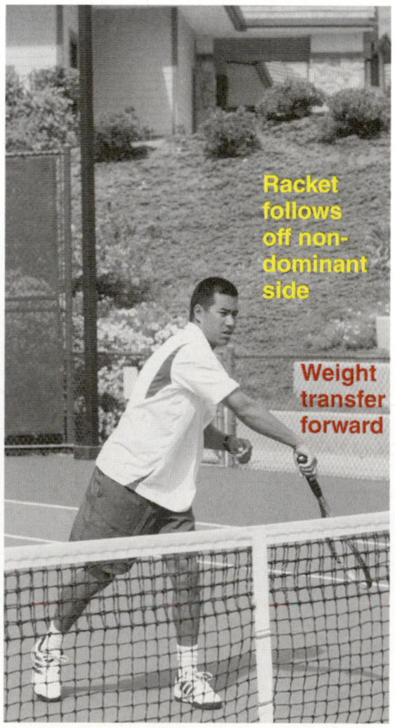

PHOTO 5.3D Follow-through.

Photography by Terrell Lloyd; assisted by Anna Symonds Myers

being hit as an overhead. Lobs that have a very high loft are permitted to bounce for better timing when hitting the overhead. Lobs that are short at the net, eliminating a good set position for the overhead, also are allowed to bounce.

Hitting a high lob following a bounce is similar to hitting the overhead from a midair position following a lob. The additional time created when permitting a bounce gives the opponent an opportunity to reposition in anticipation of returning an overhead return, and it also gives the player hitting the overhead a chance to place the ball more effectively.

When hitting a lob that bounces short, you need to stay low enough so that the stroke is still angled down and through the ball. The goal for the overhead return of a short ball is a short, hard-hit, high-bouncing ball that carries out beyond the baseline.

Backhand Overhead

The *backhand overhead* (also called "high backhand volley") is used when the player cannot run around the ball to hit a forehand overhead. To begin a backhand overhead, the player should use an eastern backhand or continental grip and turn the shoulder so that the racket side actually faces the net. The elbow on the racket side is up and points to the ball, and the racket head is below the hand. The weight is on the player's back foot and the head is up, eyes fixed on the ball.

The ball is contacted above the head, slightly in front of the racket shoulder, with the racket face moving through the ball, with a strong break of the wrist. The weight is transferred forward through the ball, with the follow-through carrying the racket head downward and parallel to the court surface (Photos 5.4A–C).

Backhand Overhead

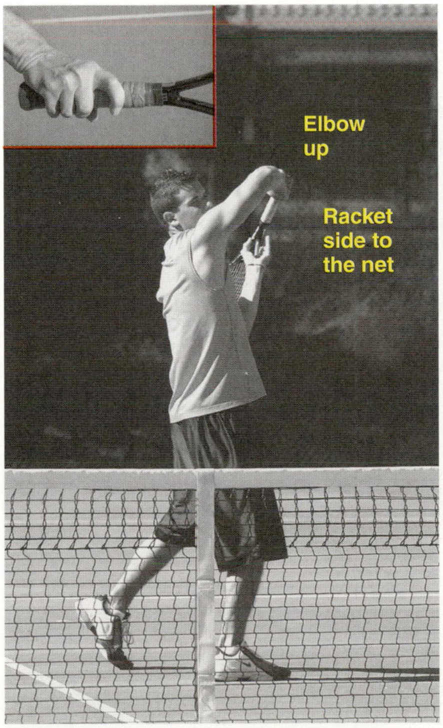

PHOTO 5.4A Preparation (eastern backhand grip)

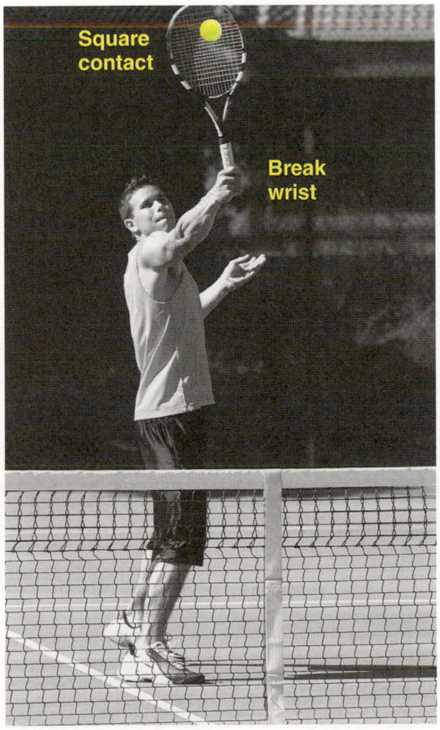

PHOTO 5.4B Contact.

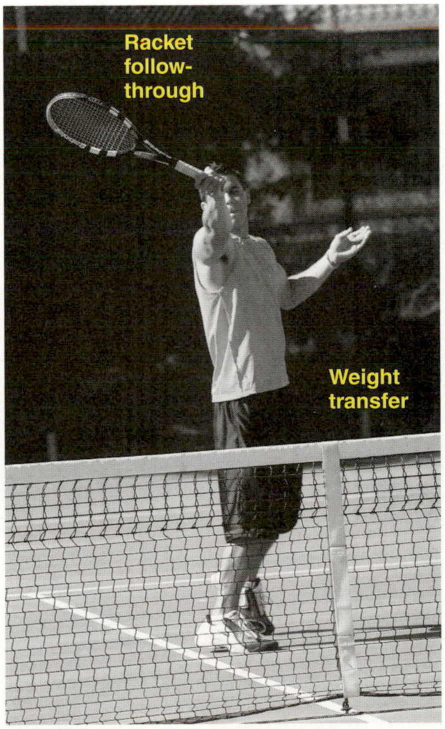

PHOTO 5.4C Follow-through.

Photography by Terrell Lloyd; assisted by Anna Symonds Myers; inset photo by Virginia Bryant

Incorporating the Overhead into Your Game

Incorporating the overhead into the total game blends favorably with the player's total game plan. Once the ball is in play the overhead is the second type of shot that is hit before the ball bounces, thus joining the volley shot as a stroke hit in the air near the net. When a player is at the net, the opponent must hit either a groundstroke that the net player hopefully can volley or a lob that the net player can return as an overhead.

Players with improving skill and confidence can hit an overhead from any location on the court, while beginning players should hit overheads when lobs land short between the service court line and the net. Beginning players also would be wise to let the ball bounce before executing an overhead so that timing can aid in the stroke. As you develop skill, the transition to a complex overhead can occur by hitting on the fly and using the scissors kick.

Regardless of skill development, the player has to remember that the overhead is an offensive shot that must be hit under control and with confidence. The player also should remember that the overhead is the first in a series of overheads if the opponent returns the first overhead. Returns of overheads tend to be shorter lobs than the first lob hit, consequently setting up the player at the net for an eventually "easy" overhead.

POINTS *to* REMEMBER

ORTHODOX FOREHAND OVERHEAD

1. Use an eastern forehand or continental grip.
2. Keep in mind that the forehand overhead is consistent with a basic throwing action that imitates the flat serve.
3. Place the racket head between your shoulder blades on the backswing.
4. Point your nonracket arm at the ball for a reference point to the ball.
5. Keep the base of the feet wide throughout the stroke.
6. Bring the racket through the ball, with a wrist snap and a downward follow-through.
7. "Bounce" the ball when it is lobbed extremely high or is hit short to the net.

POINTS *to* REMEMBER

BACKHAND OVERHEAD

1. Use an eastern backhand or continental grip.
2. Point the racket elbow at the ball on the backhand overhead, and turn the racket side to the net during the preparation phase.
3. Bring the wrist through the ball forcefully at contact.

COMMON ERRORS & HOW TO CORRECT THEM *(Forehand Overhead)*

The Error	What Causes the Error	To Correct the Error
Hitting into the net.	Ball too far out in front of the lead shoulder, or hitting the ball too forcefully downward. Or ball is not positioned above your head.	Get directly underneath the ball. Keep your chin up. Focus on a target on the other side of the net. Make sure the ball is above your head.
Hitting out beyond the opponent's baseline.	Hitting too hard with poor timing, or hitting up into the ball.	Get directly underneath the ball and hit through the ball, breaking the wrist at contact.
Inconsistency in placing the ball.	Racket not placed between the shoulder blades on the backswing as a reference point, and setup is inconsistent.	Get directly underneath the ball, and always place the racket between the shoulder blades. Hit the ball off your lead shoulder. Keep a wide foot base.
Hitting the ball off the edge of the racket at the top or off the bottom edge, causing the ball to be hit long or to hit the court surface immediately.	Swinging too early or too late.	Point the nonracket arm to the ball for a reference point, check the position of the racket on the backswing, and develop a rhythmical timing to the stroke.

The Lob

The *lob* is an extension of the groundstroke, incorporating the same grip and basic swinging action. It is the defensive answer to an opponent advancing to the net when you are retreating and an offensive response to an attacking opponent when you have time to set up. Mechanics of the stroke require the racket face to open and lift the ball. Lobs are characterized by a high *flight pattern*. The flight patterns are different for each type of lob, and the differences are based on the purpose of the stroke and the amount of spin applied to the ball. The beginning player initially is simply trying to get the ball in the air, over the head of an opponent. In a short time span, however, the beginning player needs to learn to hit both a defensive and an offensive lob. These two basic lobs are discussed next and are diagrammed in Figure 5.1.

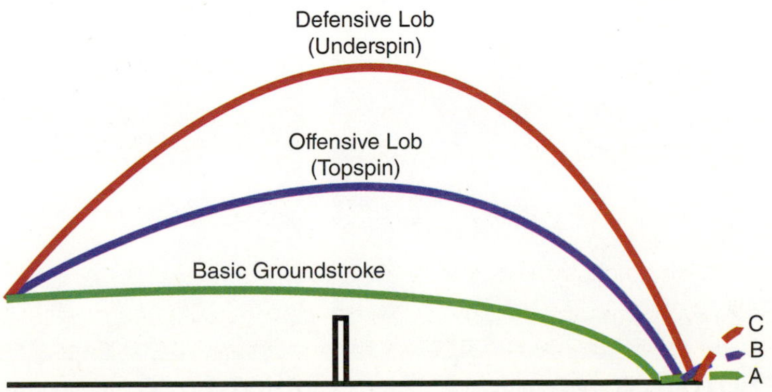

FIGURE 5.1 Flight patterns of lobs and groundstroke.

The *defensive lob* has a high flight pattern and is hit off a strong opposing-player return, with an underspin rotation. The *offensive lob* has a lower flight pattern than the defensive lob and is hit over the outstretched reach of the net player, bouncing near the baseline and kicking on beyond the baseline.

Defensive Lob

The *defensive lob* is the typical lob hit by beginning players. As they develop skills, beginners use the defensive lob as a reaction to an opponent's overhead. With a continental or an eastern forehand or backhand grip, the racket is brought straight back into a low, short backswing position with a firm wrist. The racket is brought forward at waist level to hit the ball off the lead shoulder. The bottom edge of the racket leads, opening the racket face. The follow-through is high, and the racket face remains open. The racket stays in the same plane as during the swing from preparation to follow-through. The wrist remains firm throughout the stroke, and the weight transfer, although important, is minimal compared to other strokes. The legs are bent and extended through the swing pattern, but only with a minimum amount of change. The lob is a reaction to an aggressively hit ball, so the total stroke has to be made in moderation to combat the high velocity of the ball (Photos 5.5A–C and 5.6A–C).

Offensive Lob

The *offensive lob* is really an extension of a topspin groundstroke, described in Chapter 2 for topspin forehand and backhand ground-strokes. It requires use of a continental or an eastern forehand or backhand grip.

The racket is brought back low, with an extensive knee bend and the wrist cocked. The racket then moves into the ball with a slightly open face at waist height, meeting the ball from underneath and lifting up. The wrist breaks at contact, imparting topspin to the ball. The follow-through continues, with the racket finishing at an exaggerated high position off the middle of the body, with a roll of the wrist (Photos 5.7A–C and 5.8A–C). The more speed generated by the racket head, the more topspin generated and the faster the ball will drop.

Two-Hand Offensive and Defensive Backhand Lobs

The two-hand offensive and defensive backhand lobs are executed nearly the same as traditional offensive or defensive backhand lobs, and the limitation to hitting lobs with a two-hand grip is the same as for backhand groundstrokes. That, of course, is limited court coverage, which can be significant, particularly when chasing

Defensive Lob with Forehand Underspin

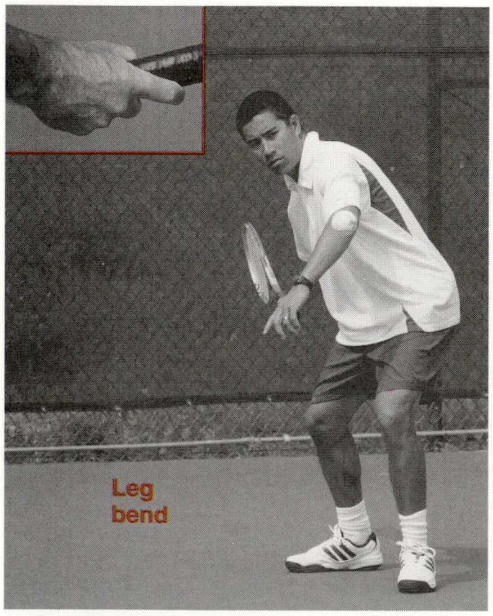

PHOTO 5.5A Preparation (eastern forehand grip).

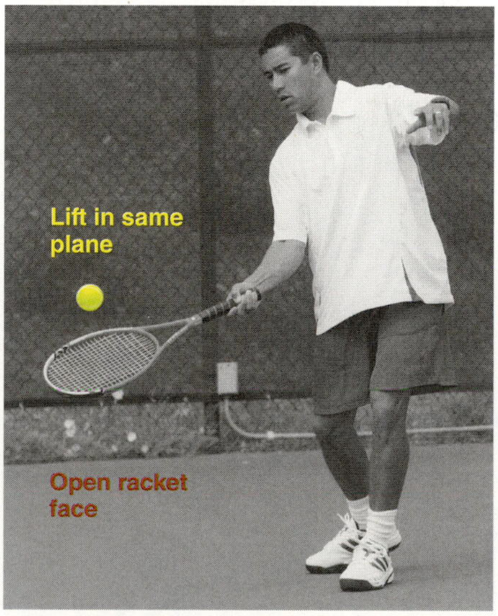

PHOTO 5.5B Contact.

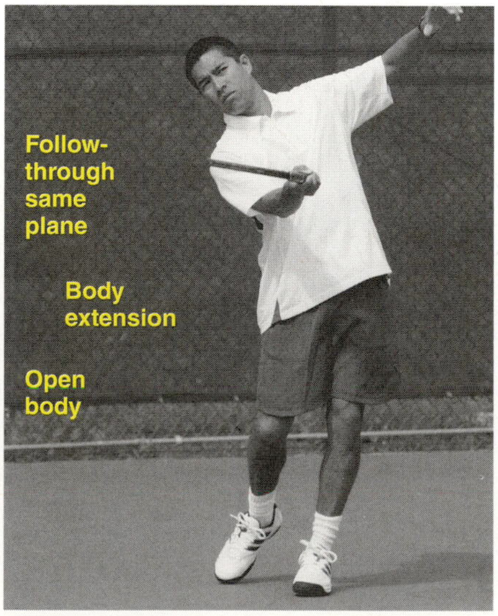

PHOTO 5.5C Follow-through.

Photography by Terrell Lloyd; assisted by Anna Symonds Myers; inset photo by Virginia Bryant

Defensive Lob with Backhand Underspin

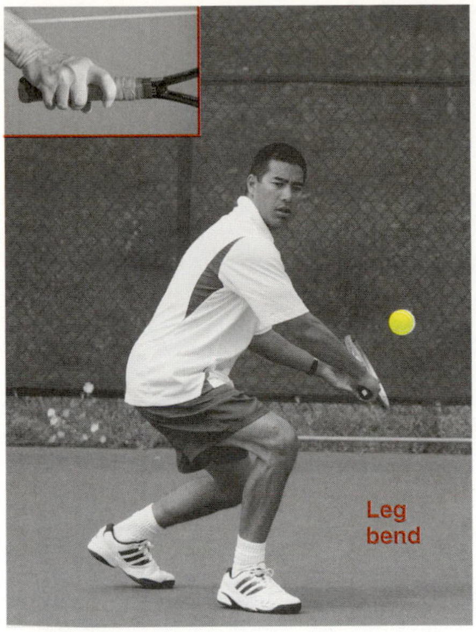

PHOTO 5.6A Preparation (eastern backhand grip).

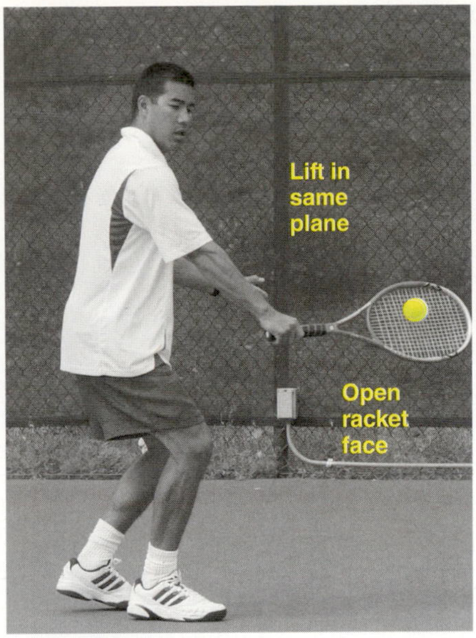

PHOTO 5.6B Contact.

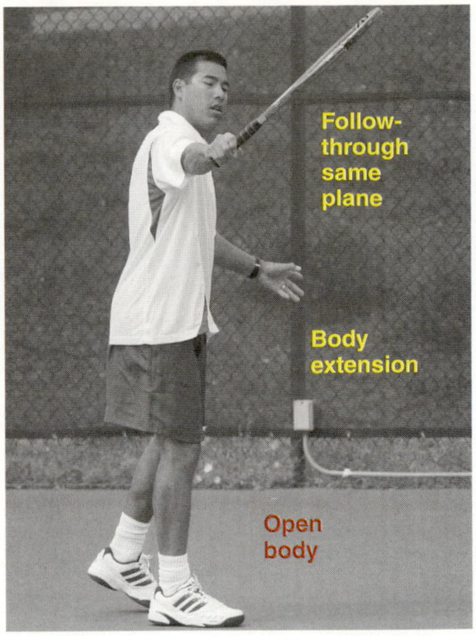

PHOTO 5.6C Follow-through.

Photography by Terrell Lloyd; assisted by Anna Symonds Myers; inset photo by Virginia Bryant

Forehand Offensive Lob with Topspin

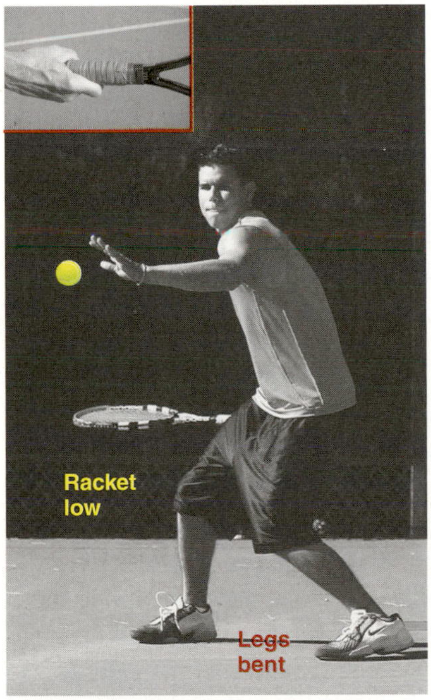

PHOTO 5.7A Prior to contact (eastern forehand grip).

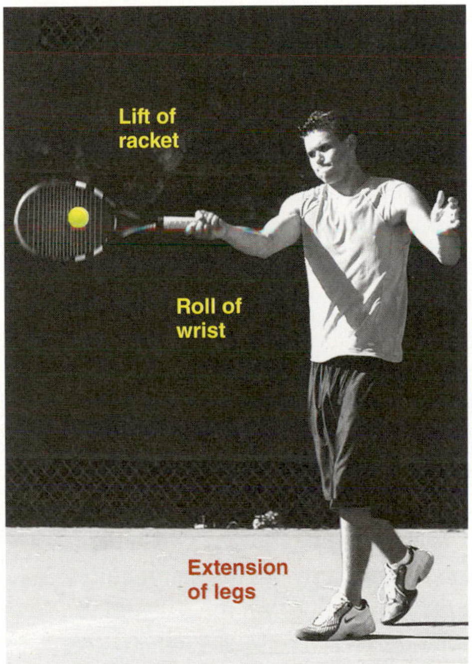

PHOTO 5.7B Just after contact.

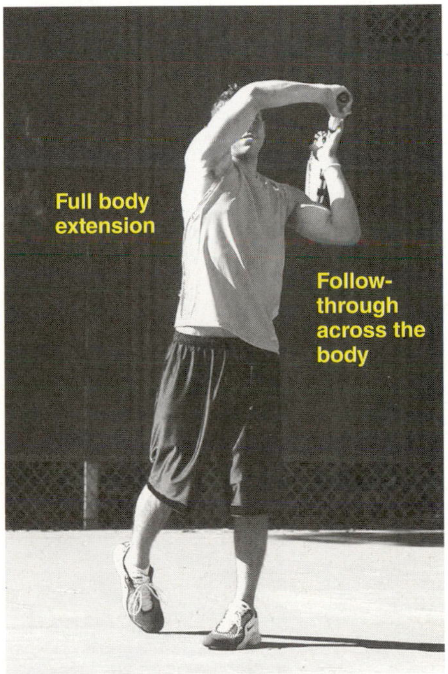

PHOTO 5.7C Follow-through.

Photography by Terrell Lloyd; assisted by Anna Symonds Myers; inset photo by Virginia Bryant

Backhand Offensive Lob with Topspin

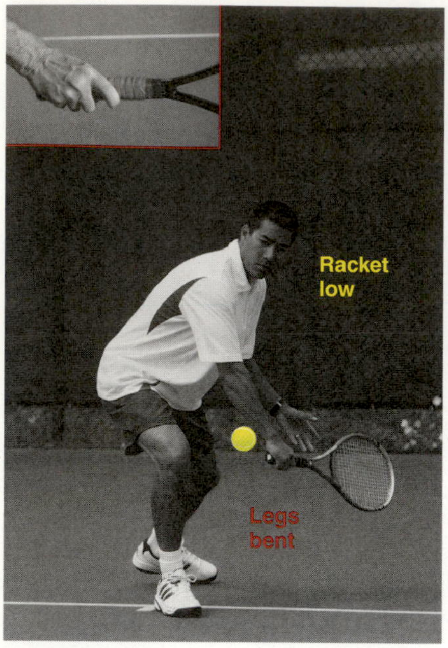

PHOTO 5.8A Preparation (eastern backhand grip).

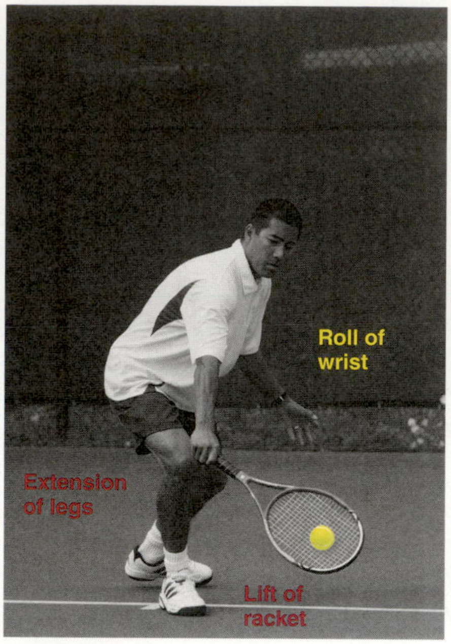

PHOTO 5.8B Contact.

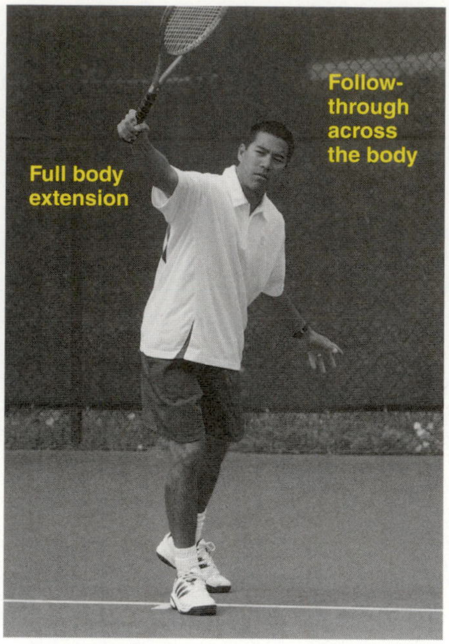

PHOTO 5.8C Follow-through.

Photography by Terrell Lloyd; assisted by Anna Symonds Myers; inset photo by Virginia Bryant

down a well-hit shot that requires a defensive lob return.

The *two-hand defensive lob* is quite similar to the traditional one-hand lob. The main focus is on leg bend and extension and on maintaining a follow-through in the same plane as the flight of the ball. This is a defensive lob, which requires a high loft to the ball. A deep leg bend and extension are required to accomplish a high lift. The follow-through must be in line with the flight of the ball rather than rolling over in a wrap-around position (Photos 5.9A–C). The critical aspect of the two-hand lob is when a shot is hit that requires a player to run down the ball and to extend to reach to hit a defensive lob return. If a player can't reach a shot of this type, the return is compromised and a weak or ineffective return results. Consequently, anticipation and speed are prerequisites for hitting a two-hand defensive lob.

Like the groundstroke, the *two-hand offensive lob* requires a low-to-high swing path which imparts topspin to the ball. It is important to remember to bend the knees and lift at contact. It is also important to remember not to wrap the racket around your head on the follow-through but, rather, to lift and then stop the follow-through off the nonracket-side shoulder (Photos 5.10A–C).

Incidentals of Hitting a Lob

Racket control, weight transfer, and movement of the feet are essential to hitting lobs. These skills require extensive work on the part of a beginning player. Racket control is used to apply topspin of varying degrees, underspin, or a simple block of the ball.

Weight transfer, as with all shots, is important with the lob, but the transfer has more to do with the hips and a little step transfer than with a long step into the ball. It is more of a center-of-gravity movement forward.

Most lobs are hit on the move rather than from a stationary position. The player either is retreating from the net to hit the ball or is moving laterally along the baseline. As

Two-Hand Defensive Lob

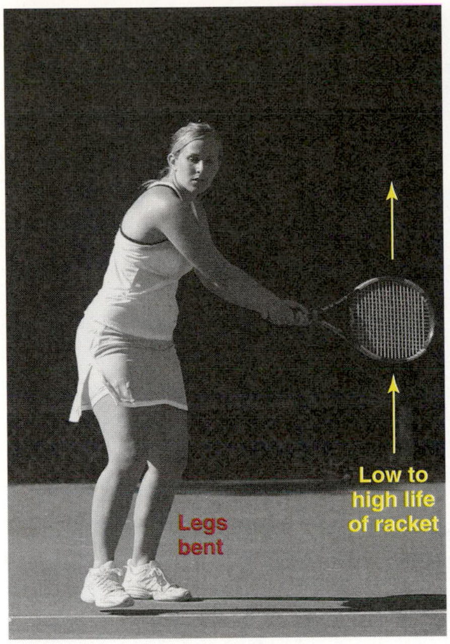

PHOTO 5.9A Preparation.

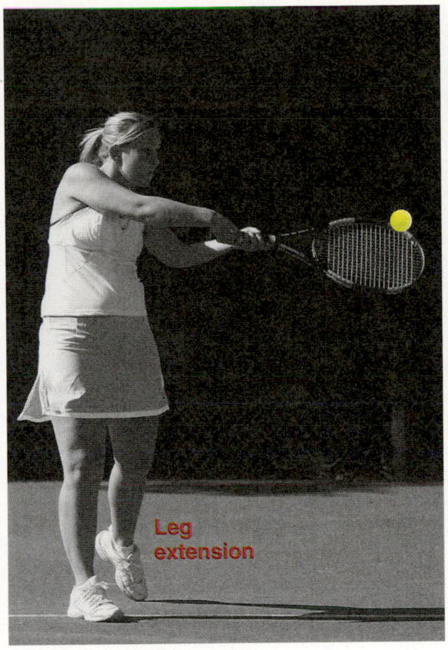

PHOTO 5.9B Contact.

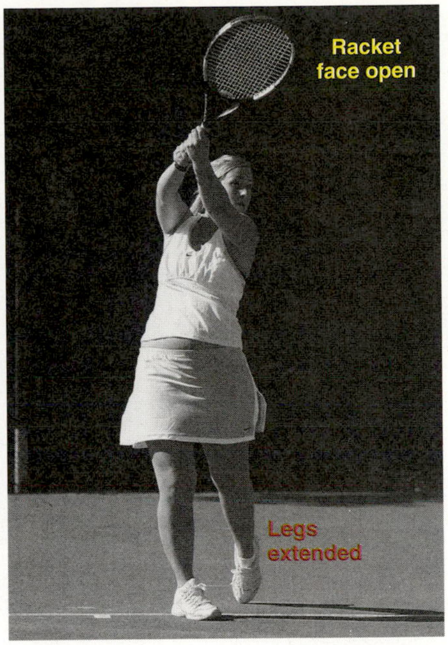

PHOTO 5.9C Follow-through.

Photography by Terrell Lloyd; assisted by Anna Symonds Myers.

Two-Hand Offensive Lob

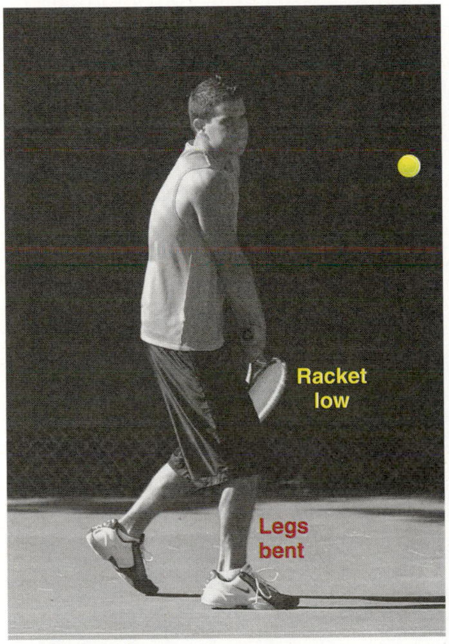

PHOTO 5.10A Preparation.

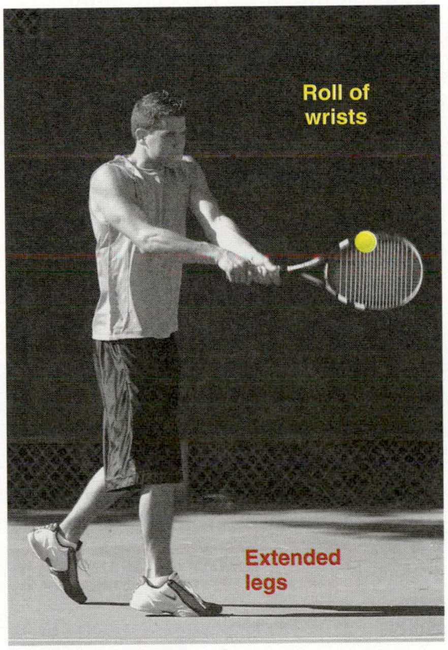

PHOTO 5.10B Contact.

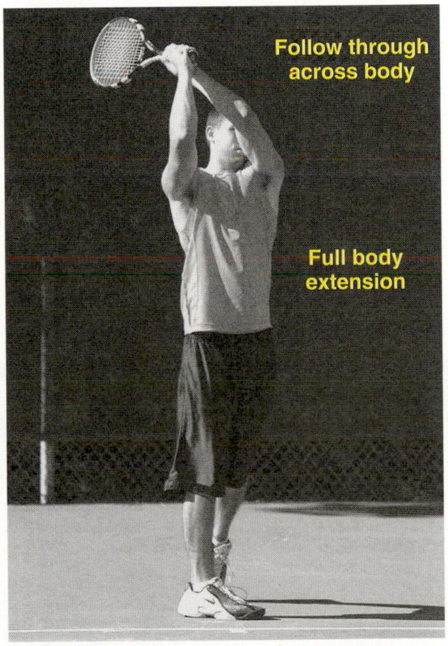

PHOTO 5.10C Follow-through.

Photography by Terrell Lloyd; assisted by Anna Symonds Myers.

a result of having to hit a lob on the run, the lob isn't always a nice setup from a ready position that permits easy execution of the stroke. Moving the feet to get to the ball and then recovering enough to place the racket on the ball while attempting to hold form are all based on the initial foot movement and anticipation as to the location the opponent has intended for a target.

The key with lateral movement along the baseline is to cross-step and then step away from and slightly behind the ball (Photos 5.11A–C). Retreating to hit a deeply hit lob

Moving Laterally to Hit a Lob behind the Baseline—Forehand

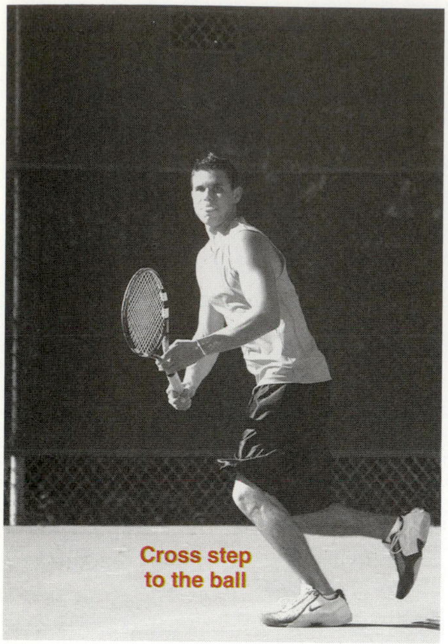

PHOTO 5.11A Preparation.

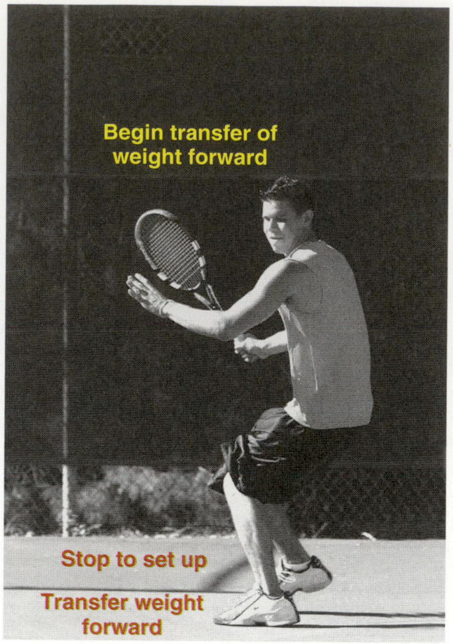

PHOTO 5.11B Backswing.

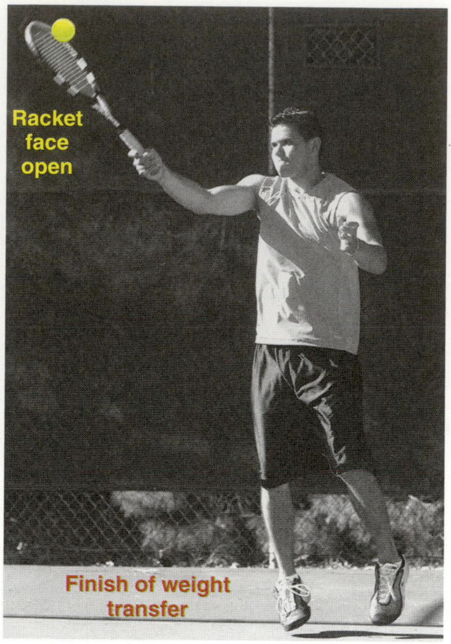

PHOTO 5.11C Contact.

Photography by Terrell Lloyd; assisted by Anna Symonds Myers

requires a similar cross-step, going back to the anticipated hitting position of the ball, which positions you away from and to the side of the ball (Photos 5.12A–C). If you can arrive early enough to step back into the ball when hitting the ball, your chances for success increase. But often, when chasing down a ball, your momentum will carry you in a continuous backward stride. In that situation, you need to compensate for the backward movement by targeting the ball a little deeper than you would normally.

Incorporating the lob into the total game is important to the developing

Retreating to Hit a Lob behind the Baseline—Backhand

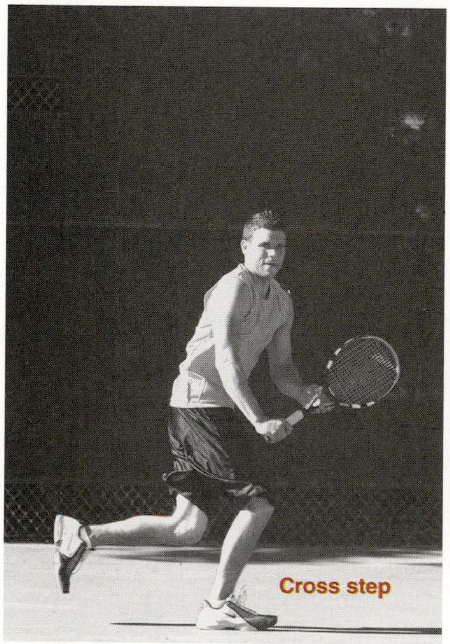

PHOTO 5.12A Preparation.

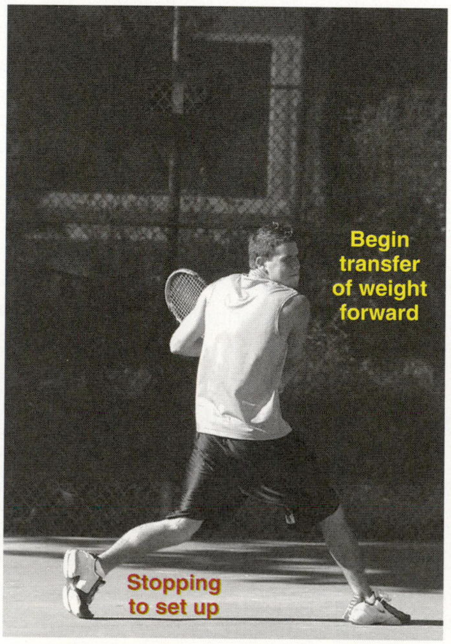

PHOTO 5.12B Backswing.

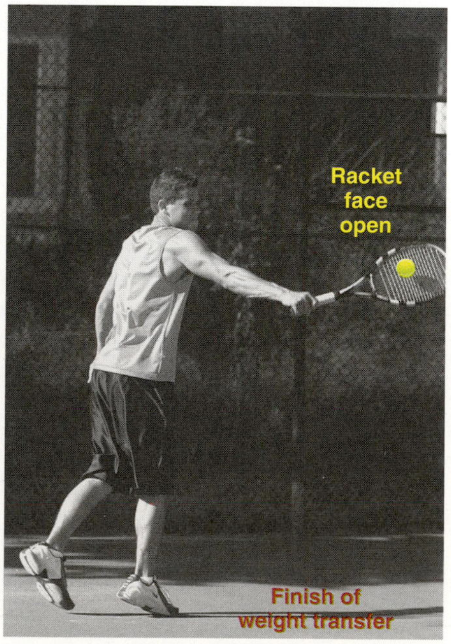

PHOTO 5.12C Contact.

Photography by Terrell Lloyd; assisted by Anna Symonds Myers

player. Without the lob, there is no response to the over-head smash and the options for hitting a ball when the opponent is at the net decrease by one. The lob also serves as an occasional change-of-pace stroke, and it can be frustrating for the opponent who likes pace associated with the game or who cannot hit an overhead effectively. Remember, the lob is an extension of a groundstroke, and developing the skill is a transition rather than development of a totally new stroke.

POINTS *to* REMEMBER

LOBS

1. To produce an offensive lob with topspin, roll the forearm from contact through follow-through.
2. Strive for all lob follow-throughs to finish high and in line with the flight of the ball.
3. Follow the principle that the more defensive a lob and the more change from some topspin to an underspin, the more firm the wrist and the shorter the backswing.
4. To regulate topspin in an offensive lob, vary leg bend and extension. The more topspin, the more leg bend and extension.
5. Open the racket face on lobs at contact.
6. Move to the ball as quickly as possible to incorporate form into the stroke.
7. The height of a defensive lob is high, with backspin; the offensive lob is lower, with topspin, just clearing a net player's racket extension.
8. If you use a two-hand backhand lob, remember to anticipate early in order to compensate for limited reach.

COMMON ERRORS & HOW TO CORRECT THEM *(Lobs)*

The Error	What Causes the Error	To Correct the Error
Lobs hit long beyond the opponent's baseline.	Too much velocity and lift applied to the ball.	The lob requires touch and feel. Focus on a shorter target. Adjust the upward angle of the racket.
Balls hit short, just over the net.	Usually not enough backswing and follow through, and/or weight transfer.	If stroking the lob, the backswing and follow-through should be equal in distance; and the more distance, the farther the ball will travel. Transfer more weight forward.
Lobs that are blocked without much follow-through. Rebound at different angles.	Racket face isn't square to the ball at contact.	Provide a firm arm and wrist base, with an open racket face, and lift.

CHECKPOINTS

1. Positioning to hit an overhead requires the body to
   a. be positioned behind the ball.
   b. be positioned in front of the ball.
   c. be positioned underneath the ball.
   d. adjust depending on the height of the lob.
2. The overhead should be hit after allowing the ball to bounce when
   a. a lob is hit short at the net.
   b. a lob has a very high loft.
   c. situations in both *a* and *b* exist.
   d. the player is unsure of how to hit the ball.
3. When hitting a backhand overhead, the position of the elbow is
   a. up, pointed at the ball.
   b. out, pointed in line with where the ball is to be hit.
   c. down, positioned to allow the racket to swing through the ball.
   d. none of the above.
4. Overhead shots hit long are caused by
   a. hitting the ball too hard.
   b. hitting the ball with an open racket face.
   c. hitting the ball with the ball positioned behind the head.
   d. all three examples above.
5. When hitting an offensive lob, the follow-through pattern requires the racket
   a. to cross the upper body and finish high.
   b. to stay in the same plane as with the backswing and contact positions.
   c. to stop following contact with the ball.
   d. to cross the upper body and stay low.
6. The ball action off a defensive lob is
   a. underspin.
   b. topspin.
   c. slice.
   d. no spin.
7. The movement pattern of the racket for a basic groundstroke, offensive lob, and defensive lob is
   a. high, middle, low.
   b. middle, high, low.
   c. low, middle, high.
   d. middle, low, high.
8. The keys to hitting successful defensive lobs include
   a. leg bend and extension, open racket face, and fast racket movement.
   b. leg bend and extension, open racket face, and high follow-through in line with the flight of the ball.
   c. leg bend and extension, closed racket face, high follow-through, follow-through off nonracket shoulder.
   d. leg bend and extension, closed racket face, and fast racket movement.
9. When retreating or moving laterally to hit a lob, it is important
   a. to keep on running as part of the follow-through.
   b. to make contact with the ball and fall back with your weight going backward.
   c. to make contact with the ball and follow through toward the back fence of the court.
   d. to stop your momentum to the side and back of the ball, and at weight transfer, move your weight forward, following contact and into the follow-through.
10. The trajectory for an offensive lob, defensive lob, and groundstroke from lowest flight pattern to highest is
    a. defensive lob, offensive lob, ground stroke.
    b. offensive lob, ground stroke, defensive lob.
    c. ground stroke, offensive lob, defensive lob.
    d. ground stroke, defensive lob, offensive lob.

Answers to Checkpoints can be found on page 167.

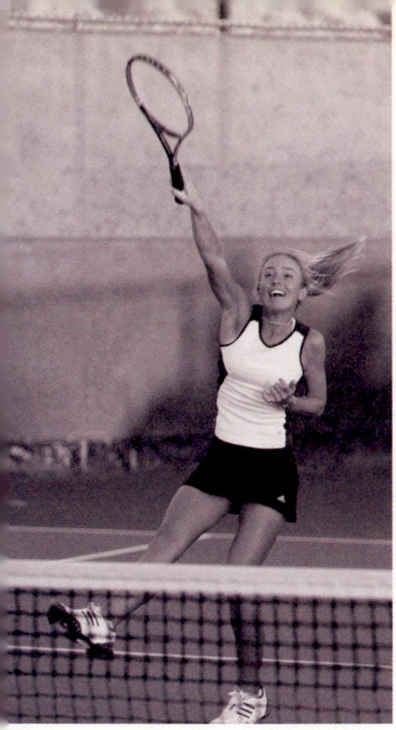

Photography by Terrell Lloyd; assisted by Anna Symonds Myers

6

Mental Aspects of Tennis Competition

This is the chapter that tends to be the most overlooked of all the chapters in the book, yet it is perhaps the most important or critical chapter with regard to playing tennis effectively.

At every level of tennis play, physical skill and mental strategy must be combined to be successful. Mental effort is the intangible that supports and reinforces the physical effort on a tennis court. Beginning tennis players tend to focus almost entirely on the physical skill aspect. Developing groundstrokes, volleys, serves, overheads, and lobs requires tremendous concentration and effort. The early mental focus for a beginning tennis player is on how and where to hit a ball and then on what the opponent is doing on the other side of the net. These are certainly important aspects in learning to play tennis, but a whole mental frame of mind is crucial to truly enjoying the game and to ultimately achieving success.

People play tennis for many reasons, including an interest and willingness to compete, a desire to play a social game, an interest in developing fitness, a way to gain college academic credit, or simply to participate in an activity to add to quality of life. Whatever the reason for playing tennis might be, the most overriding one should be the sheer joy of playing. To play tennis effectively requires that the player feel the game, feel the aesthetics, and appreciate the execution of skills related to the game. A successful tennis player plays for the enjoyment of physical movement and the fun that goes along with playing the game.

Tennis, as a game, includes sounds of ball striking racket and the wind, and those a player makes when striving to hit a ball or move to the ball. Tennis is truly a life experience that can enhance the quality of life.

This chapter is about learning how to play tennis effectively. It is about gaining an understanding of what competition really means, eliminating negative thoughts and attitudes, developing the ability to concentrate and relax to reduce anxiety, and learning how to acquire mental toughness. The focus here is on playing tennis with a strong mental outlook. If you do that, all the other parts of the game, including winning, will fall into place.

Execution and Competitiveness

Competition and winning often are confused as being the same, but they are barely related. There is a concept attached to competition that will enable you to flourish and develop as a player. That concept allows you to play within yourself and place execution of tennis skills ahead of winning. And through this process, success in terms of winning will emerge.

The Competitive Concept

Tennis competition really does not pit opponent against opponent. It pits player against barrier. There is a thought process that needs to be acquired that reduces the importance of the opposing player. If you can visualize the player on the other side of the net as setting up barriers as a challenge to you, you are beginning to understand the nature of competition. The opponent, through a serve, volley placement, or groundstroke, is creating a barrier for you to react to. If you buy into this concept, your match is reduced to a nonpersonal situation. And by establishing a nonpersonal situation, you have placed yourself in a position that allows you to concentrate on meeting the barrier challenge and ignoring the personality and effort on the part of your opponent. You are basically competing within yourself. The opponent is secondary.

Execution and Being Competitive

You need to learn to emphasize *execution over winning* in order to establish a competitive edge. If execution is the important aspect of your play, the winning will take care of itself. Worrying about winning or losing interferes with both execution and winning. Thinking about appearance (how you look) or pleasing others also interferes with execution and winning. The emphasis is on execution, the concentration is on execution, and the goal is execution.

When using the term *execution*, a clarification is in order. The emphasis is not on thinking about executing a skill pattern; it is on completing the skill pattern. The mind should focus on feeling a barrier and responding to it by a reflex action, and that reflex action is execution. If a player begins to analyze movement and strokes or begins to think of ulterior motives behind execution, skilled play collapses.

The beginning tennis player may not have been exposed to this concept before and so may have difficulty understanding why thinking about winning is not acceptable. If you can accept that emphasis on winning places pressure to excel and pressure not to fail, the idea of eliminating those pressures might become palatable. If executing by *doing* provides the realization of the long-term goal of winning, execution begins to make sense.

Eliminating Negative Attitudes

When participating in tennis, a *negative attitude* or *negative feelings* contribute to a negative response.

Negative Self-Talk

If a player is ready to receive a serve and thinks, "Please don't make the serve; double fault—please," a negative attitude has been established. Other thoughts that are apt to enter the mind include, "What if I miss the shot?" and "If I hold my serve, I can win," and "You dummy—why can't you hit the ball?" Each of these plants a negative attitude that contributes to a less-than-successful experience.

Negative attitudes arise when a player gets upset and begins to talk to him/herself. "How could you hit such a stupid shot," or "I can't believe you're real—how could you miss such an easy setup?" If a player keeps making derogatory self-statements about performance, that player may well exceed all expectations of failure through negative thoughts.

Fear of Winning and Losing

Fear of winning or losing can be a disaster to success on a tennis court, but it can be eliminated if you remember and practice what competition means regarding the use of barriers, and if you shut out any emphasis regarding winning and losing.

Fear of winning is a problem. As a beginner, it is so easy to fear winning. When doubt creeps into your mind it can be utterly destructive. "Good grief, I'm winning. I shouldn't be doing this" sets the stage for the next thought, "How did I do this?" This in turn creates a loss of focus and confidence. This sequence of inner thoughts leads to a downward spiral that places a player in a "choke" mode. Fortunately, there is a response to a fear of winning. One means of addressing this fear, and the most important, is to focus on the process. Pick a skill goal you want to achieve, maybe concentrating on hitting each groundstroke with an excellent backswing–contact–follow-through sequence. Focus on that skill to the extent that you are not thinking about the score or who is winning. Another possibility is to perceive yourself as unbeatable, maybe identifying with your favorite tennis player who always closes out matches. There is another possibility. Establish a persona that is connected to routine. For example, bounce the ball twice before each serve, remember never to slouch, choosing instead to stand tall and exude confidence, or play with the strings of your racket after each point. Yet another technique to do before each point is to take a deep breath and hold it for a few seconds, followed by letting your breath out slowly for a count of eight or nine seconds. Whatever you do, be consistent, fit it to your personality, and stand tall.

Fear of losing contributes to negative thought. Fear places pressure on a player not to make mistakes, and that negative thought reemphasizes fear of failure. Anxiety is a by-product of this fear and contributes to tension, which restricts performance. Negative self-talk again surfaces with a fear of losing. Thoughts like "If I fail I will look bad" or "Losing to a player this bad would really be embarrassing" are examples of what not to think. Instead it is important for you to establish focus on the moment, develop a routine, and assume a confident persona.

Here's a thought: You, in all likelihood, won't die if you lose a match. What is the worst that can happen? Maybe it is your perception of how others will view you, maybe you might feel embarrassed, or maybe losing is so unacceptable that you might even cry. Well, get over it. Tennis is just a game and losing is part of the game. In actuality, hardly anyone cares if you lose or not. So don't internalize the possibility of losing as earth shattering or crisis level. Live to finish the match you are playing, and live to play another day.

Anger

Becoming angry and losing one's temper is another negative. Anger is a means of releasing energy, and by engaging in anger behavior you are expending additional energy, which will take a toll on you when a demand for extra effort is needed late in a match. Losing your temper also places pressure on you. A player who gets mad and internally vents that anger creates an anxiety similar to that associated with the fear of losing. The effect of internal anger is the creation of anxiety, which establishes the cycle of anger–anxiety that contributes to an outcome of a collapsed performance.

There are things you can do to eliminate anger. First, start by being nice to yourself. Stop attacking yourself verbally. Treat yourself with respect and dignity. Stop arguing with and embarrassing yourself, and begin to find a way to compliment yourself on a good shot or a good point played. The more *positive self-talk*, the more potential for success. Positive self-talk like "That's the way to hit with control" and "Keep pushing—I have her on the run" are examples of how to provide input to yourself that reflects absence of anger and promotes feeling good about yourself.

"Psych-Out"

Another negative associated with performance and tennis play is the opponent's behavior. A popular term in sport is "psych-out." Behavior by an opponent can be upsetting and create a "psych-out" response on your part. Body language, verbal comments, gamesmanship, and outbursts by an opponent can create negative reactions that can cause you to become anxious, resulting in a loss of focus on your part.

Typical gamesmanship behavior of an opponent is when he or she makes line calls that are inaccurate. In fact, this is more than gamesmanship; it's unethical behavior. However, the point is that this behavior becomes an irritant that may well get in your head, diverting your focus from your positive effort to play. If you fall into this trap of focusing on a bad call rather than accepting a bad call as a challenge, it will be you that fails. The bottom line is that you need to maintain your focus on playing against barriers and ignore opponent behavior.

Gamesmanship, and within gamesmanship coping with an opponent's making poor line calls, is just one of the "psych-out" situations. Opponents who exude a positive body language, verbally abuse or distract you, smile at you when you make a mistake, or even scream at themselves can contribute to your being "psyched-out." All "psych-out" situations need to be coped with by refocusing and reestablishing a competitive edge against barriers instead of against personalities. Block out behavior of an opponent, and eliminate the personalization of the person on the other side of the net. Remember that you are competing within yourself and that an opponent's only role is to present barriers for you to handle. Then use positive self-talk to bolster your own psyche.

Concentration

Concentration is an important part of tennis. Blocking out all factors other than executing a shot is a requirement for success. A focus on the ball and the task of hitting the ball helps a player to concentrate. When engaged in a rally, the player should look at the seams of the ball all the way to the racket face—if possible. Research indicates that a player can see a ball only to within 4 feet of the racket, but just the effort to look the ball into the racket improves concentration.

Concentration also is enhanced by being in touch with one's own body. The ability to synchronize breathing with each stroke and to sense the heartbeat as a body function permits you to be in touch and concentrate better.

Another sense that enhances concentration is hearing—as in hearing the tennis ball make contact with the racket strings. The kinesthetic sense is evoked when feeling the impact of ball and racket and recognizing muscle contraction and tension during the stroke. To really concentrate requires the elimination of all extraneous aspects of the environment.

Exchanging sides of the court can be a time for concentration. Your concentration should be on the game plan and on thinking positive thoughts. If a player keeps saying, "I'm playing well," that thought will become reality. In sum, concentration means focusing on the task at hand.

Anxiety and Slumps

There will be times when everything "clicks" during a game—a *flow* to movement and to the play in general. That flow might last for a few points in a match, for a larger portion of a match, for a few days, or for months. Then there will be down times, when nothing seems to work. The down time is described best as a *slump*. Slumps seem to appear for no reason, but they usually result from worry, tension, or a fear of winning or losing.

In short, slumps occur as a result of self-induced pressure, and that pressure causes anxiety. Once you become anxious, the muscles tense, which in turn forces physical errors because there is no relaxation during play. When the errors mount, tension increases and the slump continues. As long as you permit the pressure to interfere with performance, the cycle will continue.

The cure for the slump is to eliminate the anxiety by reducing muscle tension. This is done in two ways:

1. Begin to think positively.
2. Begin to relax and hit out on each ball, eliminating concern for the end result.

To reduce muscle tension, you have to rebuild confidence. Participating in a match with a player who hits at a consistent pace is a start at redeveloping that confidence. Self-talk ("good shot—way to play") aids in raising self-confidence. Self-confidence also develops or returns when you identify one stroke that you can develop that you know will be successful most of the time. Believing that the flow will return and relaxing are keys to coping positively. As a means of relaxing, the player must work at minimizing the number of times the muscle groups will be permitted to tense, which lessens interference through relaxed performance.

Relaxation

The ability to relax contributes greatly to physical performance. Learning how to relax in a tennis match requires first recognizing muscle tension. If you grip the racket too tightly (an exception is when hitting volley shots), the muscles tense too much. With a little practice, shoulder and arm muscles that are tight can be recognized. A check of the shoulders will reveal tenseness in that area. This is true with each muscle group. The whole body can tense during the pressure of a point or game, and shortness of breath, excessive sweating, and mental confusion are signals that the stress is too great. Relaxation during play can be attained in several ways:

1. By immediately responding to tension on the court.
2. By preparing to play through mental rehearsal and mental imagery.
3. By relaxing before the match.

The *immediate response to tension on the court* is to learn how to recognize the tension and then to relax those muscle groups. If you feel tension in the shoulders, a rotation of the shoulders, held for a few seconds and then released, will relax that area. Tension in the arms and legs can be eliminated by running or skipping in place. Another exercise that aids in total body relaxation, as mentioned earlier, is to take a deep breath and hold it briefly, finally expelling the air slowly for a count of eight or nine seconds.

Mental Preparedness

Preparing to play by using *mental rehearsal* or *mental imagery* requires practice, but it can be learned in a fairly short time. The idea is to prepare so well mentally that your confidence is enhanced, which, in turn, reduces anxiety and tension. A skill problem can be corrected by identifying the mistake and then repeatedly visualizing the proper skill.

Sometimes a skill problem is related more to the sequence of shots or a game plan. The corresponding mental practice should be to use imagery emphasizing the acceptable shot or sequence of shots in a game plan. This mental imagery is a foundation for the actual tennis match and will assist the player in recognizing specific situations. Mental rehearsal helps during a match when a player visualizes a positive picture of the next sequence of serves or a strategy for moving.

Prematch Relaxation

One technique for prematch relaxation is called progressive relaxation. It involves developing a process by which you can recognize muscle-group tension and counter that tension with muscle relaxation. This process allows a player to transfer a prematch relaxation experience to the match itself. The carryover to a match allows a player to recognize pressure during the match and immediately relax a muscle group that is too tense, thus preventing deterioration of performance.

Imagery practice, as mentioned earlier, contributes to prematch relaxation by setting the tone for how a player plans to play the match. Using imagery requires visualizing a game plan that can include staying on the baseline and rallying, using offensive lobs continually to force an opponent who can't hit an overhead effectively to try to hit overheads, or possibly visualizing a serve–volley strategy.

Other forms of prematch relaxation include meditation, yoga, and self-hypnosis. These forms, including progressive relaxation and imagery, require additional study in order to become accomplished. But if a tennis player wants truly to use all skills available, they are part of the total tennis development package.

Mental Toughness

Players with mental toughness generate positive support for themselves and reject negative emotional distress. Those who lack mental toughness are shy about pumping a fist in the air, or looking an opponent in the eyes or make a line call too softly. Emotional strength is displayed on the court through body language, voice patterns, and general attitude. Opponents sense weak behavior and uncertainty. The key is to assume a court presence: Stand up straight, move with a purpose, use a firm voice in your calls, and don't complain.

Finally, a mentally tough player maintains alertness and intensity. Behaviors such as playing in a daze, being too casual, forgetting the score, and not caring contribute to a negative attitude. A responsive player focuses on the event and maintains a standard of expectation for a high performance level.

A great deal of mental toughness is involved when playing tennis. Understanding what competition really is, eliminating negative attitudes, and being able to play in a relaxed mode are extremely helpful.

Putting It All Together

Beginners and more experienced players alike would do well to apply the suggestions discussed in the previous pages. Think a little about how you might be most effective against another player in terms of mental outlook.

1. Don't be intimidated by an opponent. You are playing a barrier, not an opponent. Just worry about your side of the net.
2. Establish a plan of attack. The next two chapters offer the opportunity to develop strategies to compete in singles and doubles play. Think through what you are going to do—make it a mental plan.
3. Establish a mentally tough persona.
4. Have a positive self-talk attitude.

Confidence breeds confidence. Believe in yourself and what you have learned as a player up to the point of the most recent match you have played. Focus on your task. Think about what you have to do. It helps to have a desire to play well and to be mentally and emotionally ready. You also must focus on the *process*, not the result. Enjoy the moment. Hit each ball as if it is your best shot. Have fun. And play for the sheer joy of playing.

POINTS *to* REMEMBER

THE MENTAL GAME

1. Competition is not opponent against opponent; it's player against barrier.
2. Emphasize execution over winning.
3. Eliminate negative attitudes, including fear of winning or losing, becoming angry, and self-defeating negative conversations with yourself.
4. Concentrate by blocking out extraneous interference.
5. Dispel anxiety.
6. Learn to relax on the court through relaxation techniques.
7. Develop a mental toughness that includes resilience, emotional strength, flexibility, and responsiveness.
8. Establish a strong mental outlook, with confidence, match planning, and readiness.
9. Use mental imagery in preparation for how you are going to play.

CHECKPOINTS

1. Competition associated with tennis is most closely preceived as allied with
   a. winning.
   b. execution.
   c. thinking about execution.
   d. opponent against opponent.
2. Negative responses associated with tennis include all but one of the following:
   a. Anger
   b. Fear of winning
   c. Psyching out
   d. Shutting out emphasis on winning
3. Concentration associated with tennis includes all but one of the following:
   a. Focus
   b. Synchronized breathing
   c. Competing
   d. Hearing the tennis ball bounce

(continued)

4. Slumps when playing tennis are caused by all but one of the following:
   a. Anxiety
   b. Flow
   c. Muscle tension
   d. Self-induced pressure
5. Relaxation during play can be attained by
   a. recognizing tension and applying relaxation techniques immediately.
   b. immediately responding to tension on the court.
   c. preparing to play through mental rehearsal.
   d. relaxing before the match.
6. A mentally tough tennis player meets all but one of the following profiles:
   a. Resilience
   b. Emotional strength
   c. Anxiousness
   d. Flexibility
7. Mental imagery requires
   a. emphasizing an acceptable shot.
   b. visualizing a positive picture of a skill sequence.
   c. visualizing a correction to a mistake.
   d. all of the above.
8. Muscle tension relates negatively to
   a. enhanced performance.
   b. failure to execute properly.
   c. focus on fundamentals.
   d. all of the above.
9. When confronted with stress and a fear of winning and losing, a critical technique is to
   a. focus on skill execution.
   b. take a deep breath, hold, and release slowly for an eight to nine second period.
   c. focus on a routine behavior such as bouncing the ball twice.
   d. do any of the above.
10. Competition as described in this chapter is defined as
    a. player against barrier.
    b. player against player.
    c. winning at nearly any cost.
    d. personalizing the opponent's role playing against you.

Answers to Checkpoints can be found on page 167.

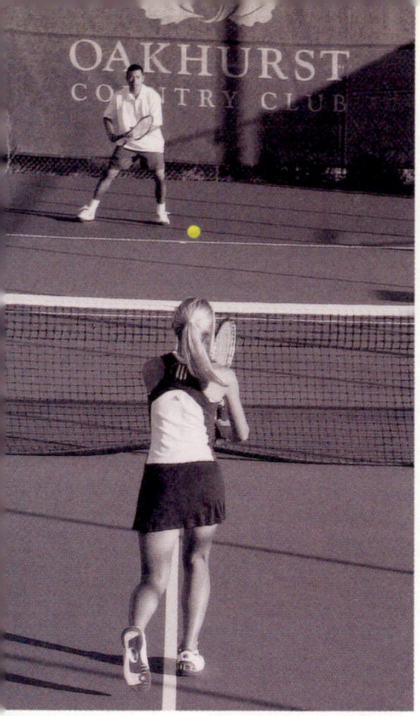

Photography by Terrell Lloyd; assisted by Anna Symonds Myers

7 Singles Strategy

Strategy in singles is part physical and part mental. The physical provides the mechanics to execute what the mental suggests be done to win a point. The mental is divided into two parts: (1) thinking and broadening thought to plan for the whole match and (2) using the mind to control the match. This chapter is concerned with the physical or mechanical execution of what the mind suggests and requires in developing a game plan.

Percentage Tennis

Tennis is a game of mistakes. The player who makes the most mistakes loses. To win at tennis requires a system of play called *percentage tennis*. Percentage tennis is specific to hitting every ball deep and within the lines of the tennis court. This sounds easy, and actually it is, if you are devoted to the system of play. The problem with percentage tennis is that players would rather hit the one spectacular shot than play the ball methodically. A percentage player is one who plays within the limits of skill, hitting only the shots that skill development will permit. In addition, the percentage player hits the appropriate stroke for a given shot. A percentage tennis player should grasp two concepts.

1. Comprehend what shot should be hit from what position on the court.
2. Understand and be able to apply the *division-line theory of play*.

Court-Division-for-Position-Play Strategy

The tennis court is divided into three parts: defensive, neutral, and offensive areas (Figure 7.1). The backcourt, or defensive area, is where the percentage player returns all deeply hit shots from the opponent. The percentage concept requires that the player try to return every shot from the backcourt deep to the opponent's court.

The defensive area is also the area defined as *No-Man's-Land* and is the portion of the court where the percentage player must step to return a shot, after which he or she retreats to the baseline to play the next shot. A player never should stand in this area. It is a highly vulnerable area and should be avoided.

The neutral area is the general area of the service court. Shots in this area can be either offensive or defensive, depending on your setup

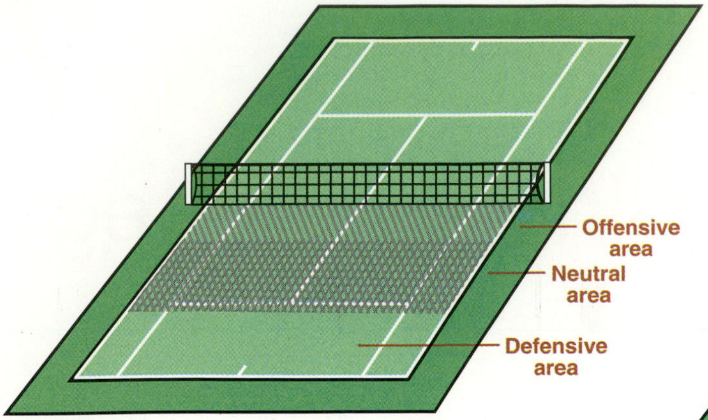

FIGURE 7.1 Court division for position play.

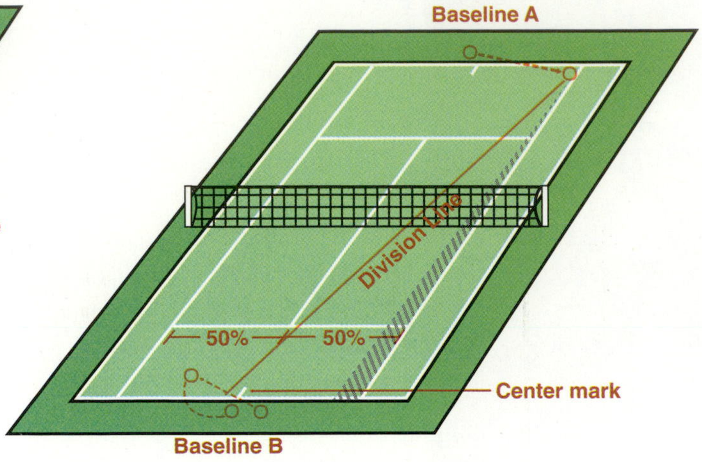

FIGURE 7.2A Division-line theory of play.

position on the court, the type of shot hit to you, and your skill level.

The offensive area is the area the player should enjoy, because a ball hit in this part of the court often represents an opponent's error and permits the percentage player to control the net area. This is where you may hit a volley shot, an overhead in response to a short lob, or an approach shot that carries you on to the net.

Understanding and Applying Division-Line-Theory-of-Play Strategy

A second consideration in percentage tennis is to understand and apply the *division-line theory of play*. This involves dividing the court into two equal parts on every stroke. If two players are rallying from the baseline and the ball is coming straight back to each player, the court is divided at the center mark on the baseline (Figure 7.2A). If Baseline A player hits a ball angled to the left of Baseline B player and then the return is a comparable cross-court return, a division line has to be established. This division line is established for the Baseline B player by that player's setting up to return the shot on the baseline a step and a half to the left of the center mark. The intent is to maintain an equal court coverage for a forehand or backhand return. The shaded area in Figure 7.2A helps illustrate this equal court balance, by balancing the coverage of Baseline B with a 50 percent coverage between the left sideline and the shaded area on the right sideline.

If the percentage player can stay out of the defensive area also called No-Man's-Land except to return a shot, can apply the division-line theory, and can hit each return deep at least three times in a row, the percentage that the opposing player will lose the point is quite high. When hitting from the baseline, the percentage player should use the increased skill shot of the topspin groundstroke when possible because of the high, safe trajectory and the deep, abrupt drop of the ball at the far baseline.

Service Strategy

Using the *service as a part of strategy* (Photo 7.1) is a necessity. Most beginners breathe a sigh of relief when their serve strikes the appropriate

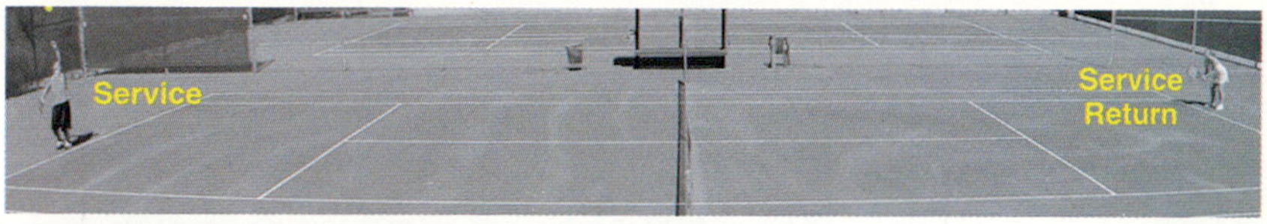

PHOTO 7.1 Service and service return position.
(Photography by Terrell Lloyd; assisted by Anna Symonds Myers)

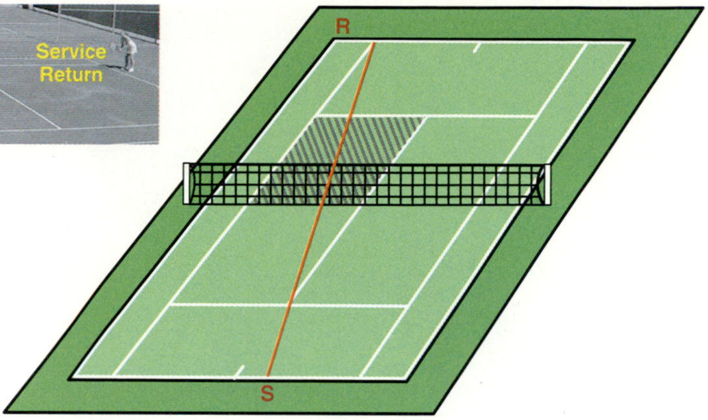

FIGURE 7.2B Receipt of serve division-line theory.

service court. Strategy comes into play when the serve strikes the service court because the server had confidence, hit the ball with velocity, and had a plan as to where to place the ball in the service court.

If a server can hit a serve repeatedly with modest speed and place the ball deep and/or in the corners of the opponent's service court 70 percent of the time, the chances for success are enhanced greatly. If spin can be applied to the ball during service, with accuracy, a variety of serves can be used to confuse the receiver. In addition, the server can capitalize on the receiver's weakness in returning a serve if those weaknesses can be recognized.

Return-of-Service Strategy

Return-of-service strategy is crucial. The server's role is to place the ball in play and force the receiver to respond to the serve defensively. The return player's role is to keep the ball in play. The strategy is not only to hit the ball back with pace, but to hit it deep into the center of the court to eliminate the server's initial advantage. Players returning serve need to apply the division-line theory, this time by dividing the court with a line from the server's position that splits the service box in half (Figure 7.2B). From this position a receiver can return serve with a backhand or forehand groundstroke. If you are successful when returning serve, the server who relies on the serve to win points will begin to lose confidence if the ball keeps coming back.

Increasing Beginner Skills: Placement and Service Strategy

Placement of the service should be deep (Figure 7.3). Then choices can be made as to where to direct the ball to cause the most problems for the receiver. Typically, when beginners play, targeting a receiver's backhand works very well. Then as beginner skills improve, the server needs to focus on three deep targets to the corners or to the center. From position S1 (Figure 7.4) a serve may be

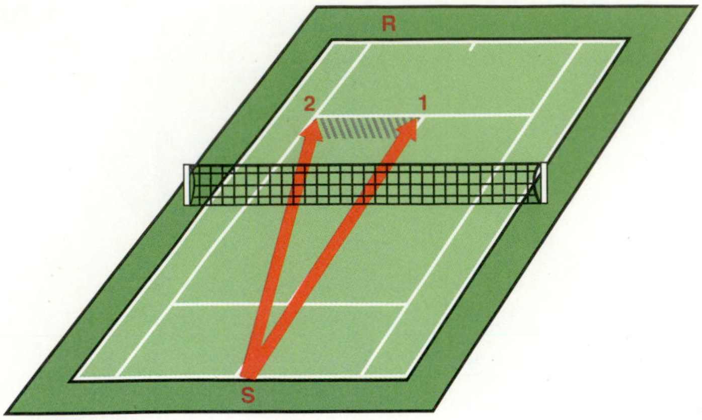

FIGURE 7.3 Hitting deep serves.

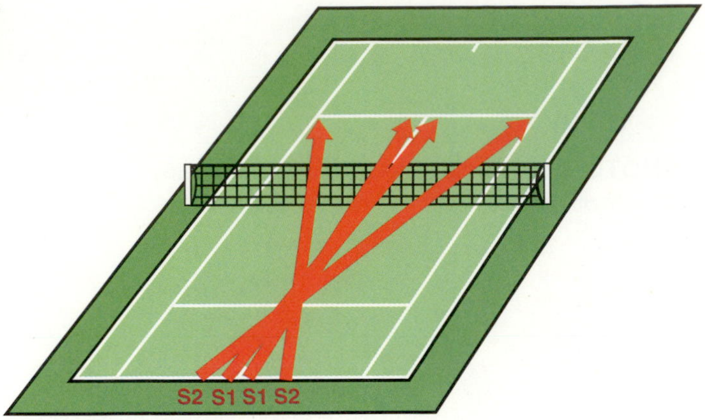

FIGURE 7.4 Hitting the corners on the serve.

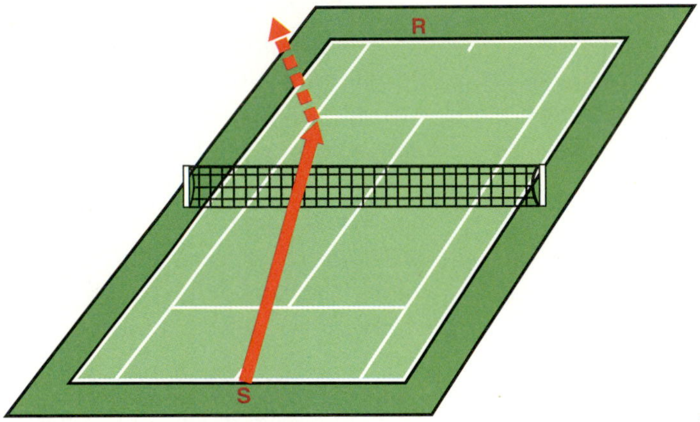

FIGURE 7.5 Placing slice serve.

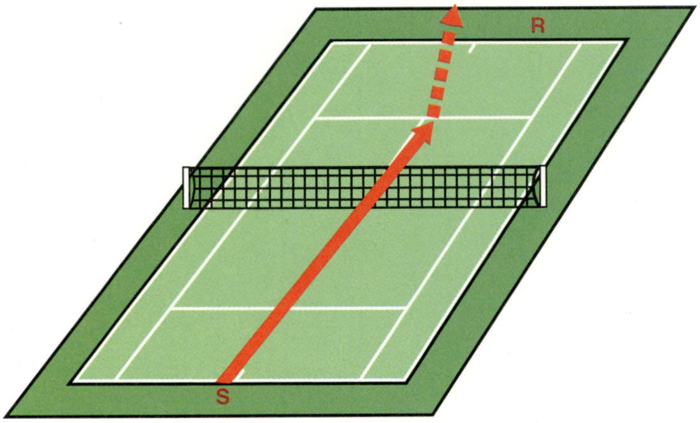

FIGURE 7.6 Placing slice serve to the "ad" service court.

directed to the inside corner of either service court. From position S2, a serve is hit wide to either service court. These placements are excellent spots to place a service. In addition, if a server puts reasonable velocity on a flat serve, the receiver will have problems even if the ball is placed directly down the center of the service court.

A more advanced slice serve can be hit wide to the right side of the "deuce" service court, pulling the receiver off the court and consequently opening the whole court for the next shot by the server (Figure 7.5). A slice service to the right corner of the "ad" service court pulls the receiver to the middle of the court, causing a down-the-middle return (Figure 7.6).

Increasing Beginner Skills: Second-Service Strategy

The second service is even more important, in the sense that if it is not placed accurately in the appropriate service court, the point is lost without a response from the receiver. Not only must the second serve be reliable and accurate, but it also should have some pace. Many servers make the mistake

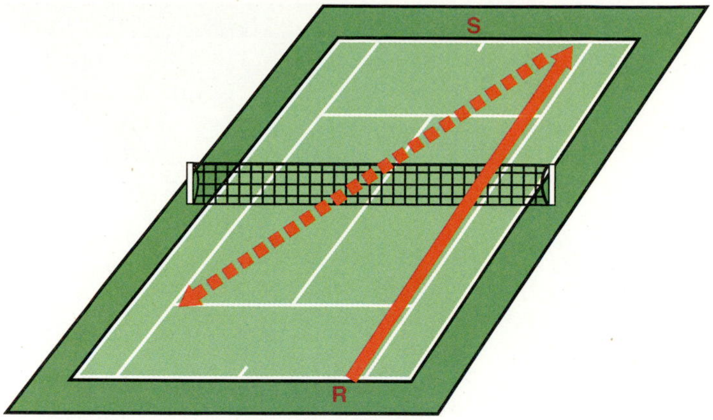

FIGURE 7.7 Consequences of return of serve down the line.

of pushing the ball into the service court rather than hitting with good form. Here are the three requirements of a sound second serve:

1. The serve must have accuracy coupled with pace.
2. The serve needs to have spin to ensure accuracy.
3. The serve must never be pushed or blooped into the service court. Accuracy is enhanced by a slice service, as mentioned in number 2 above, with attention to the placement and pace of the ball.

Increasing Beginner Skills: Return-of-Service Strategy

Once the beginner gains enough skill to return the ball to the server, it is time to establish an expanded strategy. A cause–effect relationship indicates that the receiver should respond to the server's pace and depth of serve by standing beyond the baseline to return serve. This thought must be dispelled. If the serve has a strong spin, it is best to step inside the baseline and cut down the sidespin or high bounce before the effect can occur. A serve that is pushed over the net should be returned firmly and deep, with the receiver avoiding the tendency to "kill" the ball.

When returning the serve, the receiver can use various return placements. Returning *down the line* is usually a mistake when the server has the ability and court position to move easily down the baseline to reach the ball, for it will leave the court open for a cross-court winner by the server (Figure 7.7). It is also a mistake because returning down the line requires hitting the ball over the highest part of the net, thereby creating a high-risk shot.

Service returns are most effective when hit back along the line of flight of the serve and at the feet of the server. When serves are hit with little pace, the receiver has more options, including down the line, cross-court, and angled cross-court. The effort off a weak serve should be either to hit a winner under control, forcing the opposing server to hit while moving to the ball, or to miss the ball entirely.

Increasing Beginner Skills: Attacking the Net and Beating the Net Player

Judgments a player must make include when to go to the net and, once there, when to stay and when to leave.

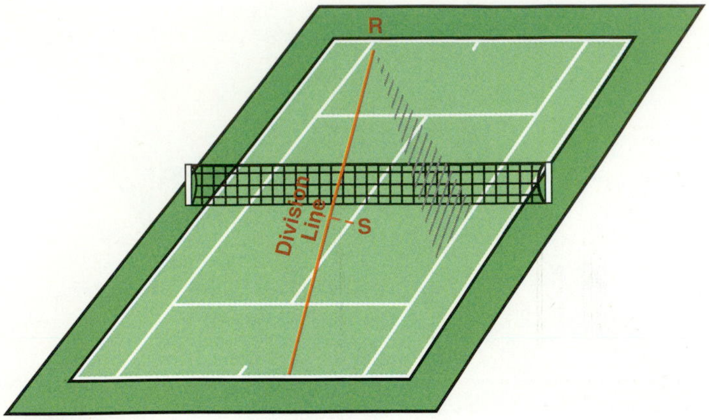

FIGURE 7.8 Division-line theory.

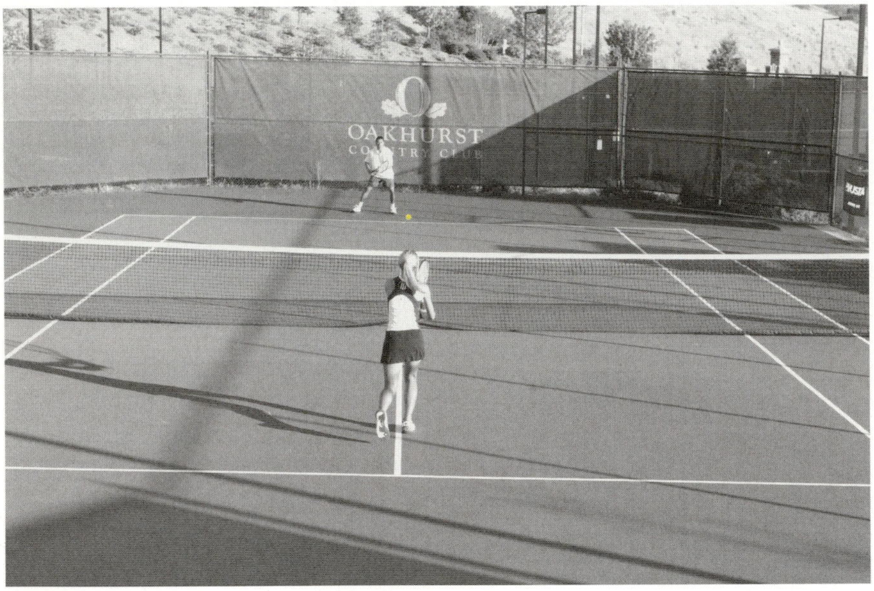

Photography by Terrell Lloyd; assisted by Anna Symonds Myers

PHOTO 7.2 Server going to the net.

A player should go to the net in three situations:

1. Off a serve.
2. Off an approach shot.
3. Off a firmly hit groundstroke that forces the opponent to move behind the baseline when returning the shot.

When at the net, there are two times to stay and continue play at the net:

1. When following one volley with another.
2. When hitting an overhead from between the service court line and the net.

The player should retreat in only one situation: when a lob is hit deep to the baseline, compelling the net player to leave the net to return the lob. The player attacking the net should apply the *division-line theory* by following the path of the ball to the net, dividing the court in half between the two players.

The division line will enable the net player to cover all territory equally between the forehand and the backhand and give the opponent only one possible winning shot. If, as an example, the net player hits to the opponent's deep, right baseline corner and takes a step and a half to the left of the center of the net, the only possible return for a winning shot is an angled far right corner shot (Figure 7.8).

Going-to-the-Net Strategy

Going to the net following a serve requires the execution of an accurate serve (Photo 7.2). In fact, an accurate serve with pace provides the opportunity to advance effectively to the net. If the serve is returned with pace, penetration is as close as it is going to be if the server can get to the service court line (Figure 7.9, Position 1). If the return of the serve is a mishit, the server can pounce on the return with an efficient volley from the net position (Figure 7.9, Position 2 or 3). If the return of serve is at the feet of the server, who has advanced on the net, a 20-foot return distance from the net may become a liability. The server now has to be an exceptional volleyer because the ball at the feet creates vulnerability. A slice service permits the server to advance closer to the net before being forced to stop and respond to the opponent's return of serve.

Going to the net following an approach shot is an ideal time to advance on the net (Figure 7.10).

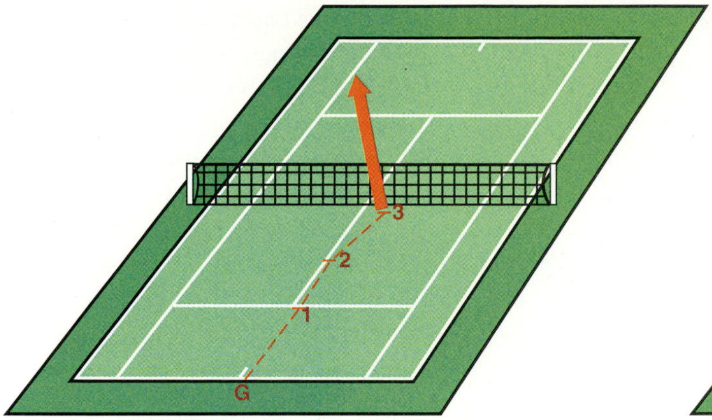

FIGURE 7.9 Going to the net following a serve.

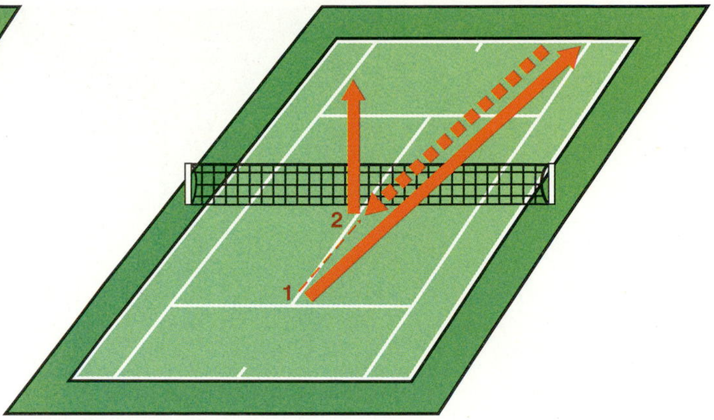

FIGURE 7.10 Going to the net following an approach shot from the middle of the court.

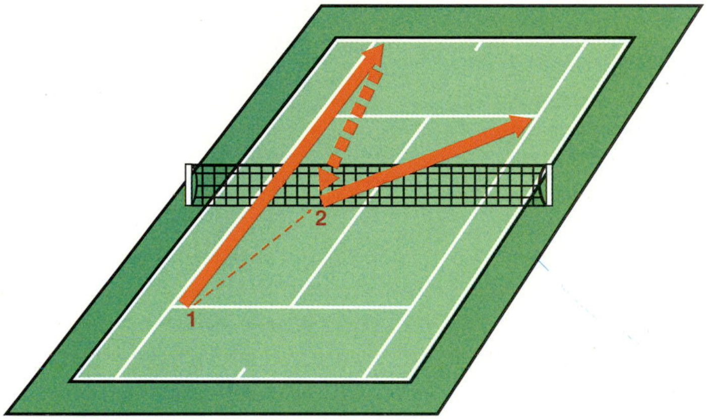

FIGURE 7.11 Going to the net following an approach shot from the sideline area of the court.

If the return from the opponent is short—at the service line in the middle of the court—the approach shot can be played to a corner (Figure 7.10, Position 1). Once the ball is hit to the corner, the player advances to the net, in line with the ball, and volleys cross-court (Figure 7.10, Position 2). If a return shot is hit to the service line, close to and parallel to a sideline, the approach shot has to be down the sideline (Figure 7.11, Position 1), followed by a short, angled volley cross-court as the player advances on to the net (Figure 7.11, Position 2). Hitting down the sideline from Position 1 does present a problem, since the net is higher and thus there is a greater possibility for error.

Going to the net off a groundstroke must be done with some prudence. It is inadvisable to go to the net when your groundstroke

1. has not been hit with authority,
2. has not been hit deep to the baseline, or
3. has not forced the opponent to return the shot while moving away from the net.

If you hit an effective groundstroke, however, you must learn to *close in on the net.* As you advance to the net from the baseline, you must assume a ready position prior to the return shot crossing the net. Once you hit a return, you need to continue on to the net in line with the ball and again stop in a ready position before the return shot crosses the net.

Between two and three stops are required to gain control of the net and to be in control of hitting a winning shot if the opponent is able to respond with some authority in returning the shots hit by the advancing player. Three thoughts should be on the mind of the player advancing from the baseline:

1. Volley and advance.
2. Punch the ball deep to the baseline.
3. Hit at the feet of the opponent so the return is "up."

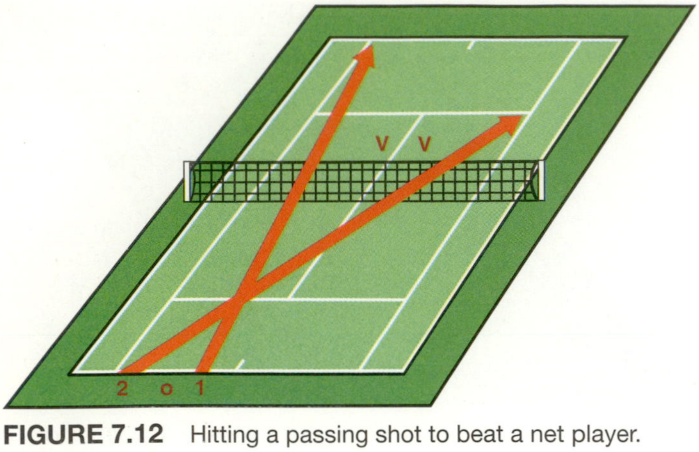

FIGURE 7.12 Hitting a passing shot to beat a net player.

Advancing to the net is an adventure and a reward if the end result is a winning shot. The choice of going to the net is based on the advantage that it will give the player to advance. Here are some final thoughts associated with attacking:

1. The volleyer always must stop and assume a ready position prior to the return shot's crossing the net.
2. When attacking, the volleyer should follow the path of the ball to provide the division line.
3. The volleyer has to get close to the net to hit a volley. A beginning player needs to be a racket-and-a-half length away from the net, whereas a skilled player can volley from as far back as the service court line. All players who volley must remember to stay low and punch the ball.

Beating-the-Net-Player Strategy

A *threefold strategy to beat the player who attacks the net* is to: (1) hit at the feet of the net player, (2) hit a passing shot, and (3) hit a lob.

Hitting at the feet of the net player forces the player to hit the ball up in the air, providing a setup to hit a winning return. Two shots are most often used to hit at the feet of a player at the net. A topspin stroke usually is hit from the baseline to the feet of a player at the net; and from a return of serve a ball often is blocked back to the feet of an advancing net player.

Hitting a passing shot to beat a net player is a second means of defeating the volleyer at the net. The passing shot may be hit down the line or as a short-angled cross-court shot. As an example, if a player is to the left of the center mark at the baseline, a shot down the net player's right sideline could pass that player (Figure 7.12, Position 1). A ball hit farther to the left of the baseline player can be played as a short-angled cross-court passing shot, because the net player has moved to the right of center to establish the division line (Figure 7.12, Position 2).

The third method of *beating the net player is with a lob.* A net player tends to get too close to the net to avoid balls returned low to the net. This diminishes the ability to retreat and cover a deep lob. If the players are beginners, any form of a lob that gets over the head of the net player will be effective. The important point is to drive the opponent back from the net, ensuring that the net player returns a shot on the move, with the back to the net.

Increasing Beginner Skills: Lob and Overhead Strategy

Lobs and overheads are an integral part of overall court strategy. The lob can be either a defensive or an offensive shot, and the overhead is a reward for effective serve or groundstroke play.

Lob Strategy

The questions when hitting a lob in singles play are *when to hit a lob*

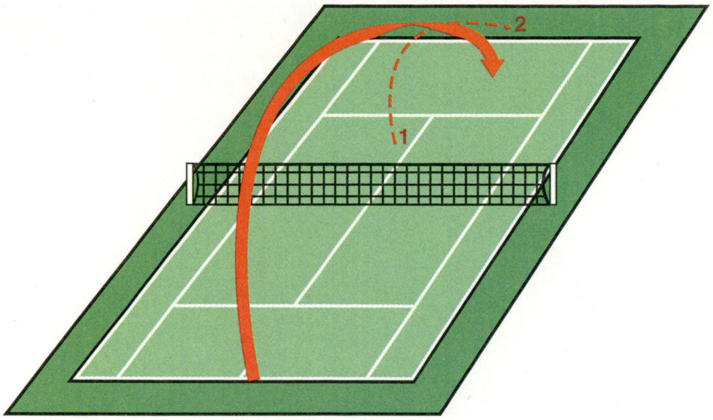

FIGURE 7.13 Retrieving a lob.

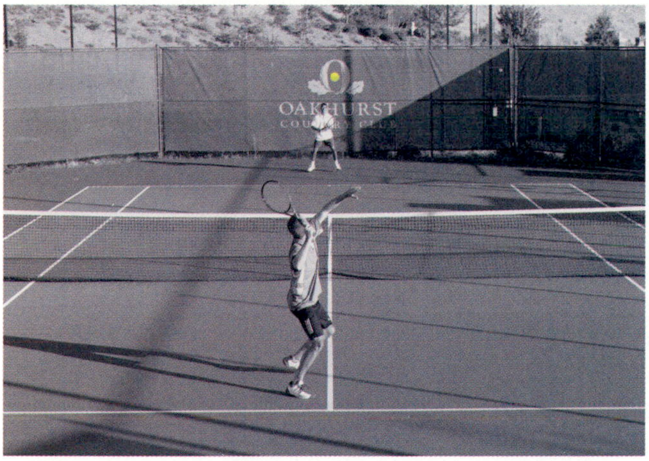

Photography by Terrell Lloyd; assisted by Anna Symonds Myers

PHOTO 7.3 Overhead setup.

and *what kind of lob.* Defensive lobs should be hit whenever the opponent has forced the play and whenever you need to "buy time" to recover from a strong offensive shot. The important part of a defensive lob is to hit the ball deep to the opponent's backhand, forcing the opponent to run around the ball to hit an overhead. An offensive lob is hit when you have time to set up and when the opponent is at the net. Remember, an offensive lob is hit lower with topspin, creating a situation for the opponent that requires retreating to return the lob, placing you in an advantageous offensive position.

When retrieving a lob, the player, instead of running in a straight line, should run to the outside of the ball and come from behind it to hit a return lob, a forceful groundstroke, or an overhead (Figure 7.13, Positions 1 and 2). A lob that has the effect of an offensive shot should, of course, be hit when the opposing net player is too close to the net.

Overhead Strategy

Overheads are used in singles strategy to respond to lobs that are hit between the service court and the net (Photo 7.3). Setting up is an important part of that strategy. A crisp volley down the opponent's right sideline forces that player to execute a lob that travels to the middle of the court, which, in turn, can be hit as an overhead to the opponent's left corner (Figure 7.14). This example illustrates that a firm offensive shot creates a weak lob return, and for each lob return there is a wide variety of targets for the overhead. Balls hit deep to the opponent's baseline always are acceptable as effective overheads (Figure 7.15).

When the return lob is closer to the net, overheads can be angled and "bounced out" of the opponent's court. The angle and bounce carry the ball into a nonreturnable location (Figure 7.16). Angled and deeply angled overheads are also effective (Figure 7.17). They ensure that the opponent has to move to retrieve the overhead rather than remain stationary and hit a lob with control. An angled overhead (Figure 7.17, Position 1) is an excellent placement for a backhand overhead because accuracy in placement is more important than speed in completing the shot successfully, while a forehand overhead angled deep is often a winning shot (Figure 7.17, Position 2).

Often the first overhead is not a winning shot, nor should it be expected to be. The first overhead "softens up" the opponent, who can return the shot only from a defensive position. Strategically, if the player hitting the lob keeps the overhead consistently deep and angled, the opponent returning lobs eventually

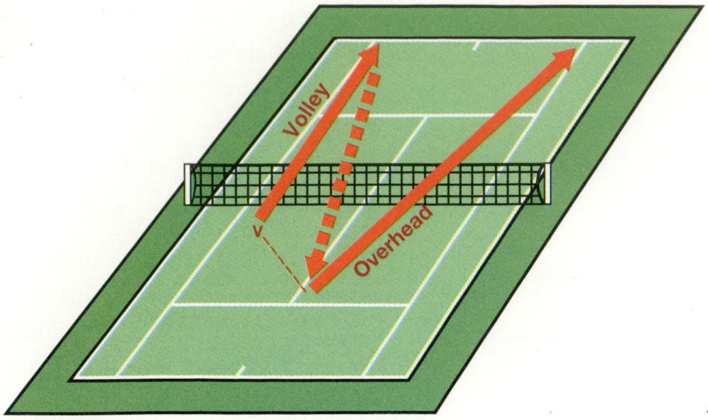

FIGURE 7.14 Setting up an overhead return with a volley shot.

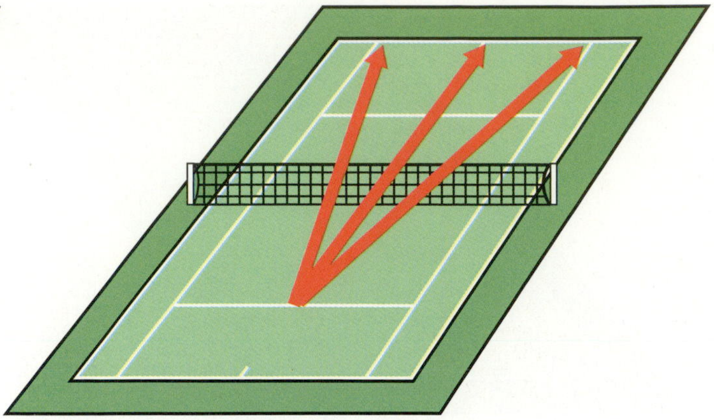

FIGURE 7.15 Hitting overheads deep.

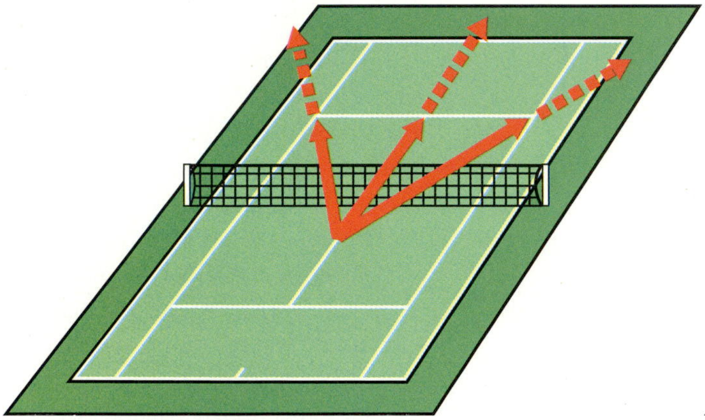

FIGURE 7.16 Hitting angled overheads.

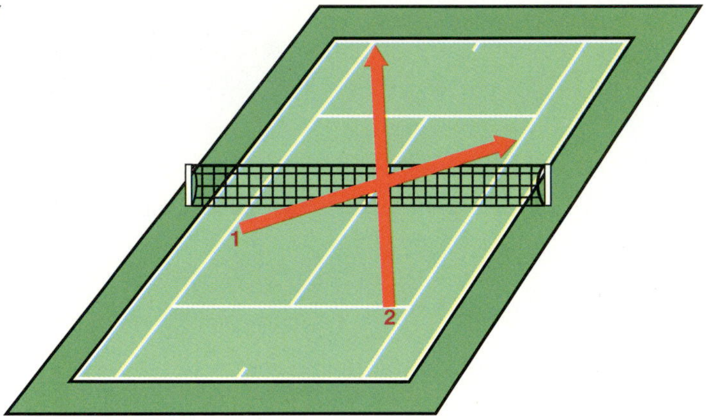

FIGURE 7.17 Angled and deeply angled overheads.

wears down or breaks down skillwise and hits a short lob that can be returned as a winning overhead.

Increasing Beginner Skills: Baseline-Play Strategy

Baseline play involves giving complete, undivided attention to hitting groundstrokes deep and relying on percentage tennis to its fullest. The idea is to force the opponent to make a mistake with a mis-hit shot or a poorly hit return. Among the several ways of forcing an error from the opponent are cross-court and down-the-line shots (Photo 7.4).

Duplicating-the-Opponent's-Groundstroke-Return Strategy

Duplicating the opponent's return is good strategy because it puts pressure on the opponent to change the direction of the ball. Singles strategy dictates that if the opponent hits cross-court, the return should be cross-court until the opponent hits down the line. At that point, the player hitting has the option of returning in duplication down the line or coming back cross-court. In either case, the advantage is with the player returning a shot rather than the opponent because the return angle favors the return player's stroke and because there is an element of the unknown in the return direction (Figure 7.18).

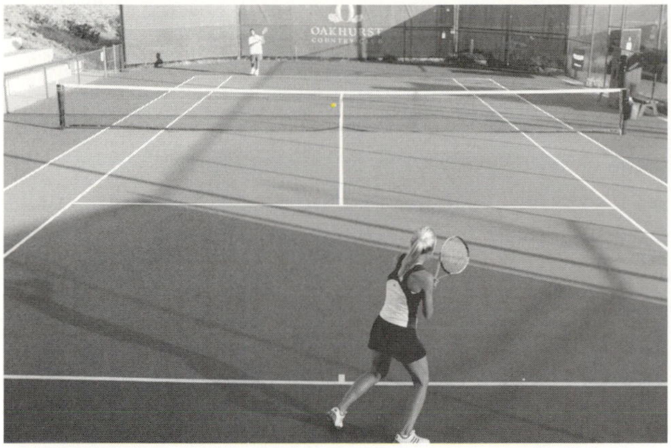

PHOTO 7.4 Baseline-play setup.

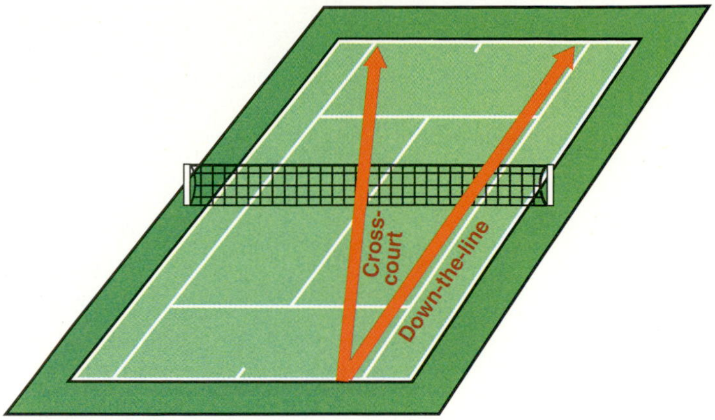

FIGURE 7.18 Duplicating groundstroke returns.

Moving-the-Opponent Strategy

Another strategy is to move the opponent back and forth across the baseline, forcing alternate forehand and backhand returns. If the opponent can be driven from one side of the court to the other, reaching for shot returns, the ball eventually will be returned short or "up" so that an approach shot, volley, or overhead can be used as a follow-up to good baseline play.

With skill and experience, the baseline player can develop strategy using varied strokes, always coming back to hit with depth and angle, which will cause the opponent to make a mistake. Sometimes varying the stroke is disguised by hitting down the sideline with a groundstroke to the opponent's backhand for a succession of shots and then switching to a cross-court shot that pulls the opponent out of a groove and requires a totally new stroke in the rally. Hitting the groundstroke again and again to the same side also will wear down an opponent's confidence, and the skill of the stroke will weaken as belief in winning the point lessens.

Scoring-Situation Strategy

Although scoring is discussed in more detail in Chapter 11, certain *scoring situations* in a match are vital to good strategy and success and are discussed below. In a game, a score of 30–15 is important because winning the next point will produce a score of 40–15. The leading player can use the 2-point difference as a lever to win the game within the next two points. If the 30–15 score becomes 30–30, either player may win the next two points.

A set score of 5–3 with the opponent serving is a crucial situation in the ninth game. If the opponent wins that game, the set is over at a 6–3 score. If the receiver of serve wins the ninth game, the score becomes 4–5 and the player who is behind serves, with a tie set possible at 5–5 in the tenth game. Obviously, the 4–5 set score also is important, but the player behind is serving; and with a degree of serving skill, the server has the advantage. Other scores that are meaningful are the first point of any given game and the potential last point of a game, set, or match.

Game-Plan Strategy

The *overall game strategy and plan* are only as good as the player's skill. The game plan for an early beginner is to do the best possible to return shots back across the net. By the time the player can hit with some consistency, percentage tennis becomes really important. It means the advanced beginner can work at hitting the ball back with depth and patience and begin to set up an opponent with subtle techniques to force an error.

Continual maturation permits the player to understand that the mind is the most important part of the game. The ability to outthink the opponent becomes the key to victory. Changing pace, moving a player along the baseline, and moving the opponent to the net and back away from the net all begin to make sense.

The game plan and strategy for a player starts with the warm-up and ends with the last point of the match. In the warm-up, the player begins to assess the opponent's ability, being careful not to become overly confident of or intimidated by the opponent. During the warm-up, each player should determine the skills of the opponent and what strokes that opponent is capable of hitting effectively. The player who is assessing the other player should not change the game plan only to meet the opponent's skills, though. The assessing player must be able to react normally and not play as the opponent dictates.

Here's an example of a game plan: If the opponent likes to serve and volley, the strategy might be to prepare to hit passing shots, lobs, and groundstrokes at the opponent's feet. Another example is to stay at homebase during a rally and, by continuing to hit the ball deep, force the opponent to rally from the baseline when the opponent lacks consistency hitting groundstrokes. Game plans and strategy should be a combination of your reacting to the opponent's weaknesses and playing to your skill level.

Here are some final game strategy thoughts:

1. Play every point and return every shot.
2. Look for the short ball, attack with an aggressive approach shot, and complete the attack by continuing on to the net.
3. Be consistent in play rather than hitting the one spectacular shot.
4. Use defensive lobs to "buy time," because most beginning players cannot hit solid overheads in reacting to a lob.
5. Keep groundstrokes in play and deep.
6. Hit serves with pace and accuracy.

POINTS *to* REMEMBER

SINGLES STRATEGY

1. Focus on playing *percentage tennis*.
2. Apply the *division-line theory of play*, which, simply stated, is a division of a tennis court into two equal parts dictated by ball placement.
3. Effective placement of serve requires hitting down the center or wide, using either pace and/or spin.
4. Effective second-serve placement requires accuracy with pace—no blooping the serve.
5. Return serves should be deep and back, in line with the server's position.
6. Attack at the net after an effective serve, an approach shot, or off a firmly hit groundstroke that moves the opposing player.
7. Beat the net player by hitting at the feet, hitting a passing shot, or hitting a lob.
8. Keep in mind that a game score of 30–15 and a set score of 3–5 when receiving are critical situations during a match.

CHECKPOINTS

1. Percentage tennis is considered
   a. representative of who loses the most points.
   b. representative of who wins the most points.
   c. a strategy established to stay close in a match.
   d. none of the above.
2. The No-Man's-Land area is an unofficial term used to describe
   a. a highly vulnerable area for a player to stand in while waiting for the next shot.
   b. another term for the service court area.
   c. the baseline area.
   d. none of the above.
3. The *division theory of play* means
   a. dividing the court into four parts.
   b. dividing the court into two equal parts.
   c. dividing the strategy of play into two parts.
   d. all three of the above.
4. In successful offensive service placement
   a. 50 percent of all serves must be "in."
   b. 70 percent of all serves must be hit deep, including the corners of the opponent's service court.
   c. serves must be no less than 60 percent accurate.
   d. serves must be 80 percent accurate on a second serve.
5. Service returns are most effective when hit
   a. along the line of flight of the serve.
   b. down the line.
   c. along the line of flight of the serve at the feet of the server.
   d. cross-court.
6. It is inadvisable to go to the net when
   a. a groundstroke has been returned with no authority.
   b. a ball has not been returned deep to the opponent.
   c. the opponent has not been forced to move away from the net.
   d. any of the above.
7. The three ways to beat a player at the net are to
   a. hit at the player's feet, pass the player, or lob.
   b. hit at the player, pass the player, or lob.
   c. lob, lob, and lob.
   d. rush the player at the net, pass the player, or lob.
8. Defensive lobs should be hit
   a. to attack the opponent's weakness.
   b. to "buy time."
   c. whenever the opposing player is aggressive.
   d. rarely since they are basically limited in success.
9. Offensive lobs should be hit
   a. to attack an aggressive player at the net.
   b. to "buy time."
   c. rarely since they are basically limited in success.
   d. when the opposing player is anchored on the baseline.
10. Within a game situation the most critical score requiring maximum effort is
    a. 40–Love
    b. 30–15 or 15–30
    c. Love–40
    d. 30–30

Answers to Checkpoints can be found on page 167.

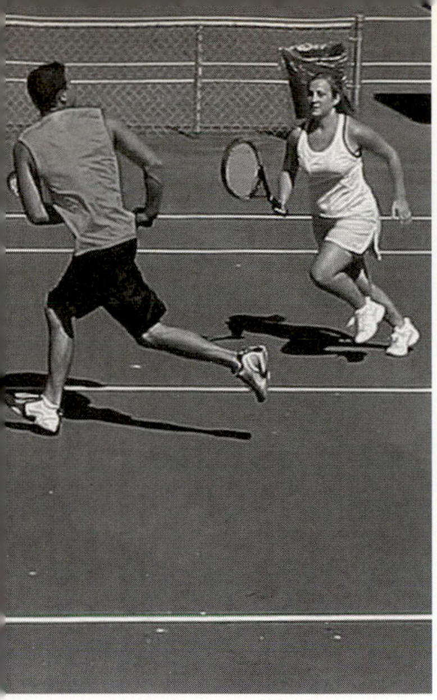

Photography by Terrell Lloyd; assisted by Anna Symonds Myers

8 Doubles Strategy

With the exception of the strokes used, doubles strategy is entirely different from singles strategy. Doubles is an attacking game, whereas singles tends to be a more passive defensive game. Doubles play is concentrated at the net or retreating from the net, whereas singles play is positioned at the baseline. The attacking concept of doubles provides an exciting type of match with quickly executed shots and good reactions. The beginner seldom experiences the challenge of doubles, yet this is the first situation a beginner may face if being taught in an instructional group.

Basic Alignments and Formations

Numerous formations are found in doubles play, including club or recreational social doubles (usually college-class doubles), conventional doubles, and mixed doubles. Choosing a partner and deciding where each partner will be aligned on the court are the beginning of a successful strategy.

Social Doubles

Beginning players should start from one of two formations, depending on how advanced the players are in executing strokes. These formations are associated with *social doubles*.

Two-Back Formation

If the players have yet to be introduced to net play, including volleying and hitting overheads, it is best to begin doubles at the baseline in a *two-back formation* (Photo 8.1). The two-back formation also is used by experienced players when the opposing team is at the net hitting overheads while the two on the baseline team attempt to return lobs to defend against the overheads.

The weakness of the two-back formation is the defensive stature of the team and the lack of control at the net. A team that controls the net has an open court that allows large areas in which to place the ball for winning shots. From the baseline, shots hit at players controlling the net have little potential for success because they involve only small target areas that the two players cannot cover at the net (Figure 8.1).

One-Up, One-Back Formation

A second social doubles formation is *one up and one back*. This alignment is used when the players' experience at the net is at least adequate for protection at the net and for execution of firmly hit volleys.

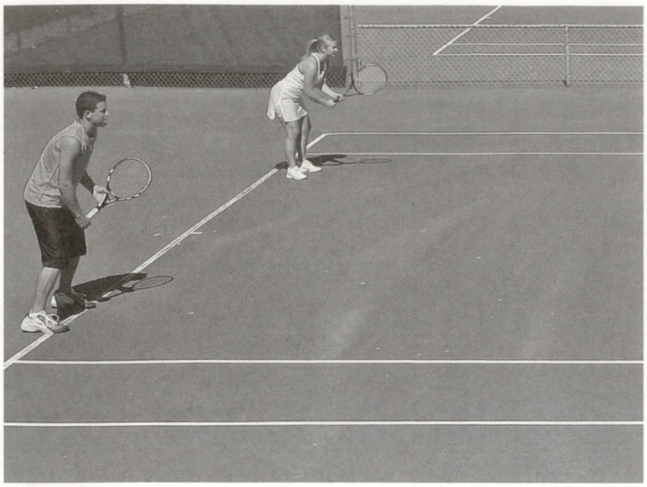

PHOTO 8.1 Two-back formation.

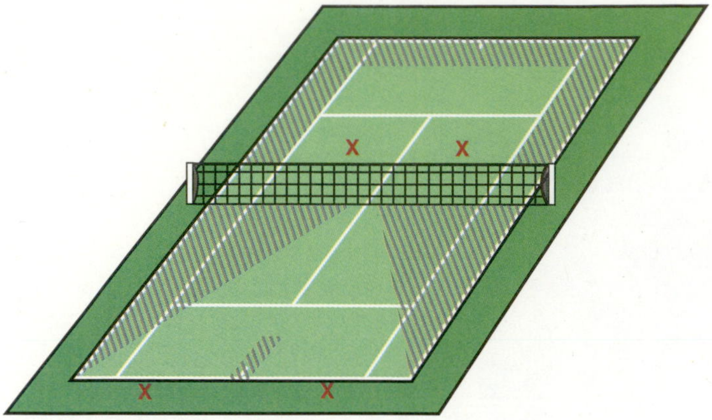

FIGURE 8.1 Target areas for two up versus two back.

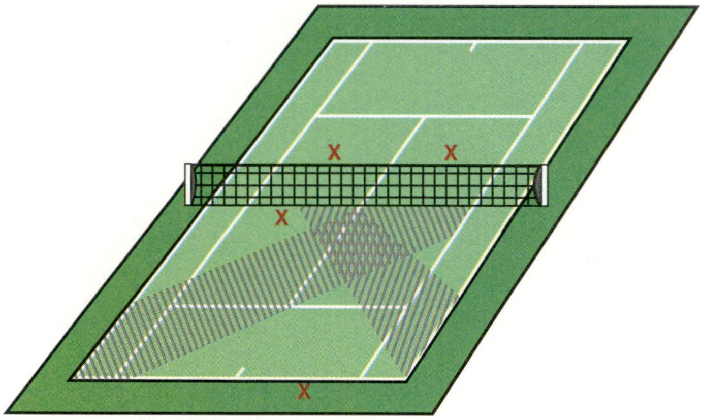

FIGURE 8.2 Target areas for two up against one up, one back.

One player up and one player back stems from the original alignment of the players in the serving and receiving positions. The problem arises when the server doesn't have the confidence to serve and follow the serve to the net or the return player does not follow the return to the net. Once the alignment holds at one up, one back, that alignment becomes vulnerable to open-area winning shots. (See Figure 8.2 and Photos 8.2 and 8.3.)

Conventional Doubles: Two Up in Tandem

Conventional doubles requires that a team attack the net and, if need be, attack face to face with the opposing team. The key to good doubles play is to work together in tandem. If the ball is lobbed deep when the team is at the net, the two must retreat together; and when one player hits an overhead from the service court line, both players must advance to the net together. Playing conventional doubles means working as a team, knowing where the other player is located, and depending on the partner to hit the appropriate shot. When controlling the net, the doubles team attacks side by side, positioned in the middle of the two service courts. From that position, as if they were on a string, the pair moves up and back and side to side in a balanced position (Photo 8.4).

A conventional formation can produce a significant number of movement patterns on the court. First, a teammate may *poach* in doubles. The definition is important. The poach means hitting a winning volley; it allows no margin for error. When poaching, the best target tends to be a volley directed at the feet of the opposing net player. A second poaching movement requires that the net player step across parallel to and at a diagonal toward the net to hit a volley directed toward the opposing player at the baseline. In both poaching situations the serving partner sees the poach attempt and veers to replace the position vacated by the poaching partner (Figure 8.3).

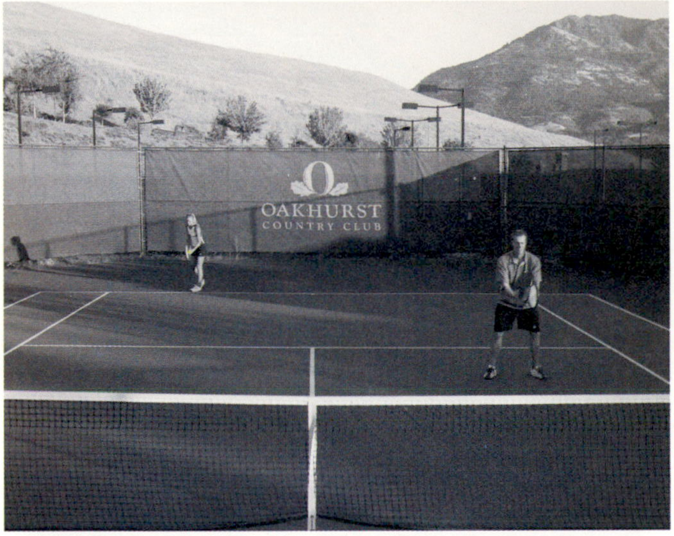

Photography by Terrell Lloyd; assisted by Anna Symonds Myers

PHOTO 8.2 One-up, one-back formation (serving).

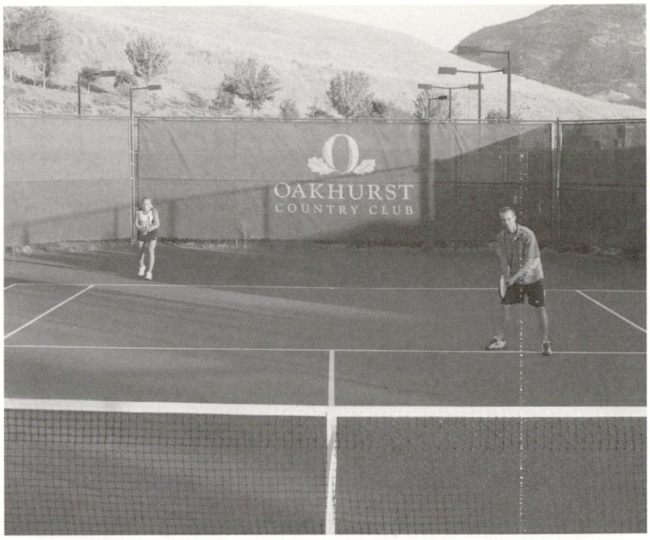

Photography by Terrell Lloyd; assisted by Anna Symonds Myers

PHOTO 8.3 One-up, one-back formation (receiving).

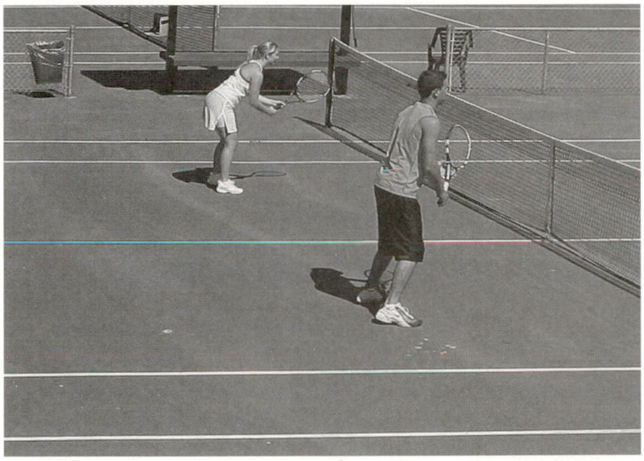

Photography by Terrell Lloyd; assisted by Anna Symonds Myers

PHOTO 8.4 Two-up formation (conventional doubles).

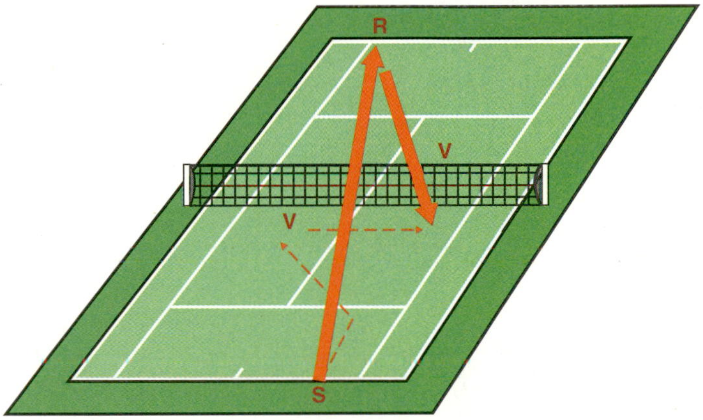

FIGURE 8.3 Poach movement patterns.

Another team movement pattern is to retreat to hit a lob and then to recover for the next shot. The retreat incorporates a cross-action by team members to reach the ball. If the lob is to the deep left corner of the baseline, the partner on the right can see the ball and react to it better than the partner who would have to retreat in a straight line with the back to the opponents. At this point, the partners are at the baseline, where they will remain in a defensive posture until they can regain an advantage and return to the net (Photo 8.5 and Figure 8.4).

Mixed Doubles

Mixed doubles combines one male and one female partner. The formation is the same as for conventional doubles. The only real change is related to the physical strength and skill of the female partner. If there is a strength and skill difference (the differences also could be between two male or two female partners), the alignment for tactic and strategy may have to be adjusted.

Mixed doubles partners may be equal in strength or skill but the

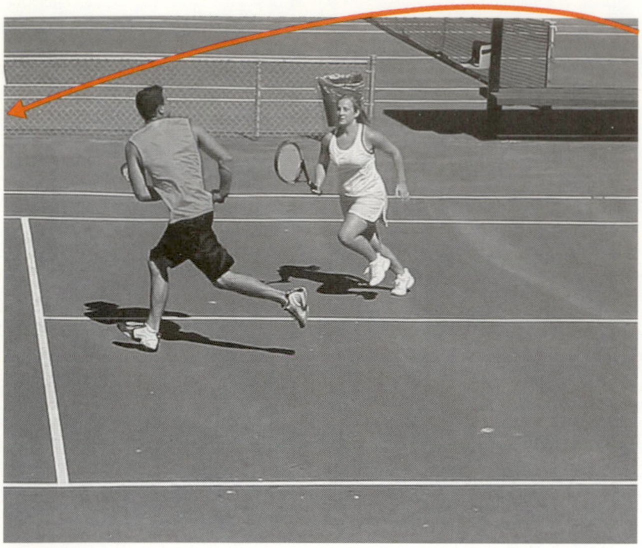

Photography by Terrell Lloyd; assisted by Anna Symonds Myers

PHOTO 8.5 Retreat to return a lob (cross-action).

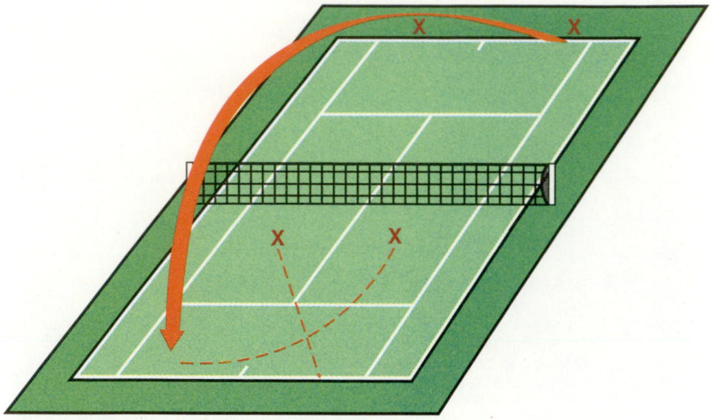

FIGURE 8.4 Movement pattern for retreating to return a lob.

opposing team typically attacks the female as often as possible. If the female player is the weaker player and a female player serves to a female opponent, the male at the net should poach whenever possible. With the female serving, the server's velocity or pace usually is not as fast as when the male partner serves; consequently, the female server may stay in an up–back alignment. That alignment already has been identified as a weak formation, and it is the reason for the male partner's poaching. A serve to the backhand of the return player will aid the serving team by making it easier for the male partner to poach and easier for the female partner to respond to a groundstroke return.

When receiving against the female server, one response might be a direct return to the male net player. If successful, the male partner eventually will retreat to the baseline to avoid being hit by a return of serve.

A second important strategy is to return serve cross-court. This subjects the server to returning a groundstroke from a defensive position, and it avoids the male partner at the net.

Mixed doubles is a delightful game, and it can be highly competitive. Each partner has a role to play and a responsibility to fulfill. Strategy for mixed doubles can be enlarged to cover any doubles in which the characteristics are similar.

Special Formations

Variations of formations can help a team in special situations. Two of these are Australian doubles and the I-formation.

Australian Doubles

Australian doubles eliminates an opposing team's cross-court return. In this alignment the server and net player are situated in a perpendicular line to the net, with both players on the same side of the server's court. If the server is serving to the opposing team's right service court, the server will be to the right of the center mark and the net partner will be set up on the inside center of the serving team's right service court (Photo 8.6). This alignment leaves the left service court of the serving team open during the serve. Following the serve, the baseline server moves to the left to cover the open court from the baseline. The

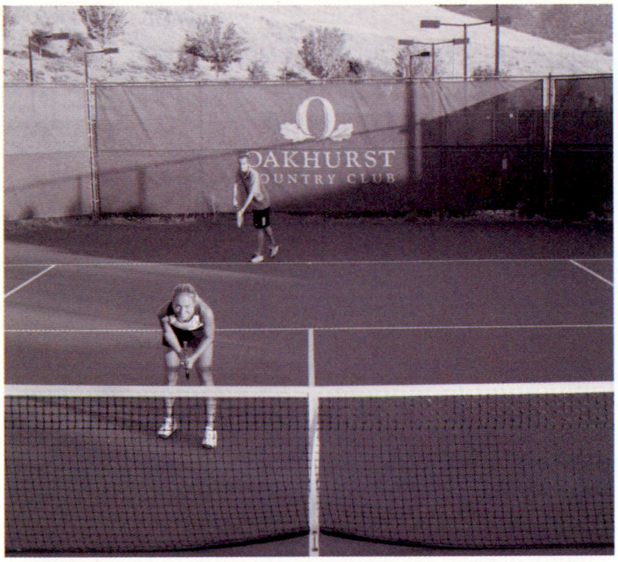

Photography by Terrell Lloyd; assisted by Anna Symonds Myers

PHOTO 8.6 Australian doubles formation.

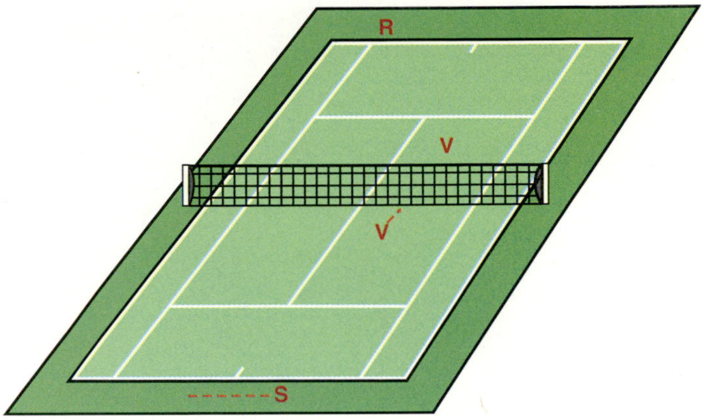

FIGURE 8.5 Movement pattern for Australian doubles formation.

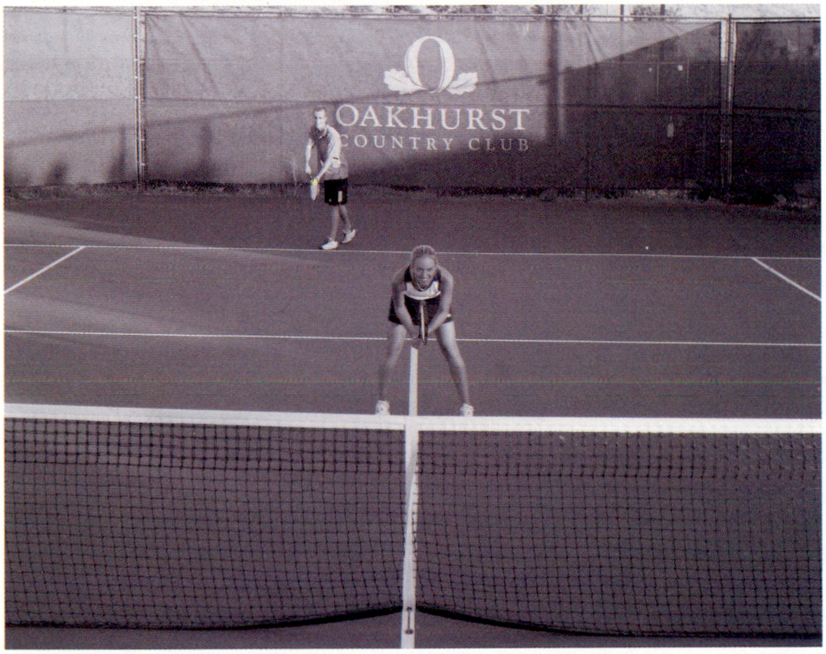

Photography by Terrell Lloyd; assisted by Anna Symonds Myers

PHOTO 8.7 I-formation.

partner at the net stays to create an up–back situation (Figure 8.5).

The Australian formation gives players several options. The first is for the net player to cross to the left service court following the serve while the serving partner moves farther to the right side of the baseline to protect that side of the court. A second option is for the team to criss-cross following the serve, with the net player moving to the left and the server going straight to the net from the right side. A variation of the criss-cross (and a third option) is for the server to follow the serve to the net on the left side, with the net player staying in the same position.

The more variations the Australian doubles formation can offer to the opposing team, the more confused those players will become. This formation is ideal for a team with one weak serving partner or a team with one partner who has a major skill weakness that this alignment can hide. Since the doubles alignment is perceived strong down the middle of the court, it is important for the receiving team to respond by returning serve down the line.

I-Formation

Another special service formation is the I-formation (Photo 8.7). It positions the net player at the net, straddling the middle service court line. Its strength is down the middle; and if the server serves wide, forcing a cross-court return, the net player is positioned to respond with a potential winning volley. Actually, any serve that forces a return down the middle is advantageous to the doubles serving team. The vulnerability with this alignment is that the receiving team can hit shots down the lines for winners.

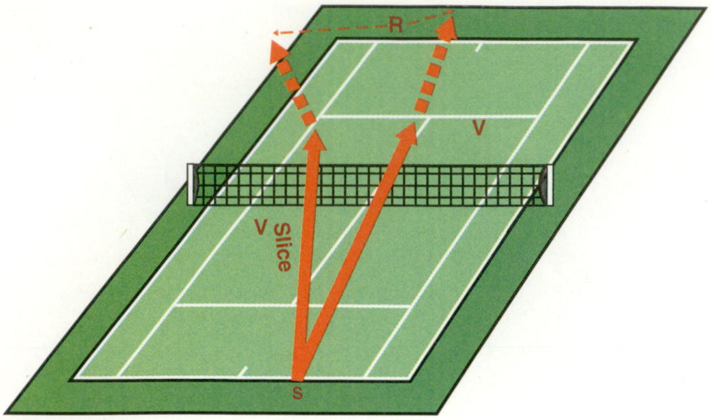

FIGURE 8.6 First-serve targets.

The I-formation gives the receiving team a look that is different from the serving team and forces the opposing team to make adjustments. Sometimes even a small adjustment creates mistakes by the team that is doing the adjusting and works to the advantage of the more creative I-formation team. Response to the I-formation by the receiving team is consistent with response to the Australian doubles formation. That is, with the perception of strength down the middle of the court, the target for return of serve should be down the line.

Service and Return-of-Service Strategy

Doubles play strategy is based on effective service and return of service. In addition, players can fully enjoy doubles play when they are consistent in executing serves and returning service.

Service Strategy

Where to stand when serving is the first aspect of serving strategy. The nonserving partner stands in the center of the service court. It is appropriate to crouch in order to stay low during the serve. The server should stand halfway between the center mark and the sideline to provide court coverage after the ball is in play and to allow for a serve placement from an angle.

The first service in doubles is extremely important. Three-fourths of all first serves should be hit successfully to give the serving team the leverage of moving to the net as a team in a two-up volley situation. Once the developing player has progressed beyond hitting flat services with pace to areas of the opponent's service courts, spin serves should be used more extensively.

A slice serve can be effective when serving to the opposing team's deuce service court, to force the receiver off the court and to allow the attacking serving team to overplay to the left to control the net. A flat serve hit wide to the ad court also pulls the receiver off the court. Another effective serve is a serve placement into the deuce or service court inside corner. To reiterate, the service must be consistently accurate, and the placement, with spin, must be thoughtfully considered (Figure 8.6).

In addition, the beginner must work hard at protecting the partner at the net during service. A soft, pushed serve will endanger that partner and compel the team to play two back on the serve, thereby defeating the advantage of the serving team in controlling the net.

Return-of-Service Strategy

The first point of discussion regarding return of serve is where to stand. The receiver of serve uses the division line theory, just as in singles. The partner of the receiving team needs to stand in the back of the service court. The responsibility of the partner is to assist in calling a serve out if served out and then to refocus on the serving team, and the ball once in play.

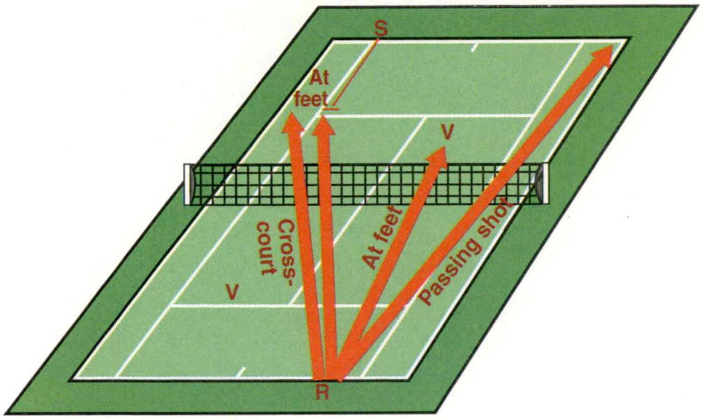

FIGURE 8.7 Options for return of service in doubles.

Three considerations are attached to a *return of service* in doubles:

1. Get the ball back over the net at the serving team's feet.
2. Hit a cross-court return.
3. Select the best target placement of the return, and then complete that task.

The first consideration is an obvious strategy related to self-preservation. The second consideration requires a mind-set to drive a return back across the net, angling cross-court. The third consideration requires more planning and assessment of at least three options for target areas (Figure 8.7):

1. Return the ball to the feet of the net player or the advancing server.
2. Pass the net player.
3. Hit cross-court, angled toward the server.

Hitting at the feet of a net player in singles or doubles creates a ball that is returned "up," allowing you to cover the return effectively.

Passing the net player requires that the player at the net lean to the middle in anticipation of poaching, with the return shot directed down the alley. Being able to pass an opponent at the net down the alley is demoralizing, for that is the one area the net player must protect. It is also a difficult, low-percentage return, since the net is higher on the ends than for the middle of the court.

Angled cross-court returns and cross-court returns at the on-rushing server's feet are exceptional choices for hitting winning shots. The server cannot reach angled cross-court shots unless the server anticipates the shot or the angled return lacks crispness. Cross-court shots at the feet of the server moving to the net catch the server in a tentative position, and the final result is often a ball hit up, for an easy return volley.

The choice of which return to hit is controlled to a large extent by placement of the serve in the service court and by the velocity of the serve. A serve hit to the inside corner of the deuce service court usually eliminates the passing shot because of the central location of the ball. All other choices of service returns from that location remain possible.

The best choice is a return at the attacking server's feet. A serve placement to the inside of the ad service court has the same response as the serve to the inside corner of the deuce service court. Serves hit wide to the respective service courts permit all three service return options to be used.

A major lesson to be learned is that a good server will give the receiver only a limited number of options from which to select during any given service situation. If a serve is well placed, the receiver will return serve to anticipated areas on the serving team's side of the court.

One last consideration of return of serve is for the receiving player always to get the racket on the ball. All strategy for a return of serve collapses if the receiver mishits the return.

Doubles Game Plan and Strategy

The doubles plan of strategy is to (1) execute strokes in an attacking manner and (2) work to gain control of the net. All players at all levels of skill must do these two things. One of the easier skills in tennis is the volley shot. If a beginner can get to the net, play will be highly enjoyable from that position.

Once the concept of taking control of the net is ingrained, the doubles team must remember to protect the alley and the middle of the court. The two must learn to move as a team, in tandem, supporting each other and retreating or advancing together. The receiving team must return serves on a low trajectory with pace and attempt to hit a predetermined target area. The serving team should establish a relentless plan of attack, with the server coming to the net following a well-paced serve.

Doubles play also requires specific responsibilities of each player during the serve. The server has the responsibility to get the first serve in play consistently, to establish a flow and to put pressure on the receiving team to return service effectively. The receiver of a serve in doubles must get the ball back across the net in play.

Once a beginner has developed the confidence to hit the ball back as receiver of a serve, it helps to think through a tactic or placement of the ball in advance and to select a target for the return of the ball. Net players on both the serving and receiving teams have similar responsibilities. Both have to be active and willing to poach. The players at the net also must have the courage to stand up and face a return of a shot and go on the attack rather than respond passively.

A final strategy is to communicate with the partner, outthink the opposing team, and outreach the opponent. Communication is of particular importance. Teammates in doubles have to move in sync with each other. They need to verbally, or through hand signals, indicate what they are going to do. Today, more often than not, advanced players communicate verbally what type of serve they are going to hit and to what part of a service court. The net player conveys strategy at the net, including a preconceived plan to poach. Beginning players are not ready to be this sophisticated in their communication, but simple verbal responses on what to do next can aid doubles strategy.

POINTS *to* REMEMBER

DOUBLES STRATEGY

1. A two-back doubles formation is a defensive alignment that positions players behind the baseline when net skill is weak or the opponents are at the net hitting overheads.
2. Although a one-up, one-back formation is often used, it is highly vulnerable to open-area cross-court winning shots.
3. A two-up doubles tandem provides the most effective offensive alignment in doubles.
4. The Australian formation and I-formation provide a different alignment for the opposing team to cope with strategywise.
5. Getting your first serve in is critical in doubles.
6. Return of service requires hitting at the feet of the net player or the in-rushing server, passing the net player, lobbing the net players, or hitting cross-court, angled toward the server.
7. The key to successful doubles is gaining control of the net.

CHECKPOINTS

1. With the exception of one choice below, the two-back doubles formation is used
   a. as an offensive strategy by experienced players.
   b. as a defensive strategy by experienced players.
   c. as a beginning player alignment in doubles.
   d. by unskilled net players.
2. With the exception of one choice below, the one-up, one-back doubles formation is used by
   a. experienced players.
   b. social players.
   c. novice players.
   d. mixed-doubles players.
3. A poach shot is a movement pattern in doubles defined as
   a. attempting to hit a winning volley shot.
   b. hitting a winning overhead.
   c. hitting a winning volley shot.
   d. attempting to hit a winning overhead.
4. Tandem play in doubles requires that
   a. players move to the net together in an attacking mode.
   b. players move to the baseline in a defensive effort to retrieve a lob.
   c. players cover for each other but remain balanced on the court.
   d. All three strategies are accurate.
5. The strength of using an Australian doubles formation is to
   a. protect the baseline.
   b. protect against the lob.
   c. eliminate a cross-court return by the opponents.
   d. eliminate a down-the-line return.
6. Return of serve requires the receiver in doubles to
   a. hit at the feet of the server.
   b. pass the net player.
   c. lob the net player.
   d. hit cross-court.
7. A two-up doubles formation is
   a. an offensive alignment.
   b. a containing alignment.
   c. a defensive alignment.
   d. all of the above.
8. When a doubles team is at the net, the appropriate reaction to a lob is to
   a. retreat straight back to return lob.
   b. designate one player who will retreat back and return lob.
   c. initiate a cross-action movement, with the partner who can see the ball retreating to hit the return and his teammate crossing over to the other side.
   d. Any of the three are acceptable.
9. When playing mixed doubles, the perception of the female as the weakest player creates a strategy of
   a. attempting to be "fair" and not hit to the female player.
   b. playing every shot to the female player.
   c. lobbing the mixed doubles team.
   d. all of the above.
10. The main responsibility of a server in doubles is to
    a. get the first serve in even if the server has to "bloop" it in.
    b. hit the second serve with high velocity to confuse the receiver of the other team.
    c. be consistent in getting the first serve in with enough pace to force the return player to work at a good return.
    d. hit the first serve with pace and, if the serve is missed, "bloop" the second serve to make sure the ball will be in play.

Answers to Checkpoints can be found on page 167.

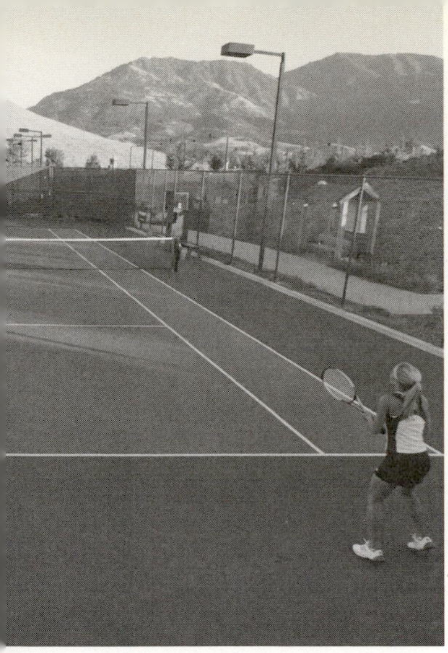
Photography by Terrell Lloyd; assisted by Anna Symonds Myers

9 Tennis Practice

Practice in between playing matches is good for developing tennis skills and applying them. Any group-instruction class uses numerous drills to develop skill. Reinforcement comes from playing in class and from suggestions during the performance of each drill-and-play situation. The beginning tennis player needs more work than can be provided in a group-instruction situation, however, and that work or practice can be achieved in additional practice time.

Development of muscle memory by hitting lots of balls correctly is critical to skill development. Two types of drills can be of particular value to a beginner. *Wall-rebound practice* drills are designed for one individual to use a systematic repetitive effort to practice specific shots that occur in both singles and doubles matches. *Cooperative practice drills* incorporate practice with one or more partners designed to simulate match play involving numerous tennis strokes and situations. Both types of drills can be intense, but there is also the reminder to add an element of fun and challenge to the practice of a tennis stroke or situation.

Wall Drills by Yourself

Most tennis complexes typically have a rebound wall. It is usually composed of concrete or wood, with a net line painted on the surface. This section is designed to allow you to focus on specific aspects of your basic tennis strokes. With these drills you are attempting to develop a groove or consistency that will enable you to visualize distance and accuracy through repetition. You are specifically trying to develop muscle memory for serves, groundstrokes, and volley shots.

Groundstroke Drill Against a Wall

From a minimal distance of 39 feet, the distance from the baseline to the net, you can simulate a groundstroke situation. In this situation your goal is to hit a series of groundstrokes in a consistent and organized fashion. The rebound of the ball will require you to hit the ball on either a first or second bounce back to you. One-bounce returns occur when you are positioned facing the wall, the

FIGURE 9.1 Checkpoint of Mechanics
Groundstroke Drill

1. Am I looking the ball into the racket?
2. Am I transferring weight into the ball?
3. Do I have a full backswing? Follow-through?
4. Am I hitting with the appropriate grip?
5. Am I turning my shoulder early?
6. Is the ball at least 5 feet high on the wall board?
7. Am I accurate? Why?

FIGURE 9.2 Checkpoint of Mechanics
Serving Drill

Counting successful serves might be insightful but total concentration on mechanics will be more productive.

1. Am I looking at the tennis ball on the toss?
2. Is my toss accurate? High enough? In line?
3. Are my feet where they belong?
4. Do I have a full backswing? Follow-through?
5. Is my grip appropriate to my serve?
6. Am I accurate? Why?

FIGURE 9.3 Checkpoint of Mechanics
Volley Shot Drill

1. Am I blocking the ball?
2. Do I have a short, compact backswing?
3. Do I have a short follow-through, with the bottom edge of my racket leading?
4. Am I making contact with the ball in front of my lead leg?
5. Am I stepping into the ball?
6. Is the racket face above my hand throughout the stroke?
7. Am I staying low on the ball?

distance from the baseline to the net. A two-bounce return requires that you back up further from the wall to allow the ball to bounce twice and rebound to a height at thigh or waist level. You should start with a two-bounce return. As you gain skill, you can move up to hit the ball on one bounce. You begin the process of hitting the ball by self-dropping and hitting the ball above the net line on the wall, repositioning into a ready position, and then hitting the ball on its rebound. When you first start, you may find that hitting the ball just one time with good mechanics is all you can do. But as you continue, you will be able to get a rhythm that allows you to hit the ball continuously on the rebound. As you hit each rebound from the wall, your job is to work on mechanics and the consistency that permits you to develop muscle memory (see Figure 9.1).

Serving Drill Against a Wall

In order to place a serve in play, you must hit the ball over the net into the appropriate service court from a distance of baseline to net of 39 feet. That is what is also required when hitting a serve against the wall. In this wall drill, you have the goal of hitting the ball from the same distance, over the line drawn on the rebound wall that represents the net. You can work on both a flat serve and a slice serve. And move the ball different distances from the center section of the net line toward imagery angled targets. At some point, in order to provide yourself additional feedback for a wall-volley drill, you need to take a bucket of balls onto an empty tennis court and repeat this drill. This provides reinforcement that the height and angles of your serves against the wall are consistent with a regulation tennis court. Again, your focus needs to be on the practice of appropriate mechanics and the consistency that will enable you to develop appropriate muscle memory (see Figure 9.2).

Volley Drill Against the Wall

You can also practice volleys against a rebound wall. In this situation you can move up much closer to the wall, close enough to permit you to hit a volley off the wall while also allowing you to be ready to hit the return rebound in a continuous and methodical manner with correct mechanics. This includes stepping into the ball and blocking the ball back to the wall. Your focus, as with the groundstroke and serve wall drills, is to develop muscle memory through proper mechanics and consistency of effort (see Figure 9.3).

Start your practice with a self-drop and just one volley shot. Then work on a repetitive series of volley shots, beginning with hitting only forehand volleys. Then switch to hitting just backhand volleys. When you are at the point where you are comfortable with both strokes mechanically, it is time to work on volleying alternately. Self-drop and hit a forehand volley, directing the shot toward a rebound to your backhand. Then go to a net ready position, followed by returning the rebound with a backhand volley. Continue this process as long as you can maintain the rhythm of alternating back and forth, forehand to backhand to forehand.

As you hit the rebound volley shots, you will find that you have to adjust your knee flexion in order to meet the height of the return of the ball. You need to do this with good form, remembering again that you also need to step into the ball and block it back. When you lose control of the rebound rally, stop and restart.

Cooperative Practice Drills

Cooperative practice drills supplement what you can practice on your own. Of the countless drills that involve two players, 15 are presented in this chapter to provide a beginning approach to practice. Six of the drills are groundstroke-oriented because groundstrokes are the basis for the game. Additional drills will reinforce lobs, overheads, volley shots, serves and return of serves and attacking the net.

Groundstroke Drills

Groundstroke drills progress from relatively simple drills designed to increase a beginner's skills.

Short-Court Drills

The short-court drill is a "touch" drill that requires the partners to stand in the service court of their respective side and hit groundstrokes with touch (Photo 9.1). The idea is to keep the ball within the confines of the service court and to assist the player in anticipation, shoulder turn, and sensing the "feel" of the stroke.

Bounce/Hit Drill

The bounce/hit drill (Photo 9.2) encourages focus and an inner feel for the groundstroke. The idea is for the partners to hit the ball from baseline to baseline without thinking about the mechanics of the stroke. By shouting "bounce" every time the ball bounces on the court and "hit" every time the ball is hit, the partners begin to focus on the ball and concentrate on the end result of hitting the ball to the other side of the court.

What is amazing is that the form and mechanics of the groundstroke come about naturally when the partners become really involved in the drill. Two points to remember when executing this drill are:

1. Both partners must verbally identify "bounce" and "hit," regardless of which side of the net the ball is on.
2. The response must be loud enough for both partners to hear. Players tend to be self-conscious when doing this drill; and if there are players on adjacent courts, the etiquette of quiet on the courts might be disrupted. When used properly, however, this drill will truly be of help in skill development, plus it's fun.

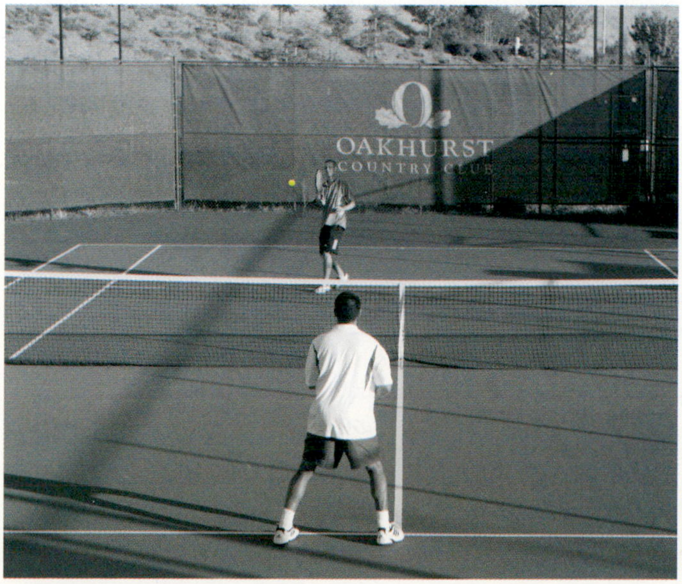

Photography by Terrell Lloyd; assisted by Anna Symonds Myers

PHOTO 9.1 Short-court drill.

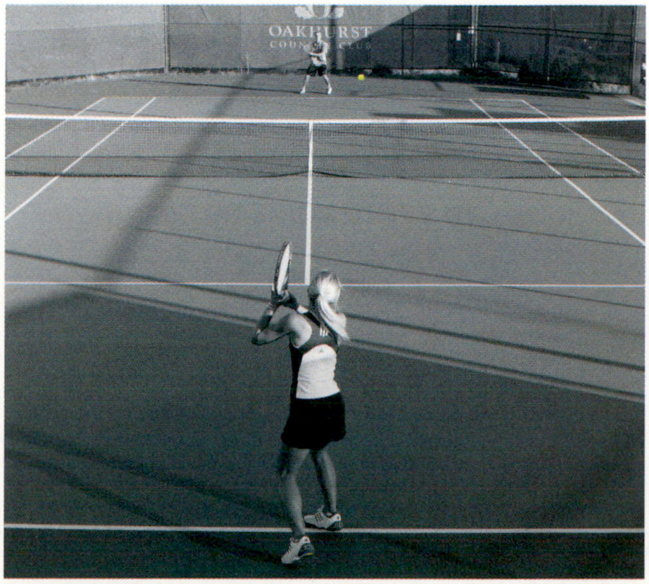

Photography by Terrell Lloyd; assisted by Anna Symonds Myers

PHOTO 9.2 Bounce/hit drill.

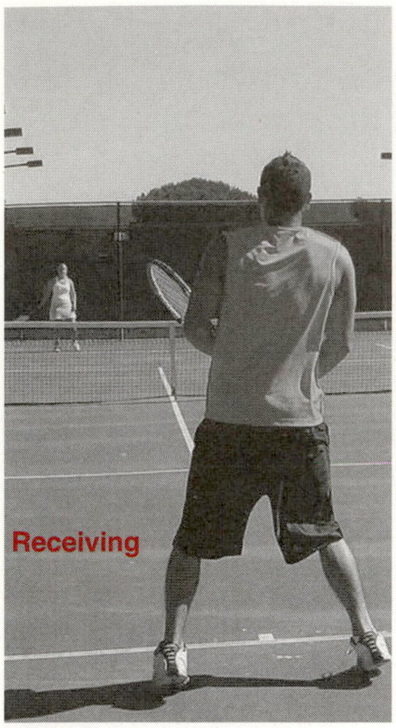

PHOTO 9.3A Receiving groundstroke.

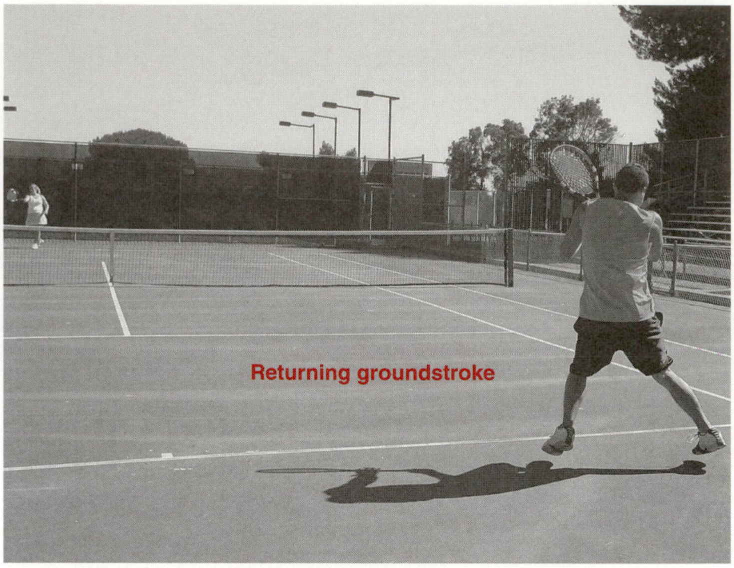

PHOTO 9.3B Returning groundstroke.

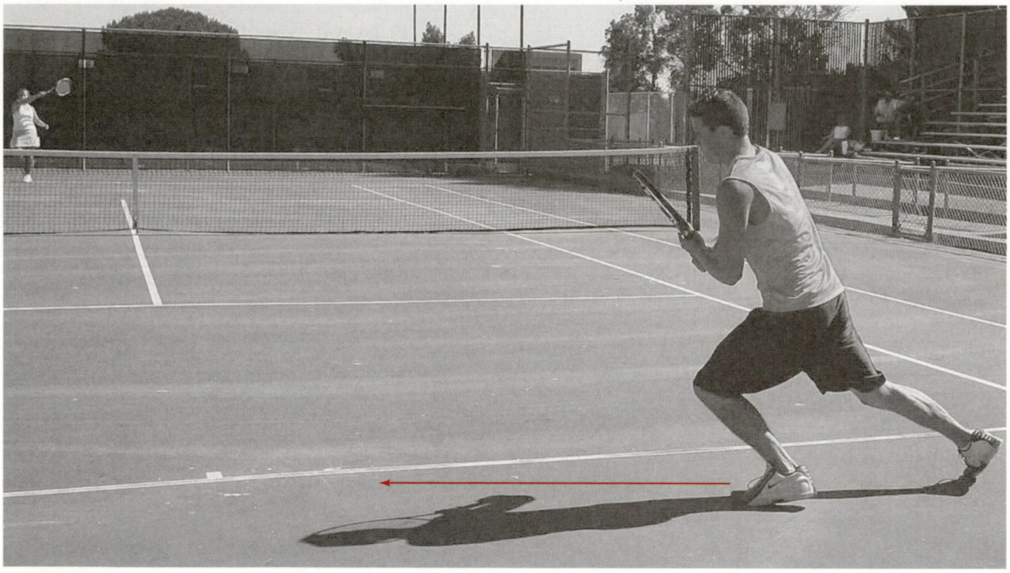

Photography by Terrell Lloyd; assisted by Anna Symonds Myers

PHOTO 9.3C Moving to homebase.

Homebase Drill

The homebase drill requires the player to return to the baseline *center mark* after hitting each groundstroke. There are two concepts associated with this drill. First, if the ball is hit deep, it will keep the opposing player pinned to the baseline, restricting the player's ability to attack the net and thereby forcing errors. Second, by returning to homebase after each shot, a player is able to maintain a balance of court coverage, enabling the player not to be out of position for the return shot. (Photo 9.3A–C).

Both players are to use the area between the service court line and the baseline as the target for each shot hit. After hitting the groundstroke, that player must return to the baseline center mark area and prepare for the next groundstroke.

The drill is played under game-like situations, in the sense that one player initiates play by self-dropping a groundstroke and hitting deep to

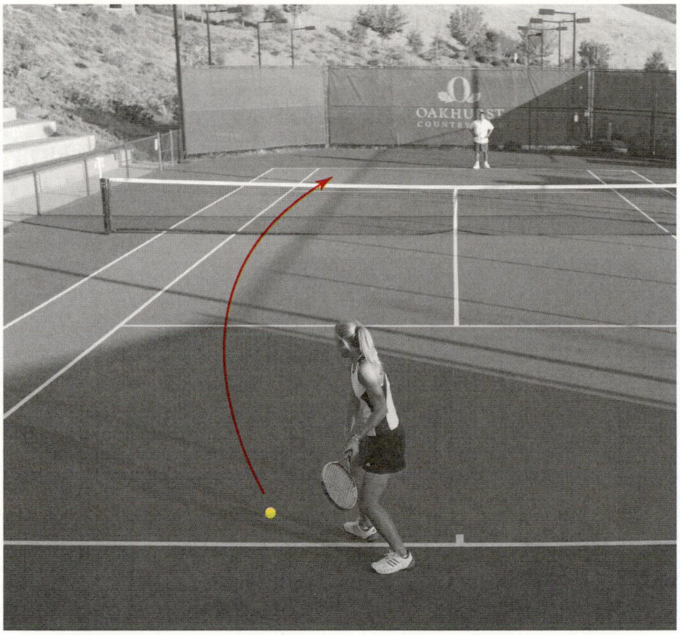

Photography by Terrell Lloyd; assisted by Anna Symonds Myers

PHOTO 9.4 Down-the-line groundstroke drill.

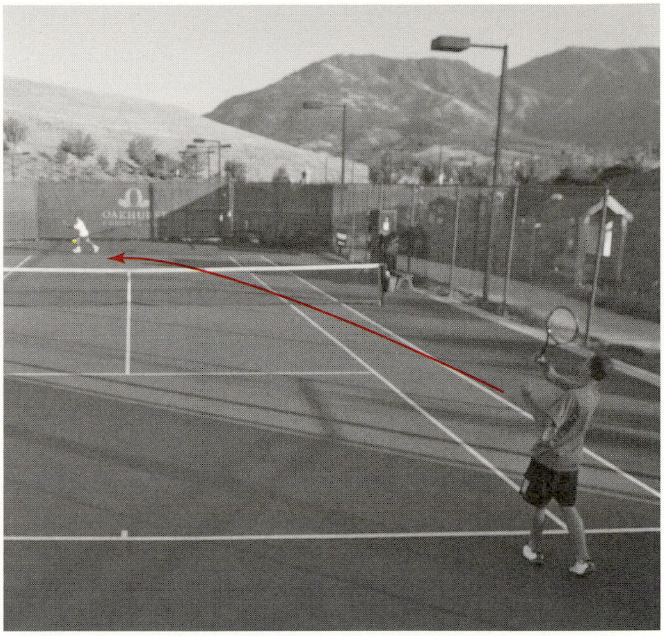

Photography by Terrell Lloyd; assisted by Anna Symonds Myers

PHOTO 9.5 Cross-court groundstroke drill.

the target area. A rally continues until one of the players hits a ball short of the target area. Play stops, and the player who hits the short shot receives a negative point.

Play then resumes with another self-drop, followed by a groundstroke rally to the target area. Play continues to a set negative score, with the player accumulating the greater negative score declared the loser (the concept with deep rallies is that it is not so much that a player is winning a point but, rather, that the other player is losing the point).

As skill develops, challenges can be added to the drill. One example is to play a homebase-approach-shot game. When a ball is hit short of the depth target, the receiving player moves up to hit an approach shot. Hitting an approach force shot earns that player 1 point. But if the shot is missed, a 2-point negative penalty is assigned the player.

Increasing Beginner Skills: Down-the-Line Groundstroke Drill

Hitting down-the-line groundstrokes encourages the player to establish a target when hitting the ball (Photo 9.4). The idea is to hit the ball down the sideline to the partner. The ball should be positioned between the player and the sideline, forcing the player to hit a forehand or a backhand, depending on which is the appropriate shot (with two right-handed players, one would be hitting with a forehand, the other with a backhand groundstroke).

After hitting the ball, the player who has just hit returns to near the baseline center mark area (homebase). The idea is to have to move to hit the ball with the appropriate groundstroke rather than to stand in one spot, and to emphasize good court balance by returning to homebase after each stroke.

Cross-Court Groundstroke Drill

The cross-court groundstroke drill has the same purpose of setting a target and the same organizational setup. But instead of going down the line, the ball is hit cross-court (Photo 9.5). Again, it is important to hit the ball and return to near the center mark (homebase).

These last two drills are somewhat difficult for beginners. Players tend to become frustrated because they are uncomfortable with hitting a backhand and reaching the intended target. Increasing the level of this skill is important, however, and you will not improve if you don't push yourself.

Increasing Beginner Skills: Down-the-Line/Cross-Court Groundstroke Drill

The final groundstroke drill adds to the progression of difficulty because it combines *down-the-line practice with cross-court*. It also requires the player, after hitting a groundstroke, to return to near the center mark (homebase) to be set up for the next shot (Photos 9.6A–D). The idea follows this sequence:

1. Partner A hits down the left sideline and returns to near the center mark.
2. Partner B returns a cross-court shot to the right-side court of Partner A and returns to near the center mark.
3. Partner A then hits down the right sideline to Partner B, who returns a shot cross-court to Partner A's left-side court. Both players, after hitting their shot, return to the center mark.

The sequence is repeated to develop consistency.

Lob/Overhead Drills

Lobs and overhead practice fit nicely together. Two drills—one incorporating a lob sequence, followed by a second, more advanced drill, consisting of a lob/overhead sequence—assist in developing these two skills.

Lob Sequence Drill

The *lob drill* simply requires the partners to exchange lobs (Photo 9.7). The emphasis should be on hitting deep, with proper height for the selected lob. You should start with a defensive lob and experiment with ball height. Then continue by hitting top-spin offensive lobs.

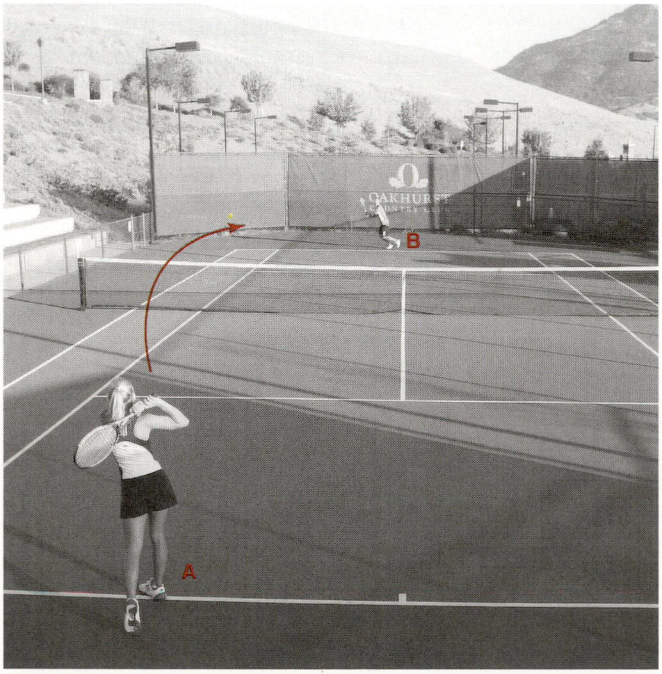

PHOTO 9.6A Down-the-line/cross-court drill sequence: Partner A hits down the left sideline.

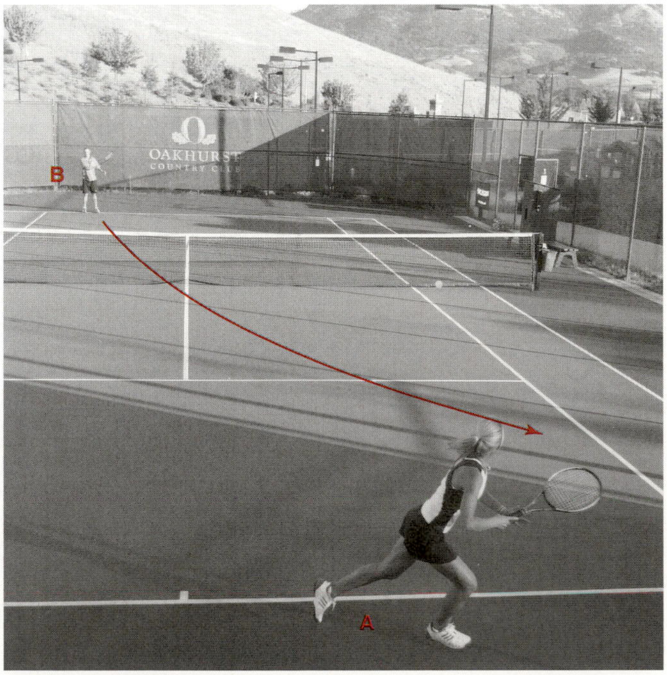

PHOTO 9.6B Down-the-line/cross-court drill sequence: Partner B returns a cross-court shot to the right-side court of Partner A.

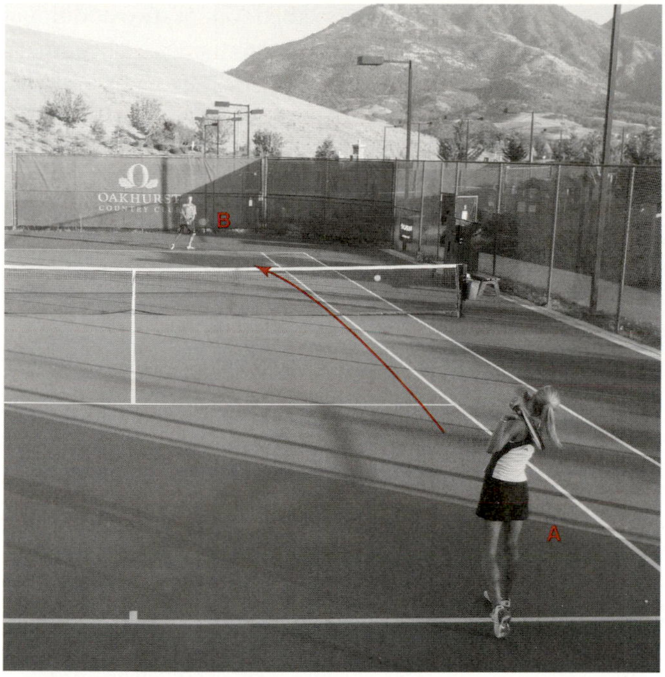

PHOTO 9.6C Down-the-line/cross-court drill sequence: Partner A hits down the right sideline to Partner B.

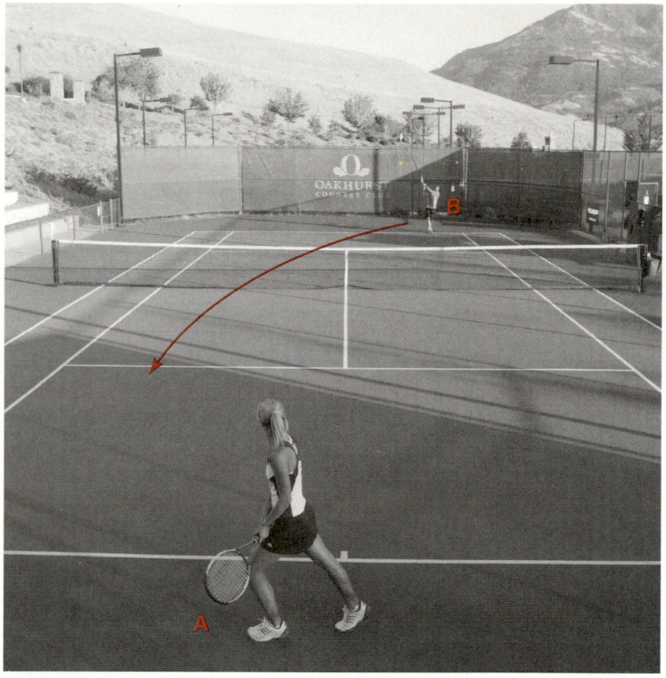

Photography by Terrell Lloyd; assisted by Anna Symonds Myers

PHOTO 9.6D Down-the-line/cross-court drill sequence: Partner B returns a shot cross-court to Partner A's left-side court.

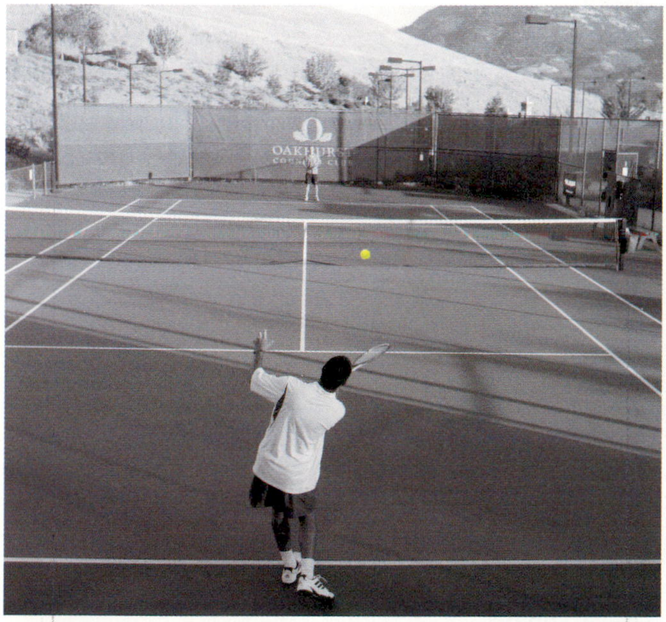

Photography by Terrell Lloyd; assisted by Anna Symonds Myers

PHOTO 9.7 Lob drill.

Work on an equal number of forehand and backhand lobs; as you progress, begin to place the lobs from corner to corner.

An element of competition can be added to the drill by awarding points for successful lobs. For example, 1 point is awarded for a lob that lands between the service court back line and the baseline. There is a 1-point penalty if the ball lands in the service court area, a 2-point penalty if a lob is hit out of bounds beyond the baseline, and a 3-point penalty if the lob fails to clear the net or lands outside the sidelines. After 10 lob attempts, players should switch roles in order to determine a winner of the "lob-depth contest."

Increasing Beginner Skills: Lob/Overhead Sequence Drill

The second drill is an extension of the lob drill. It consists of an *overhead at the end of the lob*, with one player self-dropping and lobbing short to the service court area and the partner hitting overheads (Photo 9.8). As you improve, you should work on returning an overhead with a lob rather than self-dropping to initiate the partner's overhead shot.

Competition can be included in this drill as well. Establish targets for the overhead placement, rewarding deep overheads. Overheads hit into a service court garner 0 points, overheads hit between the baseline and back of a service court line get 1 point, overheads hit deep on an

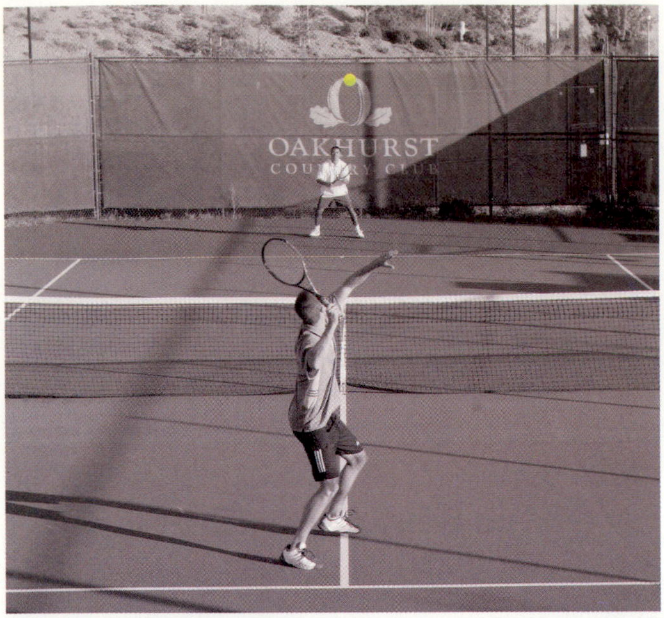

Photography by Terrell Lloyd; assisted by Anna Symonds Myers

PHOTO 9.8 Overhead sequence drill.

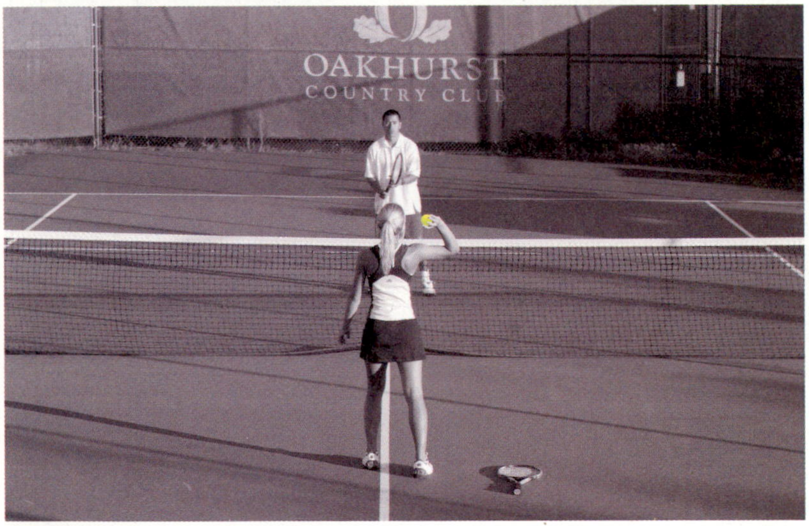

Photography by Terrell Lloyd; assisted by Anna Symonds Myers

PHOTO 9.9 Toss/Volley drill.

angle into the corner formed by the baseline and sideline receive 2 points, and missed overheads lose 2 points. After 10 overhead opportunities, players should switch roles in order to determine a winner of the "overhead-depth contest."

Volley Drills

Two volley drills can enhance the skill of all players, including beginners: the *toss/volley* and the *face-to-face volley*. As skill develops, two additional drills, designed to increase a beginner's skill, are included. They incorporate a *cross-step volley* and a *cross-court down-the-line volley*.

Toss/Volley Drill

The toss/volley drill requires that one partner toss the ball to the other partner (Photo 9.9). The idea is to toss accurately to force the volleying partner to step into the ball with a short backswing and punch the ball back to the partner. This drill encourages good form, and it can progress with variations that force the volleying partner to hit low and high volleys as well as adjust to a ball at the body. In addition, the partner's toss can force the volleying partner to cross-step and punch the ball deep to the baseline.

Face-To-Face Volley Drill

The face-to-face volley drill is a particularly fun drill because both partners face each other within their service courts and volley the ball back and forth (Photo 9.10). Progression again is important. Start with forehand-to-forehand volleys, and then volley backhand to backhand. As your skill increases, you can alternate from forehand to backhand volleys, hit volleys at different elevations of the ball, and react to each placement of the ball that comes to you.

Increasing Beginner Skills: Cross-Step Volley Drill

The cross-step volley drill is designed to force the volleying player to cross-step rather than to step with the inside foot (Photos 9.11A and B). The baseline player hits a selected number of groundstrokes wide from the back of the service court line to the forehand of the net player, and the net player cross-steps to hit a deep volley return. Then the baseline player hits the same number of

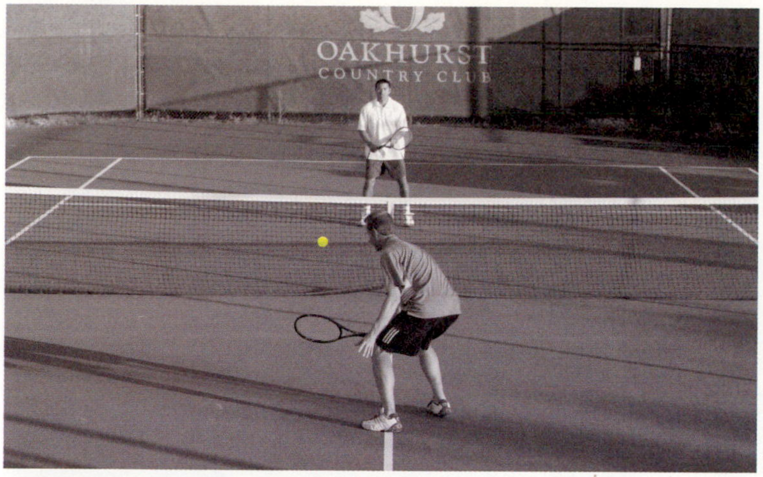

Photography by Terrell Lloyd; assisted by Anna Symonds Myers

PHOTO 9.10 Face-to-face volley drill.

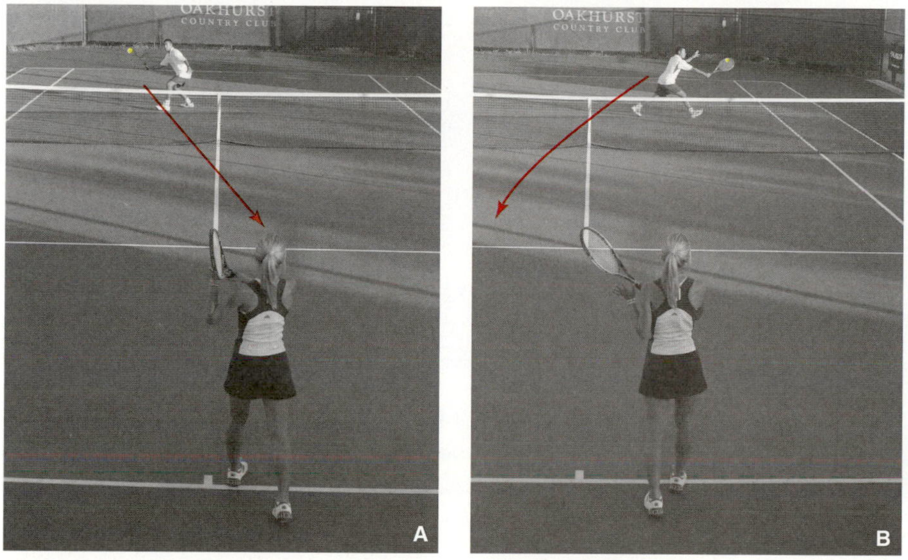

Photography by Terrell Lloyd; assisted by Anna Symonds Myers

PHOTO 9.11 Cross-step volley.

groundstrokes to the backhand side, forcing cross-step volley returns. All volley returns are to be hit deep between the service court line and the baseline.

Increasing Beginner Skills: Down-the-Line/Cross-Court Volley Drill

The down-the-line/cross-court volley drill (Photos 9.12A–D) has the same premise as the cross-step volley drill illustrated in Photos 9.11A and B. The difference is that a select number of groundstrokes are hit from the baseline to be volleyed cross-court from the forehand side, then from the backhand side, and repeated with forehand down-the-line and backhand down-the-line shots.

Service Drill

Hitting serves at spots allows the server to think target. Place markers (towels are good) in each deep, back corner of the deuce and ad service courts. In addition, stretch a towel horizontally across the back of each service court line between the corners (Photo 9.13). The problem with the drill for beginners is how easy it is to hit a lob or soft serve to one of the targets. Since that is not the goal of the drill, and thus not acceptable, a string can be placed above the net (or just an imaginary line will do) at a 6-foot height, forcing the server to serve with pace and/or spin. If competition is necessary, then assign point values to the targets. Corners are worth 3 points, the back line between the two corners equals 2 points, a serve placed in the service court allows a 1-point score, and a fault is a 2-point penalty.

Service Return Drill

Service returns seldom are practiced and, as a result, returns are neglected. The drill is simple: One partner serves and the other returns the serve (Photo 9.14). Focusing on returns should be a first priority, with the main goal to hit each serve deep to the baseline. Then service returns can become more target-oriented by hitting both cross-court and down-the-line returns, placing them deep to the baseline.

To become really skilled in return of service, the return partner should have the opportunity to return serves of different velocities with different spins. The drawback to practicing with another beginner is that neither is at the level to execute a variety of consistent serves. This drill requires a skilled partner or a ball machine to deliver the serves.

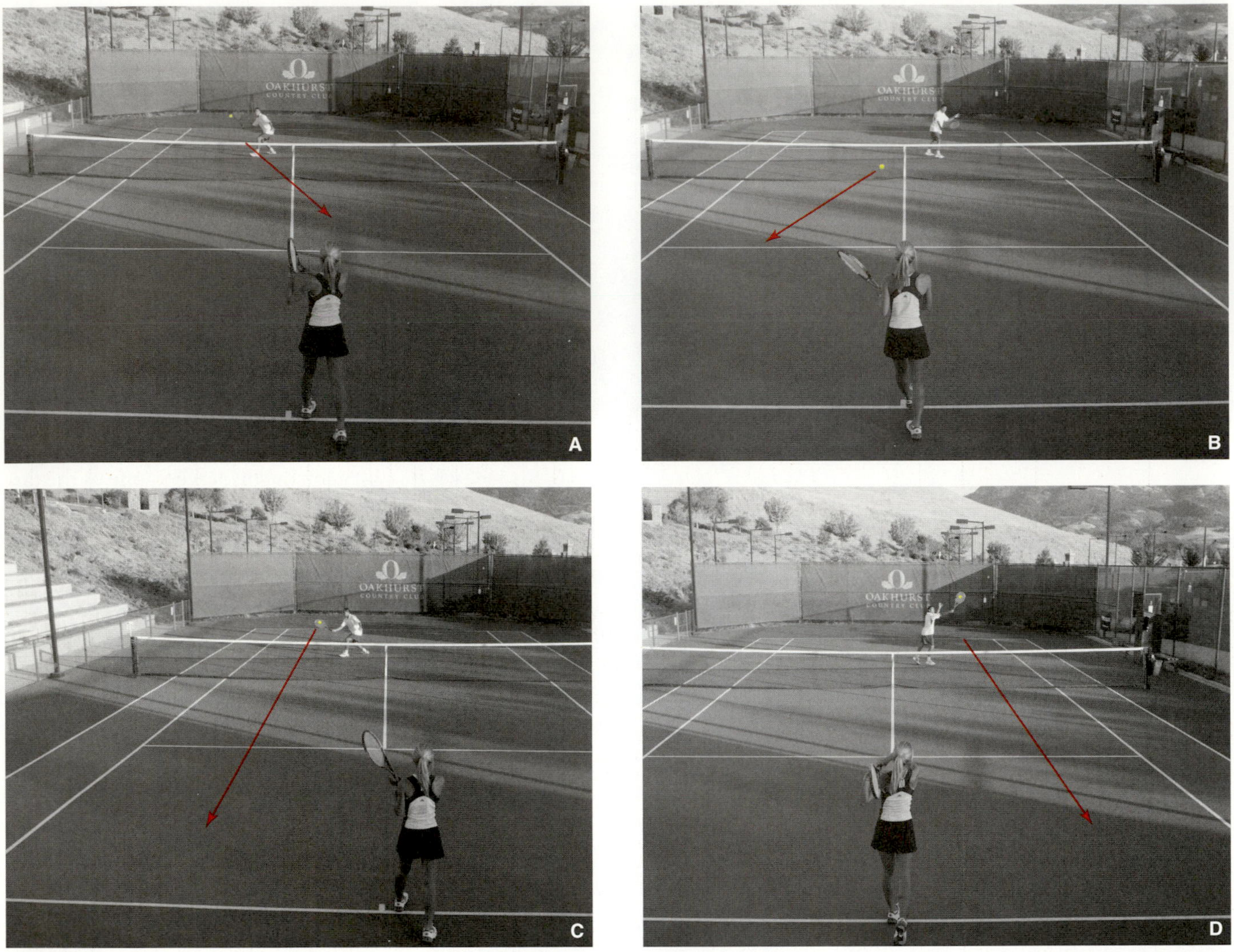

Photography by Terrell Lloyd; assisted by Anna Symonds Myers

PHOTO 9.12 Down-the-line/cross-court volley drill.

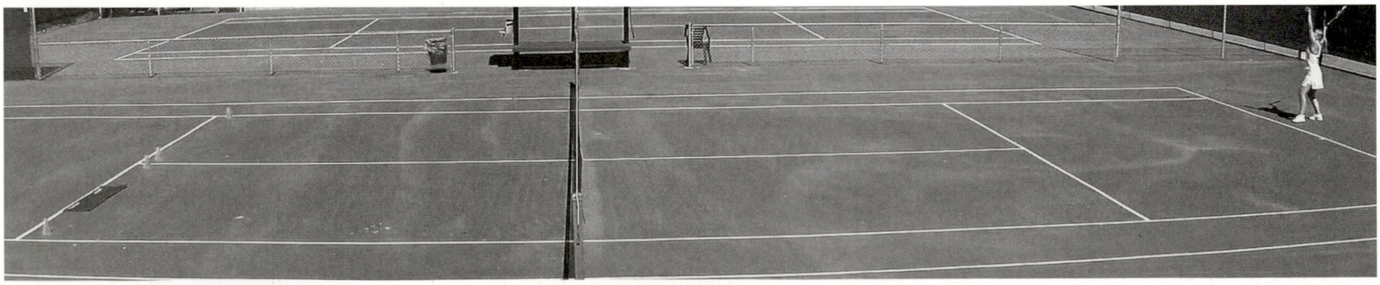

Photography by Terrell Lloyd; assisted by Anna Symonds Myers

PHOTO 9.13 Service drill.

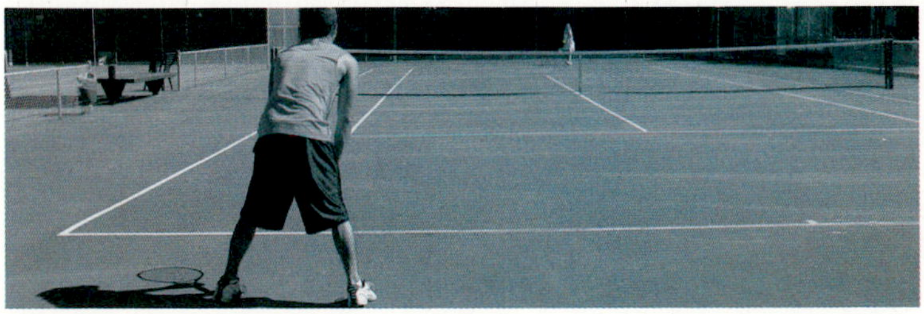

Photography by Terrell Lloyd; assisted by Anna Symonds Myers

PHOTO 9.14 Service return drill.

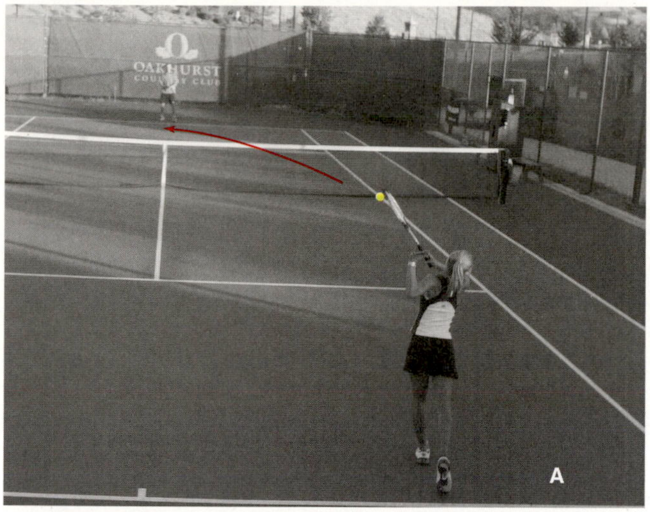

PHOTO 9.15A Attacking-the-net drill sequence: attacking Player A hitting groundstroke.

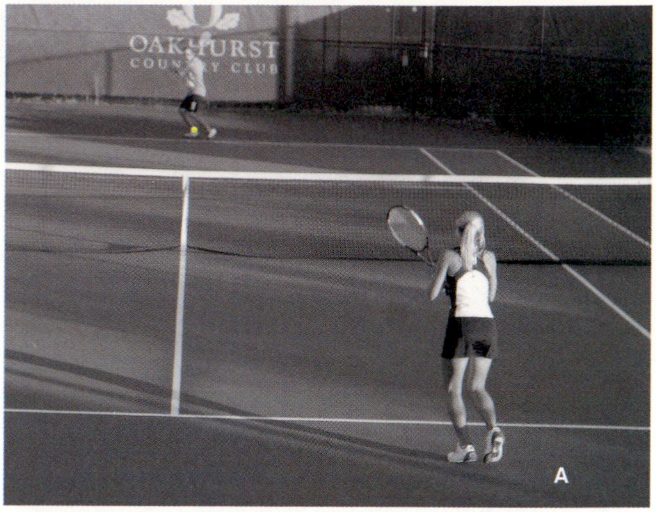

PHOTO 9.15B Attacking-the-net drill sequence: attacking Player A moving forward.

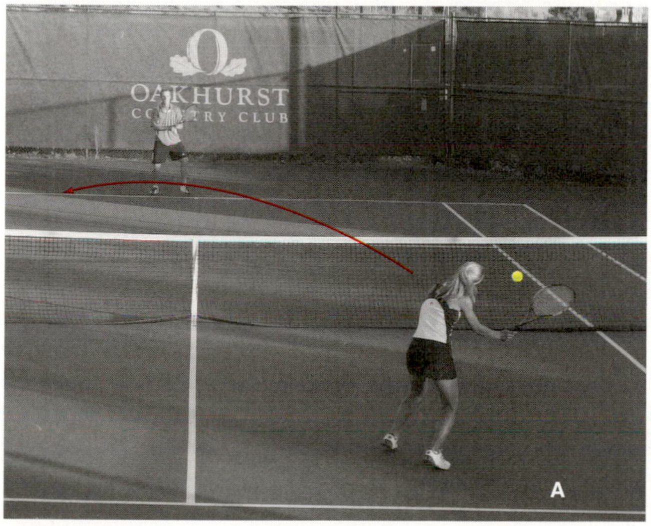

Photography by Terrell Lloyd; assisted by Anna Symonds Myers

PHOTO 9.15C Attacking-the-net drill sequence: attacking Player A returning volley shot.

Attacking-the-Net Drill

The final drill is an attacking-the-net drill designed for the beginner who is comfortable moving to the net. In this drill, one of the partners feeds the ball to the attacking partner. The feeding partner holds three balls and places the first ball deep to the forehand of the attacking partner. The attacking partner hits a deep forehand groundstroke return and begins to advance to the net. The feeding partner then places the second ball to the attacking partner's forehand, forcing a forehand approach shot deep to the baseline. The attacking partner continues to advance to the net and receives a ball to the forehand side from the feeder that then is volleyed by the attacking partner (see Photos 9.15 A–C).

The sequence can be repeated to the backhand and mixed so that the attacking partner does not know which direction the ball is being placed. Other shots, including a second volley and an overhead, can be incorporated into the drill as skill improves. The attacking player also can work on placement with depth and at angles to gain the best advantage at the net. This is not a particularly easy drill, but you will be surprised how well you do because you do not have time to think and because the ball is being placed to you. As an alternative if hitting to set up the attack shots is too difficult, the set up person may throw the ball to the appropriate spot in each part of the sequence.

Final Practice Thoughts

As you continue to develop as a tennis player, game situation drills become important. Singles strategy can be built into drill situations as can doubles strategies. The nice thing about tennis practice is that besides this series of drills, there are many more options. The use of a ball machine allows for stroke consistency when it comes to hitting groundstrokes, volleys, lobs, and overheads.

You can even design your own drills by using imagination and creativity. Practice is important. The wall volley and cooperative practice drills will enable you to progress and increase your skill level more rapidly than by simply listening to instructions and practicing only during that instructional time. Once you gain the skills to play tennis, it is an easy game. Always keep in mind that practice enables you to gain the skills so that you can have fun.

POINTS *to* REMEMBER

TENNIS PRACTICE

1. It is critical to have meaningful practice following lessons and as a supplement to playing matches.
2. The wall-volley drills require effort and motivation to be helpful. To make the drills work, be sure you read the boxes related to each skill area.
3. Cooperative practice drills require a motivated partner who can return various shots with consistency.

CHECKPOINTS

Select four specific skill-related drills and describe how each drill will enhance your specific skill development.

Answers to Checkpoints can be found on page 167.

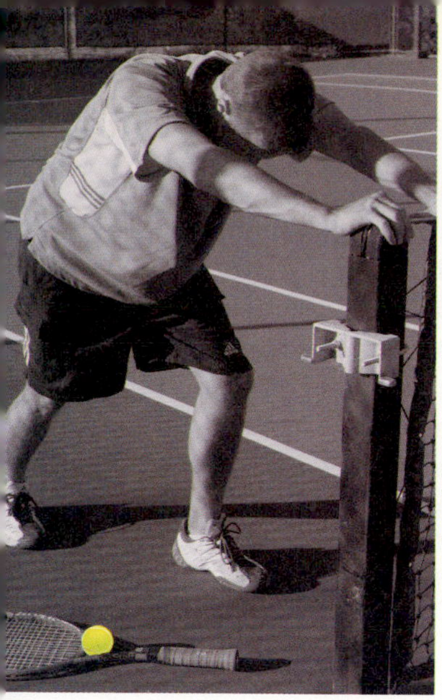

Photography by Terrell Lloyd; assisted by Anna Symonds Myers

10

Physical Aspects of Playing Tennis

The physical aspects of playing tennis begin to take on a major role in performance when you can maintain a rally—keeping the ball in play for a significant amount of time. You need to be physically fit to play tennis. To do this, you should engage in an overall fitness-development program. As part of this program, you should be aware of how to prevent and care for tennis-related injuries and how to deal with problems on a tennis court related to heat, sun, and insects. And, of significant importance, tennis playing should be preceded by a *warm-up* and followed by a *cool-down* period.

The Structured Warm-Up

In preparation for play or practice, you need to engage in physical work to prepare for an extensive tennis participation. Warm-up is divided into three parts: (1) a 5-minute aerobic activity, (2) a 5-minute dynamic stretch activity, and (3) 8–10 minutes of basic stroke warm-up. Preparing for practice requires the same attention to warm-up but when in a college class time is limited and the warm-up process will likely be reduced significantly.

Aerobic Exercise

The *aerobic exercise* structure consists of low-intensity jogging or cycling, which increases the blood flow, heart rate, and oxygen available to the muscles. If tennis courts have a fitness center as part of the complex, then riding an exercise cycle or fast walking or running on a treadmill is a really good way to accomplish the aerobic goal. If fitness equipment is unavailable, then you can simply run outdoors next to or, if feasible, inside the tennis court.

Dynamic Stretching

Stretching has been recommended for tennis players as a preparation for play for many years. Recently the emphasis has focused on *dynamic stretching* as part of a tennis warm-up. The previous static stretch used as a warm-up is now considered by exercise physiologists to be an inhibitor to muscle performance during a tennis match (or any sport activity). Static stretching involves placing muscles in tension, and it is more appropriate for the cool-down phase after a match. A dynamic stretch is more sport specific and requires a ballistic range of motion. After an aerobic warm-up and before stroke warm-up, you need to stretch dynamically for five minutes, including work for your arms, legs,

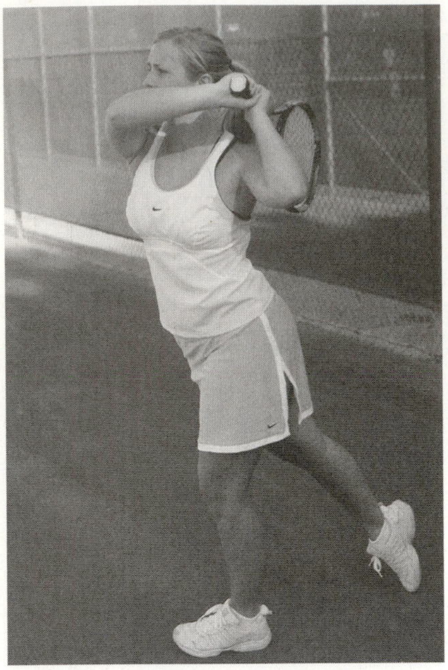

Photography by Terrell Lloyd; assisted by Anna Symonds Myers

PHOTO 10.1A Groundstroke motion rotation.

Action: Copy serve and groundstroke swings. Involve the full stroke with knee bend, arm movement, hip and shoulder rotation, etc. Swing through and back into the beginning of the stroke.

and trunk. A series of 10 dynamic stretching exercises are presented here that involve these body parts (Photos 10.1A–J). Use the stretches to ready your muscles for play, and work to develop a habitual routine that includes these stretches every time you prepare to play or practice.

Basic Stroke Warm-Up

Now you are getting there, in terms of actually hitting a tennis ball. It is time, finally, for *basic stroke warm-up*. You have worked aerobically for five minutes and dynamically stretched for five minutes, and it is now time to hit a tennis ball to complete the warm-up. This warm-up is designed to increase circulation and respiration and to provide a grooving of tennis strokes. A good stroke warm-up should follow dynamic stretching and last 8 to 15 minutes. At the conclusion you should be perspiring. When warming up, a beginning player should always work

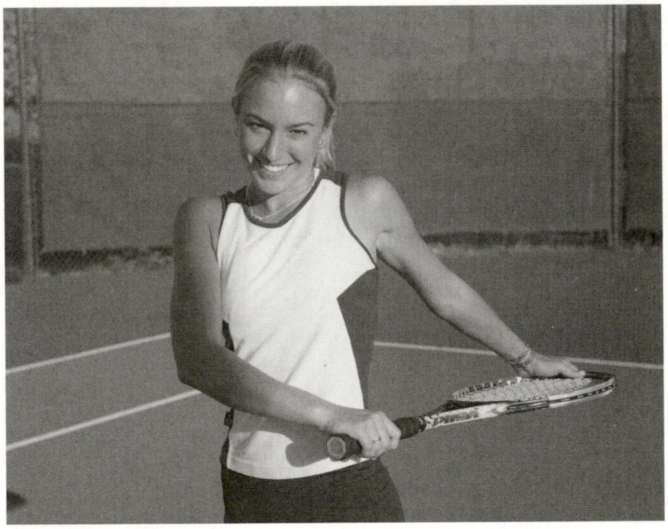

Photography by Terrell Lloyd; assisted by Anna Symonds Myers

PHOTO 10.1B Semi-groundstroke body rotation.

Action: Place the feet approximately shoulder width apart, grasp the racket with your hands, and, with the arms away from the body, rotate the trunk as far as possible and briefly hold the stretch. Repeat the rotation in the other direction, and continue to follow the same process several times.

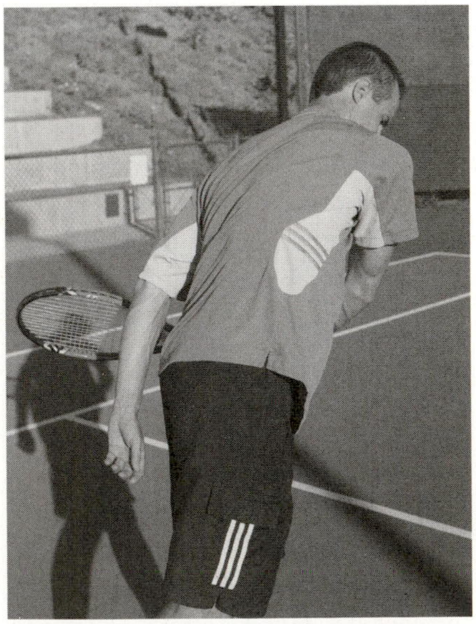

Photography by Terrell Lloyd; assisted by Anna Symonds Myers

PHOTO 10.1C Serving motion rotation.

Action: Start with the head of the tennis racket between the shoulder blades, and rotate through the service motion. Hold the stretch on the follow-through and then repeat the process.

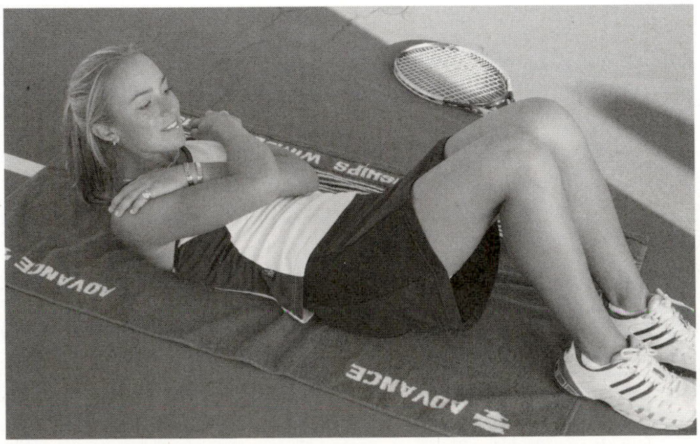

Photography by Terrell Lloyd; assisted by Anna Symonds Myers

PHOTO 10.1D Curls.

Action: Lie flat on padded surface and bend your knees at a 90-degree angle. Place the arms across your chest and curl the upper body to the knees. Repeat the process 15–20 times.

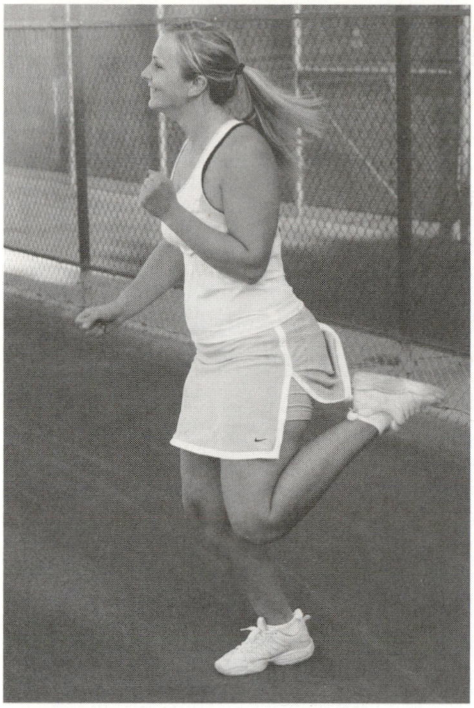

Photography by Terrell Lloyd; assisted by Anna Symonds Myers

PHOTO 10.1E Quick kicks.

Action: Jog in place, bringing heels up to buttocks.

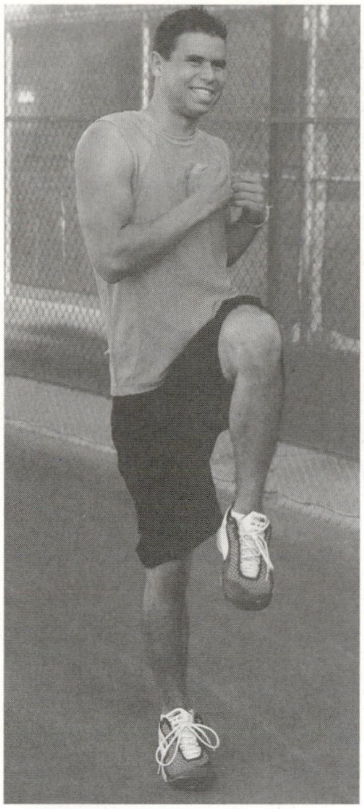

Photography by Terrell Lloyd; assisted by Anna Symonds Myers

PHOTO 10.1F High-step trunk rotations.

Action: Bring your left knee up to your right arm, which is tucked into your chest, while rotating your trunk. Repeat the process on the right side.

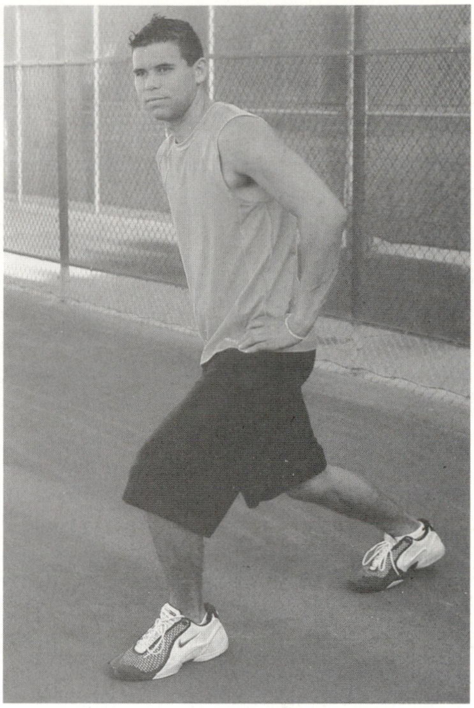

Photography by Terrell Lloyd; assisted by Anna Symonds Myers

PHOTO 10.1G Crossover lunge.

Action: From a wide base, take a step with your left leg across your body and move into a minimal squat position. Repeat the process using your right leg.

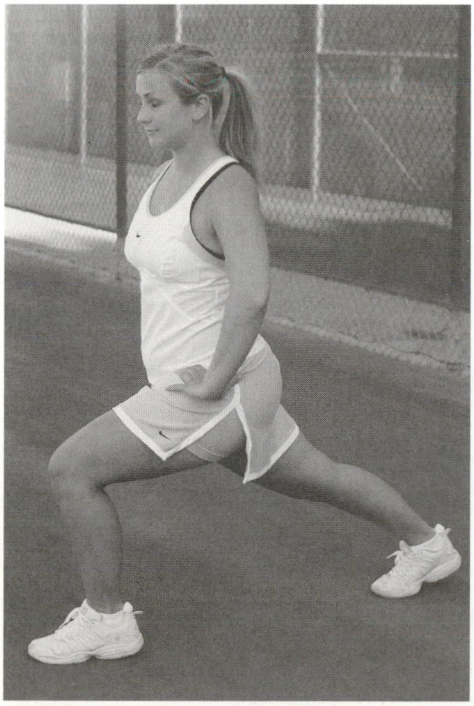

Photography by Terrell Lloyd; assisted by Anna Symonds Myers

PHOTO 10.1H Front lunge.

Action: From a wide foot base, take a step with your left leg into a minimal squat and hold for two seconds. Repeat the process with your right leg.

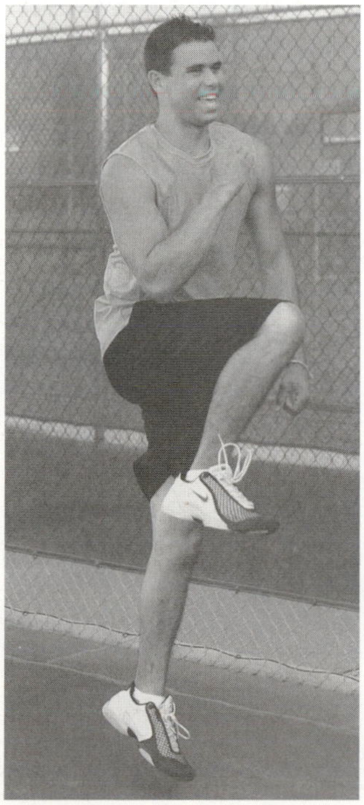

Photography by Terrell Lloyd; assisted by Anna Symonds Myers

PHOTO 10.1I High skipping.

Action: Skip 50 to 100 feet, lifting your knees above your waist. Jog back and repeat the process.

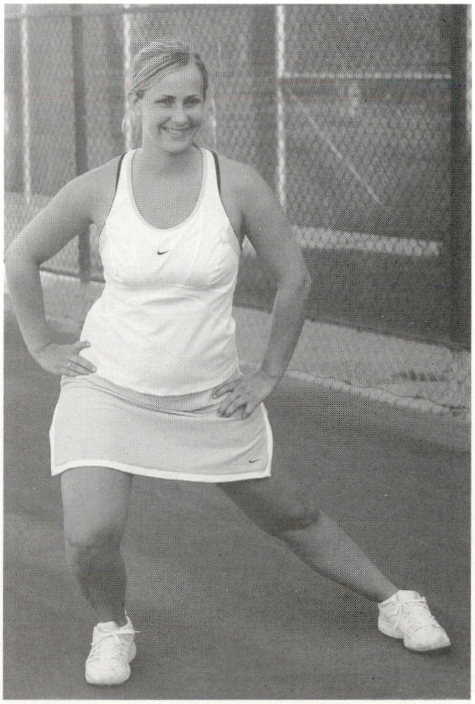

Photography by Terrell Lloyd; assisted by Anna Symonds Myers

PHOTO 10.1J Side lunge.

Action: With a wide foot base step to your left side into a minimal squat. Repeat the process with your right leg.

on strokes to be used in the match. Players should be partners in the warm-up—giving as well as receiving and attempting to ensure that the other partner has had the opportunity for a sound warm-up. The sequence for every tennis warm-up is as follows:

1. Groundstrokes.
2. One player hits groundstrokes, the other volleys; then switch.
3. One player hits lobs while the other hits overheads; then switch.
4. One player hits serves while the other player retrieves the serves; then switch. (*Note:* There is no return of service; that takes time and detracts from the total warm-up effort.)

Although the sequence may differ depending on the location of the players and the player skill level, the concept is reasonably standard.

The Cool-Down

Following a tennis match or practice, you need to accept that you are not done for the day, at least not yet. Take a brief walk to allow your heart rate to decrease and to consume water. You are now focused for stretching. Your muscles are warm and they are ready to be stretched. Now is the time to use a *static stretch* process. You are now ready to place a muscle group in tension and hold for 10 to 30 seconds being careful not to overextend your tension to the point where you are hurting yourself. This is the flexibility phase of your full tennis experience. You are now developing an increased range of motion when you use the 14 static stretches that follow (Photos 10.2A–N).

POINTS *to* REMEMBER

PHYSICALLY PREPARING TO PLAY

1. Do physical work for at least 5 minutes before dynamic stretching.
2. Dynamic stretching exercises should include both upper and lower body.
3. The tennis stroke warm-up consists of a specific sequence of groundstrokes, volleys, lobs/overheads, and service.
4. After a match, cool down by static stretching.

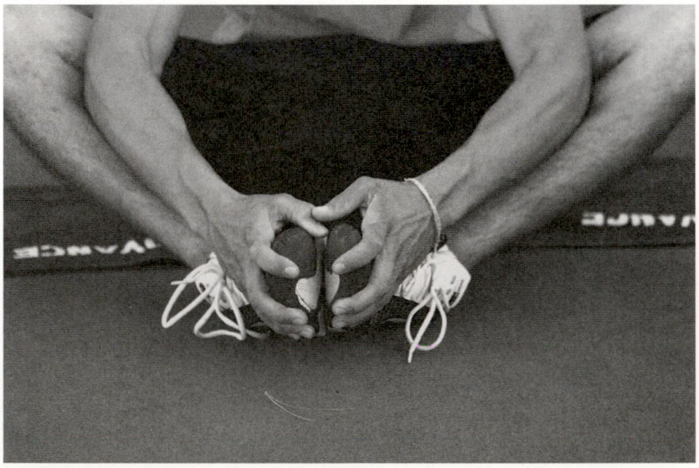

Photography by Terrell Lloyd; assisted by Anna Symonds Myers

PHOTO 10.2A Groin stretch.

Action: Sit with the soles of the feet together. Bring your chest forward toward your feet, bending from the hips. Push your knees toward the ground with your elbows.

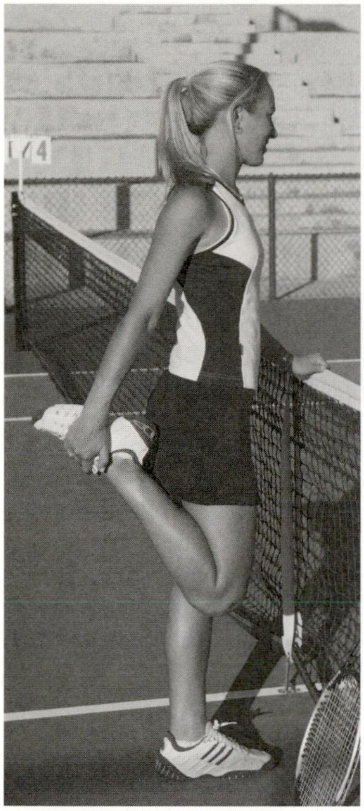

Photography by Terrell Lloyd; assisted by Anna Symonds Myers

PHOTO 10.2B Quad stretch.

Action: Stand up straight, grasp the front of the ankle, and flex the knee until the heel of the foot is touching the gluteal area. Hold the stretch, then change legs.

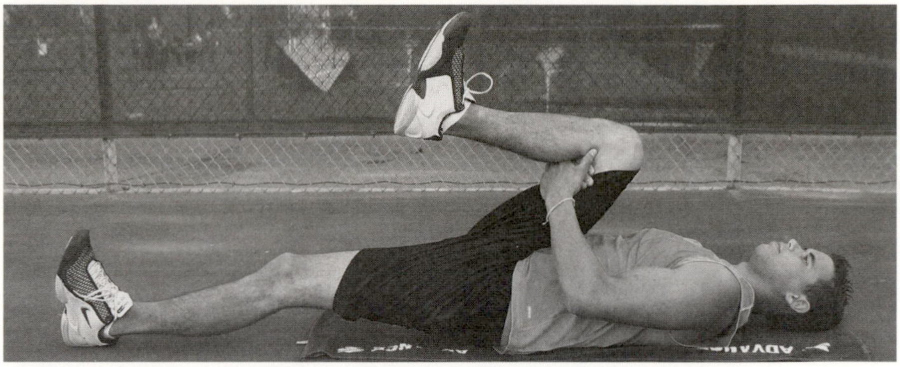

Photography by Terrell Lloyd; assisted by Anna Symonds Myers

PHOTO 10.2C Hamstring stretch.

Action: Lie on your back, with one leg on the court and the other extended above your hips. Grasp the extended leg with both hands and slowly straighten your extended leg as you pull it toward your upper body.

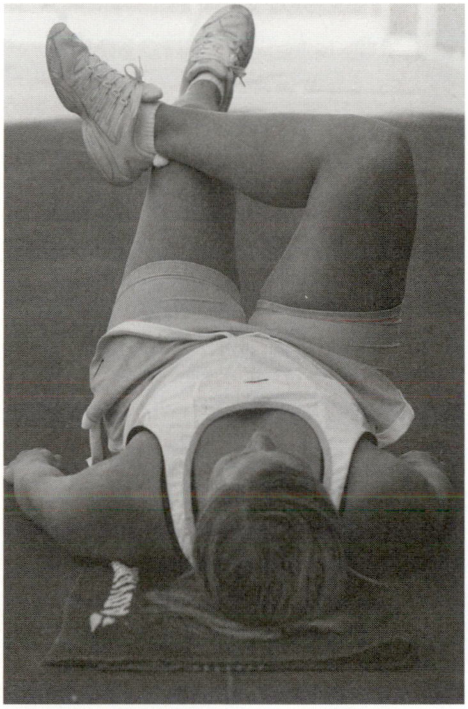

Photography by Terrell Lloyd; assisted by Anna Symonds Myers

PHOTO 10.2D Glute stretch.

Action: Lie on your back, with one foot on the court and your leg bent. Cross your opposite ankle just above the bent knee and bring that knee toward your chest. Repeat the process on the opposite side.

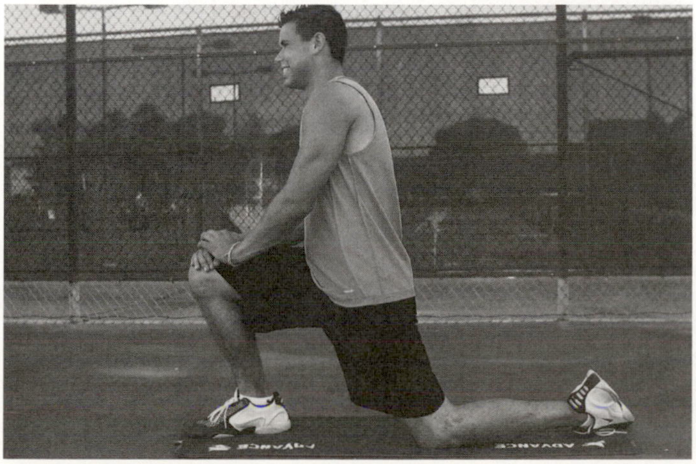

Photography by Terrell Lloyd; assisted by Anna Symonds Myers

PHOTO 10.2E Hip flex.

Action: From a standing position, lower yourself to one knee on the court, with the other knee bent at a right angle in a semilunge position. Then tilt your pelvis forward, stretching the front of your hips and quads.

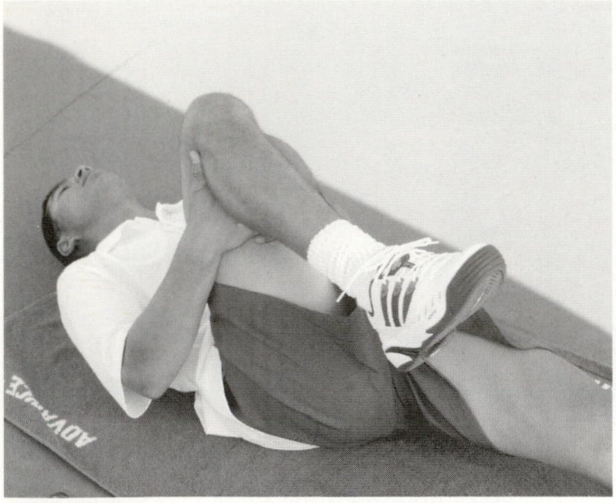

Photography by Terrell Lloyd; assisted by Anna Symonds Myers

PHOTO 10.2F Single-knee-to-chest stretch.

Action: Lie flat on a padded surface. Bend one leg at approximately 100 degrees and place both hands on the lower back portion of the knee of the opposite leg, pulling that knee toward the chest. Hold the stretch at chest level.

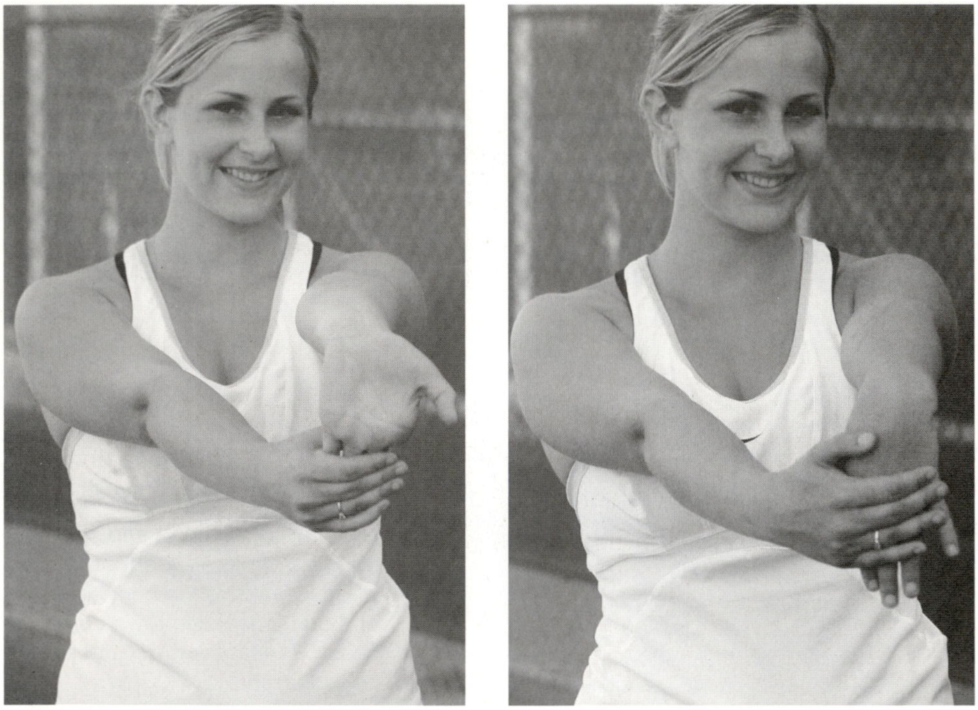

Photography by Terrell Lloyd; assisted by Anna Symonds Myers

PHOTO 10.2G Wrist and forearm stretch.

Action: Extend your arms in front of your shoulders. Turn one arm with the palm face up and the fingers directed downward. Use your opposite hand to press the fingers of the hand down. Repeat the process by switching arms.

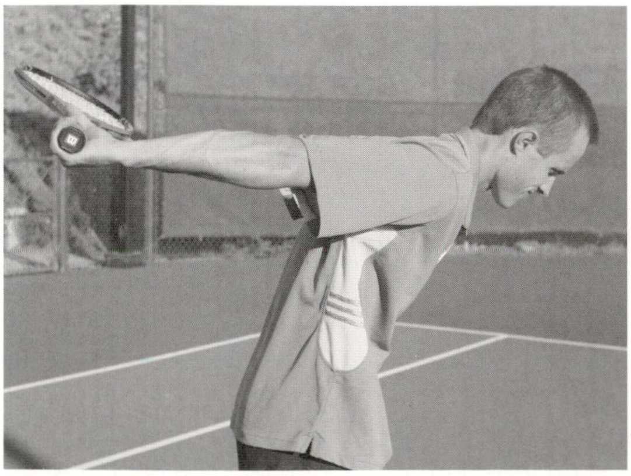

Photography by Terrell Lloyd; assisted by Anna Symonds Myers

PHOTO 10.2H Shoulder hyperextension stretch.

Action: Grasp the throat of the racket, with the hands close together. Slowly bring the arms up to as close to a perpendicular position to the shoulders as possible.

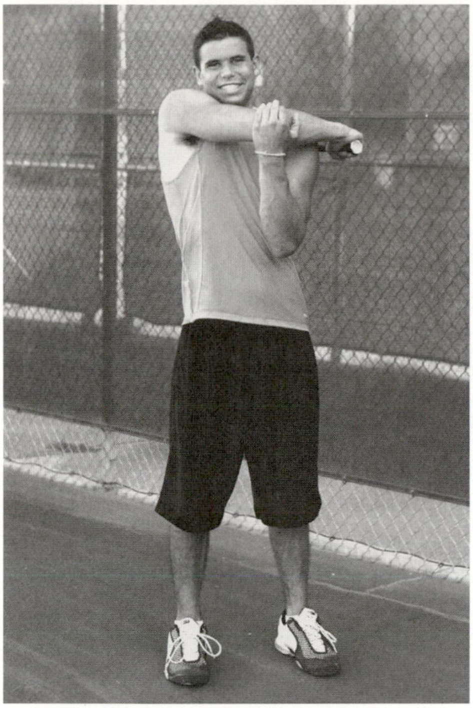

Photography by Terrell Lloyd; assisted by Anna Symonds Myers

PHOTO 10.2I Cross-arm stretch.

Action: Stand upright and place one arm across your chest at shoulder height. Place your opposite hand on the elbow of the arm across your chest. Pull your shoulder across your body, with the hand placed on the elbow. Repeat the process by switching arms.

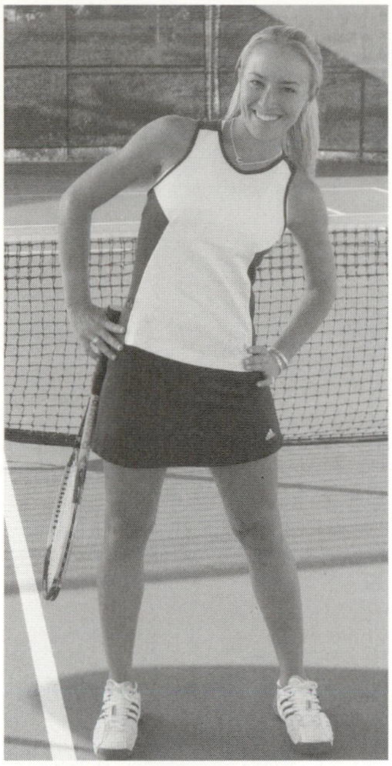

Photography by Terrell Lloyd; assisted by Anna Symonds Myers

PHOTO 10.2J Side stretch.

Action: Spread the feet shoulder width, with hands on hips. Rotate the body to one side, and repeat the process to the other side.

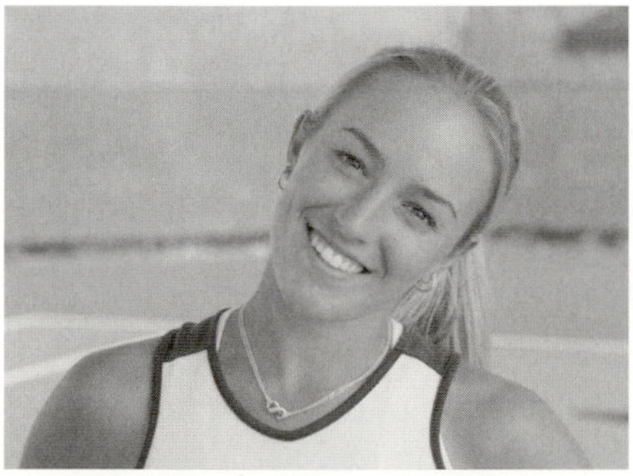

Photography by Terrell Lloyd; assisted by Anna Symonds Myers

PHOTO 10.2K Lateral head tilt.

Action: Tilt the head slowly and gently to one side and hold the stretch for a few seconds. Alternate to the other side, and repeat.

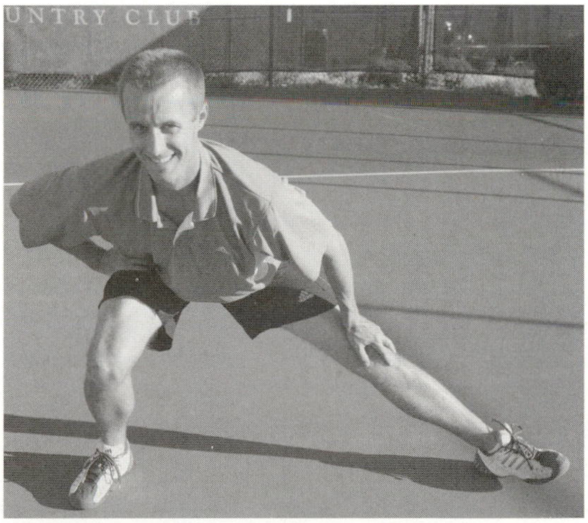

Photography by Terrell Lloyd; assisted by Anna Symonds Myers

PHOTO 10.2L Adductor stretch.

Action: Spread the feet twice shoulder width, with hands placed slightly above the knee. Flex one knee and go down to approximately 90 degrees. Hold the stretch, and then repeat on the other side.

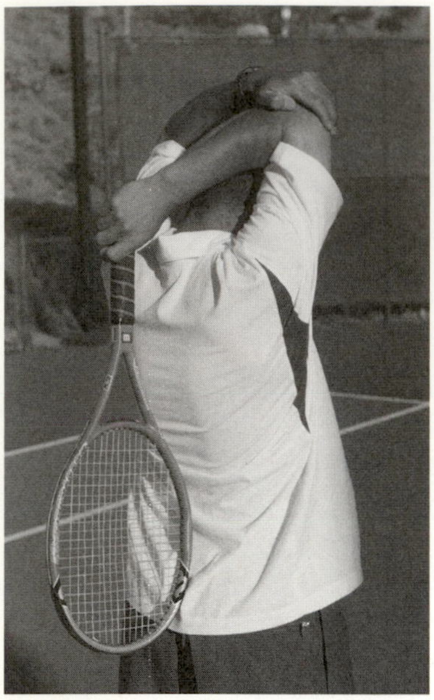

Photography by Terrell Lloyd; assisted by Anna Symonds Myers

PHOTO 10.2M Serving-shoulder-and-arm stretch.

Action: Place the tennis racket head in the small of the back, with the elbow in an up position. Place the nonracket hand below the elbow, and apply minimal pressure to place the shoulder area on stretch. Repeat the process several times.

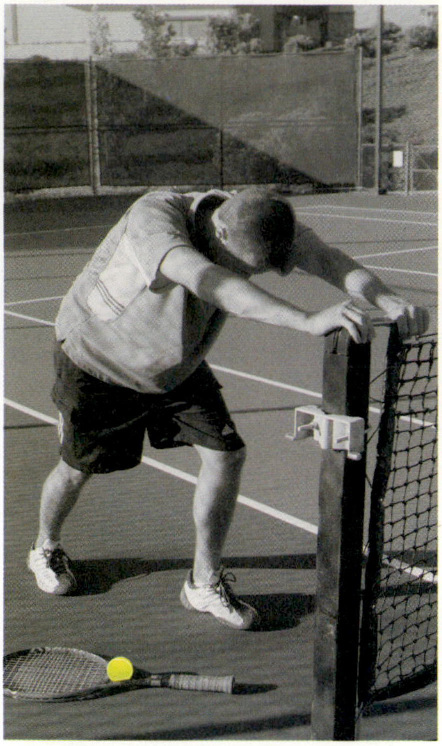

Photography by Terrell Lloyd; assisted by Anna Symonds Myers

PHOTO 10.2N Heel cord stretch.

Action: Stand against a solid object and stretch the heel downward. Hold the stretch and then change legs.

Developing Overall Fitness

Fitness development for tennis can range from basic to sophisticated through the use of aerobic and anaerobic exercise and strength-training programs. Tennis players who are willing to run, follow a sensible exercise program, and work on tennis drills that incorporate agility and quickness will establish an advantage over individuals who neglect fitness development.

Developing Aerobic Fitness

Aerobic exercise contributes significantly to success as a tennis player. You cannot use your skills and apply strategy to best advantage if you are not in good physical shape. In addition, you are at risk for potential injury. During a tennis rally, most of the energy the body uses is a product of anaerobic metabolism, the release of energy without the use of oxygen.

Therefore, although energy needs during tennis play are not primarily *aerobic* ("with oxygen"), the more oxygen that can be used during a rally, the faster you can recover and the less tired you will be during play. This means that you need to train your body to use large amounts of oxygen quickly. You can accomplish this through a number of physical activities, which can include a short-distance walk and long-distance running.

For most people under age 35, an exercise intensity between 70 percent and 85 percent of *maximal heart rate* is adequate and is called an *exercise heart rate range*. Maximal heart rate is the fastest a heart can beat when exercising as hard as you can. The typical way to predict your exercise heart rate range is to take the number 220 and subtract your age. After you have tabulated that number, simply calculate 70 or 85 percent of that number. For example:

$$220 - 20 \text{ years of age} = 200$$
$$200 \times 70\% = 140$$
$$200 \times 85\% = 170$$

Calculation of these two numbers represents an exercise heart rate range (i.e., a 20-year-old's exercise heart rate range is between 140 and 170). If you are in good health, this heart rate range will provide a guide for your level of exercise effort. Also, before starting any exercise program, it is advisable to have a physical exam.

Once you have arrived at a proper rate of exercise intensity, you have to determine the duration of your workout effort. Anywhere between 15 and 60 minutes will provide enough time to give your body sufficient practice at using oxygen. In general, 20–30 minutes is recommended as the proper workout duration. This means 20–30 minutes of constant, nonstop exercise at your exercise heart rate. If you are just starting out, you need to work progressively into a full workout. It does you no good to start at a high level of effort, only to experience discomfort or injury the first day. Start slowly and progress to a more full workout. Try to do your aerobic work at least three or four times per week. Five times per week can be tolerated, but you also need to give your body a chance to rest. A minimum of 24 hours between aerobic workouts is desirable. The less fit you are, the more time you need to set aside between your aerobic work and rest.

Anaerobic Exercise

Anaerobic exercise may also be incorporated into your fitness workout. Tennis is a game of quick lateral movement, elevated heart rate, and stops and starts. Make an effort to incorporate short sprints and change-of-direction speed work that will enhance your tennis skills as well as your anaerobic fitness level. As an example, start at the baseline and sprint to the T formed by the center line and back line of the service court, cut right to the sideline, backpedal to the baseline from the sideline, and then sprint from one end of the baseline to the other (Figure 10.1). Repeat the process, but go to the left at the T of the service court. Take a brief rest and then go again. The intensity level should be near full capacity doing this speed work, followed by what may be termed a recovery time.

If you combine aerobic work with practice time on the tennis court using the drills presented in Chapter 9, *Tennis Practice,* you will gain a positive level of fitness and you will also have improved your quickness and agility for tennis play.

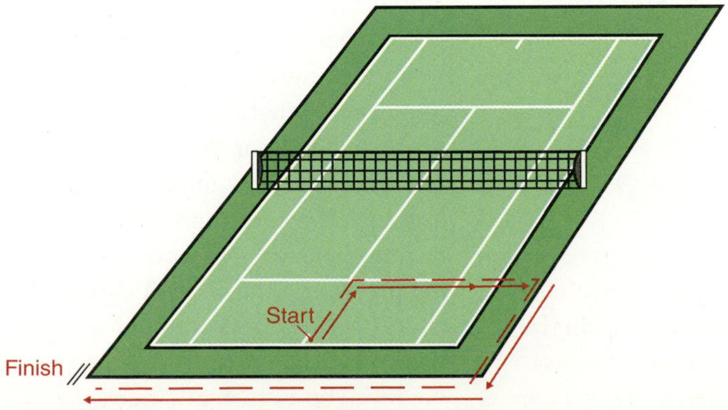

FIGURE 10.1 Court sprint to the T.

Developing Strength and Fitness

Several forms of *strength training* are designed for further development of both muscular strength and endurance, which can also enhance physical development for tennis. You can use either free weights or weight machines to accomplish this development. Each of these workouts should include weight work for shoulder strength, abdominal development, bicep and tricep strength, quadricep and hamstring strength development, and calf strength development. When you do these exercises, you should breathe, and lift, using a smooth, slow action.

Your workouts should consist of every other day or a minimum of 3 days per week, with 2–3 sets of 10–15 repetitions. One of the exciting aspects of strength-training programs is that most colleges and universities have established facilities for your choice of weight-training workout, with state-of-the-art equipment.

POINTS to REMEMBER

OVERALL FITNESS DEVELOPMENT

1. Predict an exercise heart rate range by subtracting your age from 220, then multiplying that number by 70% and 85% to determine a range.
2. Aerobic workouts should consist of 20–30 minutes for 3 or 4 times per week.
3. Anaerobic workouts can be incorporated within the aerobic workout and patterned after tennis movements.
4. Strength-training workouts using free weights or weight-training machines should consist of 2–3 sets of 10–15 repetitions each performed every other day.

Preventing and Caring for Tennis Injuries

Of the numerous injuries associated with tennis, most can be prevented. Serious injuries related to contact sports, including concussions, cartilage and ligament damage of the knee, shoulder separations, and neck injuries, are seldom found in tennis. Knee, shoulder, and back injuries, however, are increasing in number. Hard tennis court surfaces can be blamed for many knee and back injuries, and overuse or improper shoulder rotation when serving often contributes to shoulder injuries.

As a general rule, though, injuries in tennis usually are mild and seldom restrict a player's participation. The few serious injuries that do occur can be prevented in many cases.

Minor Tennis Injuries

Some common minor tennis injuries can be prevented with a little attention.

Blisters

The blisters that often appear on the hands and feet are caused by moisture, pressure, or friction. Blisters on the feet are caused by the feet sliding in tennis shoes. To prevent these blisters, wear cotton tennis socks with cushion insoles.

Blisters on the racket hand often are caused by the racket turning in the player's hand. You can prevent this type of blister by making sure you have the correct grip size. Usually a larger grip enables a player to prevent the racket from turning in the hand, although sometimes a larger grip is too large and results in a turning action as well. Blisters also develop on the racket hand from extensive play when the hand has not been accustomed to that amount of play. The wear and tear creates a "hot spot" that results in a blister. Prevention consists of being conscious of the length of playing time and placing some limit on it.

Bruises

Sometimes a player is bruised when hit by a ball or racket. The only way to avoid this injury is to avoid positions on the court that provide an opportunity to be hit, or to avoid being hit in vulnerable spots of the body. For example, if you are on the direct opposite side of the net from the opposing player and the opposing player is about to hit an overhead in line with your position on the court, it is prudent for you to turn and duck.

Also, bruising can occur when a player follows through with the racket and hits the shin when serving, or when doubles partners swing at the same ball and hit each other. These incidents can cause severe bruising, called a *hematoma*.

Cramps

In unusually warm and humid weather, when a person loses body fluid and salt rapidly, a player may get cramps. A muscle or muscle group contracts, causing spasms, usually in the abdominal area or *gastrocnemius* (calf muscle). To prevent a serious cramping problem, consume fluids in fairly large quantities. Although water is the best choice of liquids, diluted fruit juices are an excellent alternative. Sports drinks (such as Gatorade®, Powerade®, and Exceed®) also are alternatives to dealing with cramps when you play for extremely long periods in hot weather. They replace carbohydrates and electrolytes while also replenishing liquid.

More Serious Tennis Injuries

The following more serious tennis injuries require professional care.

Pulled Muscles

Pulled muscles, including the groin, hamstring, and gastrocnemius, usually occur as a result of poor stretching preparation. These injuries often can be avoided by going through a full warm-up. You will know when you have pulled a muscle simply from the pain and limited mobility following the pull.

Common remedies are rest, ice, and other athletic training modalities. If you pull a muscle, it is important to see a sports-medicine-oriented physician or athletic trainer for evaluation.

Sprained Ankles

A sprained ankle is one of the most common injuries in tennis. These injuries usually happen when the player tries to make a quick turn without the foot following in the turn. Sometimes a player jumps to hit a ball with a scissors kick on the overhead and lands on the side of the foot, or a player steps on a ball during play. Pivoting incorrectly or landing on the side of the foot is a matter of not coordinating effort and physical skill.

Stepping on the ball is controllable. Only three tennis balls should be available for play at any given point in a match. If one ball is in play during a rally, only two other balls can become a problem. Court awareness is important. You should keep your side of the court "clean" by picking up or pushing balls on the court to the net or fence. You also should be aware of a ball that comes from another court and stop play if the ball is in your court area. If a tennis player is lazy when it comes to picking up loose tennis balls, injury can be the result.

Ankle sprains are classified as Grade 1 (painful), Grade 2 (very painful), and Grade 3 (severe pain). Most ankle sprains occur to the outside of the ankle. With any significant discomfort, the player should see a physician for an x-ray; and once a sprain has been diagnosed, you will be directed to use ice in combination with rest, elevation, and compression. You don't recover from an ankle sprain overnight. Give yourself time to rehabilitate.

Foot Injuries

Foot injuries occur in three of four people. If you play long enough, you will sustain a foot injury. *Plantar fasciitis* is a typical tennis injury and it is a high-risk foot injury. Symptoms are pain in the heel or arch, usually after you have rested following playing.

Other foot injuries include inflammation of the *sesamoid* bone (the two metacarpal bones behind the big toe), *capsulitis* (an inflammation of connective tissue under the second toe), *metatarsalgia* (inflammation under the ball of the foot), tendonitis, stress fracture, and the common foot callus ("Foot Faults," by A.L. Shaffer, *Tennis,* May 2000, pp. 80–82).

Knee Injuries

Tennis players are susceptible to knee injuries because of the weak anatomical structure of the knee and the quick lateral movements and countless stops and starts required during play. Typically, knee injuries are related to overuse and don't require surgery. *Patellar tendonitis* and *patellofemoral pain syndrome* are reflective of overuse and are treated with ice, rest, compression, and elevation. This combination speeds the healing process and reduces any tissue damage.

Shoulder Injuries

One of the most likely tennis injuries is the shoulder injury. The shoulder relies on muscles, tendons, and ligaments to maintain stability, and tennis injuries tend to affect these soft tissues rather than the bones. Overuse injuries often occur in tennis when a player repetitively hits with a serving motion or overhead. This causes a pinching of the rotator cuff tendons, which can result in tendonitis or bursitis or more serious structural damage.

Symptoms suggesting a shoulder injury include pain and weakness in the shoulder (tendonitis), gradual onset of pain in the front and upper shoulder (bursitis), feeling that the arm has slipped out of its socket (dislocation), and the inability to raise the arm (torn *rotator cuff*). Each injury is treated differently. If you are only feeling some discomfort, take a day off to rest your shoulder. In addition, when you are back to playing avoid placing spin on serves and bringing the racket too far back on a serve. *Tendonitis* and *bursitis* require rest and ice application along with anti-inflammatory medication. A dislocation or torn rotator cuff requires medical intervention ("The Unknown Shoulder," *Tennis,* June 2001, pp. 65–68, and "Shouldering the Load," *Tennis*, March, 2010, p. 52.

Wrist Injuries

Wrist injuries are increasing in tennis. The most common are tendonitis of the extensor tendons of the back of the hand, trauma to the soft tissue triangular fibrocartilage that encircles the wrist, and a *carpal ligament sprain*. These injuries happen when the player is using a racket with limited shock absorption or too high a string tension. Other causes are applying too much pressure with spin strokes (i.e., slice or topspin) or swinging late.

Wrist injuries can be managed through some modifications.

1. Either lower the tension on your racket strings or get a more flexible racket for better shock absorption.
2. If you are experiencing discomfort hitting spin shots, back off and return to basic flat strokes.
3. Work on stroke timing to make solid, timed contact with the ball.

Wrist injuries "grow" on you. When you first feel pain, it is time to stop and check it out. If you let pain continue, your wrist problems will expand. Rest and ice application are advised with a wrist injury. After several days without improvement, it is time for you to seek medical advice. If you must play with a wrist injury, wrist braces are available, but you should make sure you are not developing a chronic injury before you go to a wrist brace.

Leg Injuries

The constant pounding, running, jumping, and landing on a hard court can create an inflammation of the soft tissues of the lower legs called *shin splints*. A change of tennis court surfaces, a high foot arch, tight calves, and intensity in your workouts and playing situations all can contribute to this injury. This injury is identified by pain along the front and sides of the shins.

Prevention requires being aware of the causes, stretching, and using common sense regarding playing intensity and the type of court you are playing on. Selecting the proper shoe with arch support and excellent shock absorption capabilities is also important. Recommended ways of dealing with a shin splint injury are rest and the application of ice when shin splints are in the acute stage ("How to Prevent Shin Splints," by D. Higdon, *Tennis*, June 1992, p. 102).

Stress fractures of the tibia and fibia are also relatively common. They are typically caused by overuse (too much time on hard court surfaces). This is another injury that requires rest.

Back Injuries

Back injuries occur frequently in tennis.

Tennis requires repetitive twisting and trunk rotation. The trunk accelerating through on groundstrokes and executing the overhead arching motion in a serve or overhead increase the risk for back injury. In addition, hard court surfaces can be damaging.

Preventive measures for back injury include aerobic conditioning, strength programs, and good stroke technique. Also, improving lower back and hamstring flexibility can save you from nagging back injuries. Professional help following a back injury includes rehabilitation provided by an athletic trainer or a physical therapist who specializes in sports medicine ("Oh, My Aching Back," by D. Squires, *Tennis USTA*, April 1993, p. 10).

Achilles Tendon Injuries

The *Achilles tendon* sometimes is injured by simple physical actions such as jumping and landing on the ball of the foot without lowering the heel or by pushing off the ball of the foot, thereby placing extreme pressure on the tendon. When rupturing, the tendon sounds like a gunshot, and the player becomes immobile immediately. Ridged, high-arched feet with heels that angle inward or flat feet that roll inward are most vulnerable to Achilles tendon problems.

The Achilles tendon often is chronically sore because players ignore persistent, tolerable pain and swelling and continue to play. The Achilles tendon and the sheath that surrounds it become inflamed, and soreness, swelling, and pain are the outcome. Ignoring these signs can lead to severe problems. The only way to address the injury is to decrease play to every other day or stop playing and rest. To prevent Achilles tendon injuries in the first place, the Achilles tendon should be stretched in warm-up and cool-down with the caveat of not overstretching.

Orthotics for the shoe or heel pads also are used as a preventive measure, but elevating your heel also shortens the tendon, when what is needed is to lengthen the tendon. As a result, stretching becomes even more important when using a heel pad.

Once an Achilles tendon injury has occurred, rehabilitation consists of rest and modality application. Possible modalities used in therapy include ice, massage, ultrasound, and electrical stimulation. They are used to reduce swelling and begin rehabilitation that brings the Achilles tendon back to a normal condition.

A stiff or achy tendon is a sign of an impending rupture. If you rupture an Achilles tendon, the process of rehabilitation following surgery or immobilization is lengthy

("Protecting Your Achilles," by A. McNab, *Tennis,* June 1993, p. 99, and "The Weakest Link?" March, 2010, p. 58).

Tennis Elbow

There are two types of *tennis elbow* injuries. They are lateral and medial tennis elbow injuries. Lateral injury is centered on the outside of the elbow and is usually caused by incorrectly using the backhand or by consistently being late when hitting a backhand. The medial injury is found on the inside of the elbow and is caused by incorrect service skill. The main characteristic of either type is inflammation of the elbow area, usually recognized as nagging pain of the elbow or forearm. The injury can be prevented by using proper skill techniques and strokes and selecting a racket with proper tension, weight, and grip size. Hitting with the elbow leading on the backhand or hitting numerous slice or spin serves especially invites the injury. Treatment of lateral, medial tennis elbow injury is restricted to rest. Elbow supports and splints, along with icing the painful area for 15–30 minutes several times a day and taking anti-inflammatory medication such as ibuprofen, are available to relieve minor pain from tennis elbow, but they will not eliminate the cause.

Treatment Resources

If an injury is perceived as serious, a physician should be consulted as soon as possible. Then, if rehabilitation is recommended, it is advisable to seek out a sports medicine clinic. Most metropolitan areas have centers that work closely with physicians to rehabilitate injuries, and a number of university campuses include a university hospital with a physical therapy unit.

Home treatment should be limited to minor injuries only. Blisters usually dry up on their own; the main concern is to make sure that they do not get infected. For minor injuries, athletic trainers can create devices to enable continuation of activity. For example, a trainer can devise a doughnut-shaped pad that will cover the blister, reduce pain at the pressure point, and prevent additional friction on the blister area. Bruises often can be treated with cold compresses or ice packs to reduce swelling. For injuries such as Achilles tendon injury, tennis elbow, and pulled muscles, rest may be the only solution.

POINTS *to* REMEMBER

PREVENTING AND CARING FOR TENNIS INJURIES

1. Minor common tennis injuries include blisters, bruises, and cramps.
2. Serious tennis injuries include pulled muscles, sprained ankles, foot injuries, knee injuries, shoulder injuries, wrist injuries, shin splints, back injuries, Achilles tendon injuries, and tennis elbow.
3. Overuse injuries often occur in tennis, typically rotator cuff, shin splints, lower leg stress fracture, knee tendonitis, and patellofemoral pain syndrome and injuries to the back and feet.
4. Hard tennis court surfaces also contribute to most overuse injuries due to jarring effects.

Dealing with Heat, Sun, and Insect Bites When Playing Tennis

Additional problems that arise in tennis include hyperthermia, dehydration, sunburn, and insect bites or stings.

Heat- and Sun-related Problems

Hyperthermia

Hyperthermia (elevated body temperature) may lead to *heat cramps*, *heat exhaustion*, and *heat stroke*. Any of these conditions can occur when playing in hot weather for an extended time, because large amounts of body fluids are lost through sweating. Heat cramps can be painful, but they are not life threatening. Untreated heat stroke, however, can be fatal.

Dehydration

To prevent problems associated with *dehydration*, make sure your clothing allows for good air circulation around your body. Avoid clothing that traps or absorbs heat. Dark shirts are an example of material that absorbs heat. Wearing light clothing reduces that absorption.

Maintaining intake of body fluids is important for regulating body temperature. If too many fluids are lost, the body is likely to overheat just like an automobile radiator does when its water level is low. Some sweating is necessary to keep the body cool, so you need to replace lost fluids by drinking appropriate liquids. To determine how much liquid to drink, a good guide is to drink a pint of water for each pound lost during play. Start replacing your body fluids by drinking small amounts (3–6 ounces of water) in 10- to 15-minute intervals prior to beginning a match or practice and continuing throughout the duration of playing time. Because water is being lost from the body, water is needed to replace body fluids. Most players do not need electrolyte replacement solutions (such as Gatorade®) during normal exercise, although these fluids can aid in recovery after play. Intake of water and/or an electrolyte solution is important for replacing body fluids. What should be avoided are liquid supplements, including beverages with caffeine, since they contribute to dehydration. If you are playing in hot weather for an extended period of time, electrolytes do need to be replaced and that would require an electrolyte solution.

Sunburn

Sunburn can be avoided by applying sunscreen with a sun protection factor (SPF) of at least 30. PABA sunscreen offers even better protection. That type of sunscreen blocks both UVA and UVB rays. Wearing a hat is a prerequisite for avoiding sunburn and also for preventing heat stroke. Players often reject sunscreen because the lotion is applied by hand and then is transferred to the racket grip. By simply wiping your hands, you can avoid transferring the lotion to the grip of the racket. Some players also reject wearing a hat, suggesting that they can't see the ball on the serve toss and it gets in their way generally. These are just excuses.

Eye Conditions

One last potential physical problem deserves consideration. Eyes exposed to ultraviolet rays over an extended time are at risk for at least three eye diseases:

1. Cataracts (clouding of the lens)
2. Pterygium (a fleshlike growth on the white of the eye near the iris)
3. Macular degeneration (breakdown of the retina with age)

Pterygium is of particular concern, because the incidence of developing this eye disease is relatively high for those who are in the sun extensively. A partial answer is to begin wearing sunglasses while playing tennis. New technology has produced a polycarbonate lens, in which the lens is wrapped around the head. It is recommended that the lens block 100 percent of UVA rays and 75–90 percent of visible light. A quality pair of sunglasses protects against the sun and also screens out peripheral light and wind while still providing clear visibility for the player.

Insect Bites and Stings

Depending on what part of the country you come from, insect bites and stings might bother you. Probably the most prevalent insect sting is from bees or wasps. When you are around bees and wasps, be especially alert. When you pick up a racket, make sure a bee is not lurking. Bees and wasps congregate at the opening of cans containing beverages with sugar, so check a can before drinking from it.

If you are stung, the recommended way of removing the stinger is to scrape the sac away and to extract the stinger with a tweezer. Application of ice to the site also may be required to reduce swelling. If you are allergic to stings, you may have to seek immediate medical attention.

POINTS *to* REMEMBER

DEALING WITH HEAT, SUN, AND INSECTS WHEN PLAYING TENNIS

1. Replenish lost fluid by drinking water prior to playing and throughout a match.
2. Protect yourself from the sun by applying at least a 30 SPF sunblock.
3. Protect your eyes from the sun by wearing sunglasses with a lens block of 100 percent UVA and a 75–90 percent block of visible light.
4. Be alert to insects that sting—bees, wasps, etc.—and avoid them.

CHECKPOINTS

1. Warm-up requires
   a. an increase in blood flow.
   b. an increase in heart rate.
   c. a series of stretching activities.
   d. all of the above.
2. Identify and describe a dynamic stretch action for the upper extremity.

   ____

   ____

   ____
3. Identify and describe a dynamic stretch action for the lower extremity.

   ____

   ____

   ____
4. Identify and describe a static stretch for the upper extremity.

   ____

   ____

   ____
5. Identify and describe a static stretch for the lower extremity.

   ____

   ____

   ____
6. Numerous possible injuries are associated with tennis. Three serious conditions are
   a. dehydration, tennis elbow, and back injuries.
   b. blisters, bruises, and dehydration.
   c. sprained ankles, shin splints, and Achilles tendon rupture.
   d. blisters, sprained ankles, and cartilage damage.

7. Determine your exercise heart rate by
   a. taking the number 220 and dividing by 70% and 85%.
   b. taking the number 220, dividing by your age and multiplying by 70% and 85%.
   c. taking the number 220, subtracting your age, and multiplying 70% or 85%.
   d. taking the number 220 and subtracting by 70 and 85.
8. Drinking liquids is important
   a. prior to and following a match.
   b. prior to, during, and following a match.
   c. prior to and during a match.
   d. during and following a match.
9. Tennis players usually are susceptible to knee injuries because of
   a. quick lateral movements and the weak anatomical structure of the knee.
   b. sprinting and the weak anatomical structure of the knee.
   c. jumping and the weak anatomical structure of the knee.
   d. quick lateral movements and sprinting.
10. Sunglasses should be designed to
   a. block out 15 percent of UVA.
   b. block out 75 percent of UVA.
   c. block out all UVA.
   d. decrease UVA as much as possible.

Answers to Checkpoints can be found on page 167.

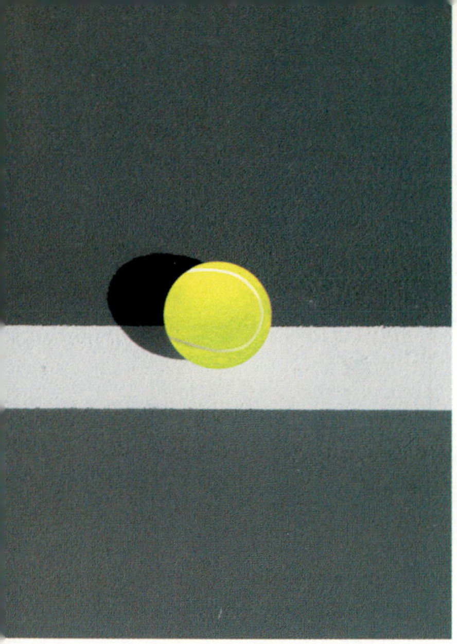
Photography by J. E. Bryant

11

Tennis Behavior and Interpretation of Rules

The game of tennis has written and unwritten rules that the player must understand to play the game. Tennis has been played for centuries, and certain ways of behaving and interpreting rules have evolved over time.

Behavior on a Tennis Court

The unwritten rules of tennis prescribe behavior on a tennis court. Most have a logical reason or purpose, and it is up to the player to respect these rules.

Clothing

Appropriate clothing for tennis does not require a major expenditure, and proper dress is part of the game. A tennis player must wear tennis shoes rather than track-type shoes or basketball shoes. Wearing proper shoes reduces the chance of injury and also prevents marring of the tennis court surface (Chapter 12 contains additional comments about shoes as equipment). Municipal, private, and college courts have basic, general rules requiring proper footwear, and, in addition, players are expected to wear shorts and a shirt to play on those courts. When playing at a private tennis club, more conventional clothing is expected: tennis shorts or skirt and a tennis shirt or blouse.

Even the act of picking up a tennis ball requires a certain behavior. Bending over and picking up the ball is, of course, one way to retrieve the ball. Other methods include a foot/racket pickup and a ball-bounce pickup.

In the *foot/racket pickup* (Photo 11.1), the ball is positioned between the racket-side foot and the face of the tennis racket. Simultaneously lift the foot, ball, and racket to midcalf level, and, as the ball becomes airborne, use the racket to bounce the ball to the court surface and catch it with your nonracket hand.

The *ball-bounce pickup* (Photo 11.2) requires you to choke up on the racket handle and place the racket face on top of the ball. Then lift the racket slightly and contact the ball with a series of quick wrist movements that lift the ball off the court and into your nonracket hand.

Walking and Talking on the Court

Most tennis facilities consist of three or more courts enclosed by a fence, with one or two gates to

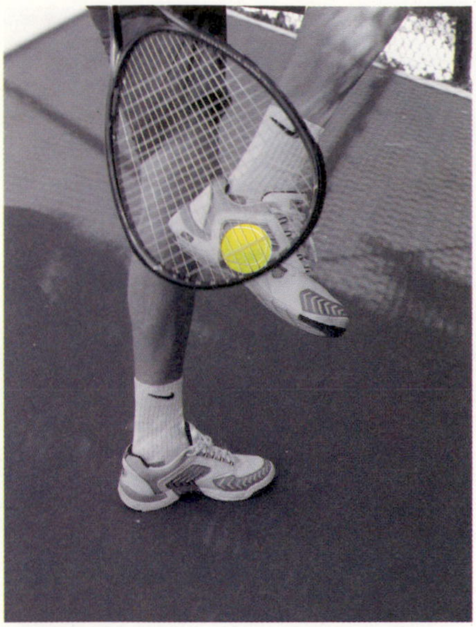

Photography by Virginia Bryant

PHOTO 11.1 Foot/racket pickup.

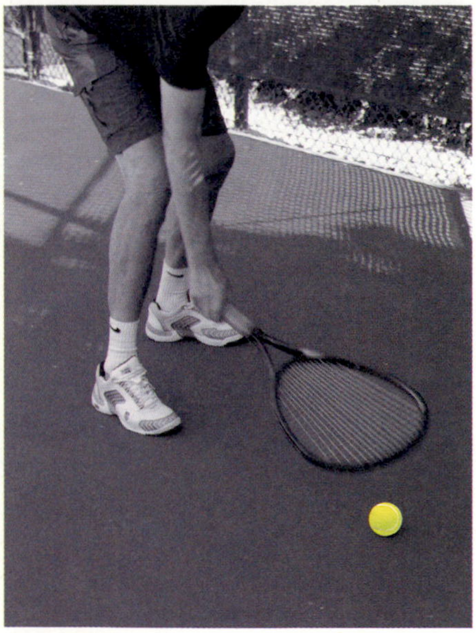

Photography by Virginia Bryant

PHOTO 11.2 Ball-bounce pickup.

admit players. When walking on a tennis court, you should wait until play on adjacent courts stops before proceeding to an assigned court, and you should walk along the fence as quickly as possible.

Talking on a tennis court should be in normal voice tones. Conversation should be limited as much as possible to the match rather than to everyday visiting.

Warm-Up

Warm-up is described in Chapter 10 as a part of physically preparing to play. Etiquette, or proper behavior, insists that players be considerate of one another during warm-up.

Return of Tennis Balls

Returning tennis balls to another court and requesting a return of tennis balls are part of etiquette. When a tennis ball rolls across a court from an adjacent court while play is in progress, action should stop, assuming that the rolling ball interferes with the play. The ball should then be returned to the adjacent court on a bounce to the requesting player and the point replayed.

If a ball is hit onto another court, the requesting player should wait until play ceases on that court and then, with a raised hand, request "ball please," followed by "thank you" upon receiving the ball.

When retrieving balls hit over the fence, players should follow the same court behavior as when entering the court for the first time.

Ball in Play

Once the ball is in play during a match, interruptions should cease. This includes practice serves. If practice serves are done during the match, they interfere with the flow of the game and are not allowed.

The server always must begin with two tennis balls. For convenience, one ball should be placed in the pocket of the tennis shorts and one in the hand for the toss. When receiving, the player should hit only a ball that is legally in play. Returning an "out" serve is poor form.

When a ball or other interference occurs during a match, a gesture of "play a let" is acceptable. In one situation the server hits the first serve as a fault, followed by a ball rolling across the court. If the receiver responds by picking up the ball and returning it to the adjacent court, the receiver should immediately respond to the server, "Take two."

Another form of court behavior is to communicate all calls to the opponents. Verbal forms of communication are "out" and "let." A ball that is "in" is assumed in by the continued play on the part of the player who is returning the shot. An index finger pointing up can be used as sign language indicating that a ball is out, and a ball hit out of reach of a player that is good is signified by a flat, palm-down motion.

Emotions

Emotion is to be left off the court! Throwing a racket, hitting an erratic shot after play has stopped, and verbal outbursts should not be tolerated or engaged in by you or your opponent. An easy way to deal with opponents who behave in such an unacceptable manner is to refuse to play them. Life is too short to accept that sort of behavior in an environment that is supposed to be fun. Other unacceptable responses include making excuses for losing while not acknowledging the good play of an

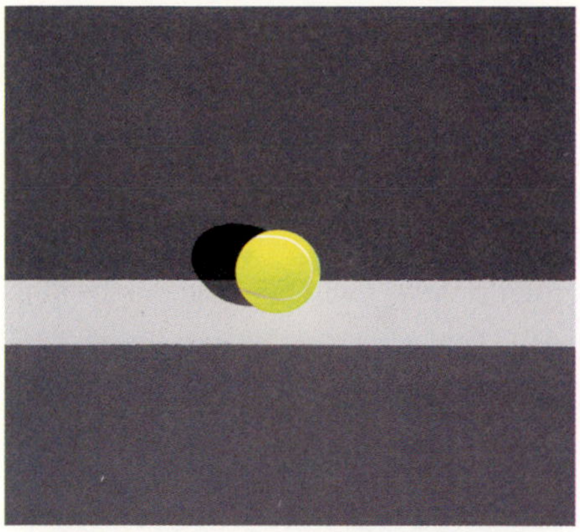

Photography by J. E. Bryant

PHOTO 11.3 Ball on the line—"in."

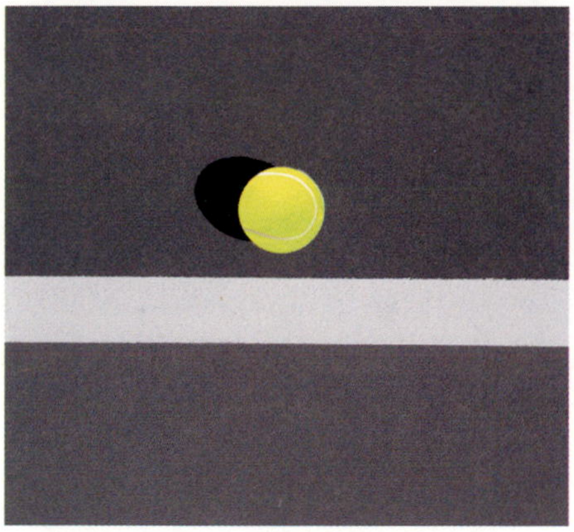

Photography by J. E. Bryant

PHOTO 11.4 Ball near the line—"out."

opponent, and not keeping score accurately.

"In" and "Out"

Perhaps the most misunderstood part of etiquette is related to rules interpretation of when a ball is called "in" or "out" on a line call. The rule and the etiquette application are simple: A ball that touches any part of a court boundary line is "in" (Photo 11.3), and any time a ball is wholly out as a result of not touching any part of a court line, the call is "out" (Photo 11.4).

The problem arises when players don't see the ball and start guessing. There is no excuse for guessing; the call is specific! If a player does not see a ball as "out," the ball must be considered playable, and it is communicated as good by continued play. There never is a guess on a line call in tennis. Bottom line: The ball is good unless seen to be out.

When it is unknown if a ball is in or out on the last play of a rally or on a serve, there is one exception to the call: If a player does not see the ball, that player can request that the other player make the call. If the opposing player was unsighted or doesn't wish to make the call, the call reverts to the original player, who then must accept the ball as being in bounds.

Viewing a Match

Besides playing a tennis match and acknowledging etiquette, viewing a tennis match requires certain behavior, for a spectator has the obligation to observe a match with respect for the players. No communication should take place between player and the spectator, including the often-asked question "What's the score?" The spectator should be quiet, watch the play, and applaud a good point. Spectator disruptions are not approved at major tennis tournament matches (such as the U.S. Open, professional tour matches, and collegiate competition).

POINTS to REMEMBER

BEHAVIOR ON A TENNIS COURT

1. You must wear appropriate tennis shoes on a tennis court.
2. *Foot/racket pickup* and *ball-bounce pickup* are tennis skills related to picking up a ball off the court.
3. Wait until play has ceased on surrounding courts before walking onto your assigned tennis court.
4. "Ball please" and "Thank you" are appropriate terms to request that a ball be returned from a court and to acknowledge the return.
5. A ball that is "in" is acknowledged by continued play.
6. A ball that is "out" is acknowledged by stating "Out" or by pointing your index finger *up*.
7. A ball is always called in on any line call unless it is observed to be out.
8. If *unsighted,* it is appropriate to ask for an opponent to make a line call. If the opponent is *unsighted,* the ball must be ruled "in."

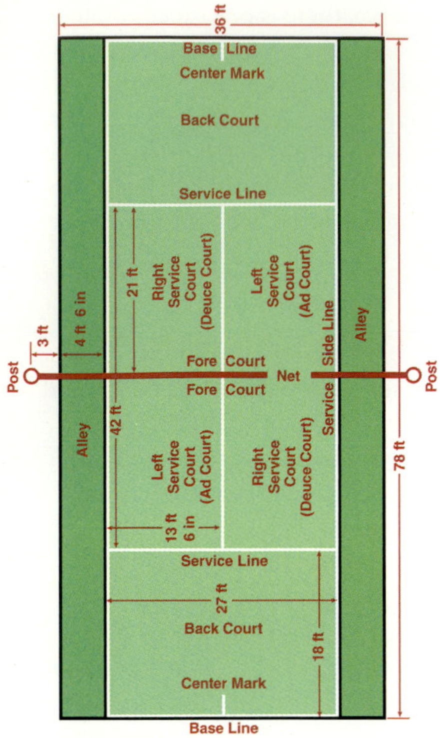

FIGURE 11.1 Court dimensions.

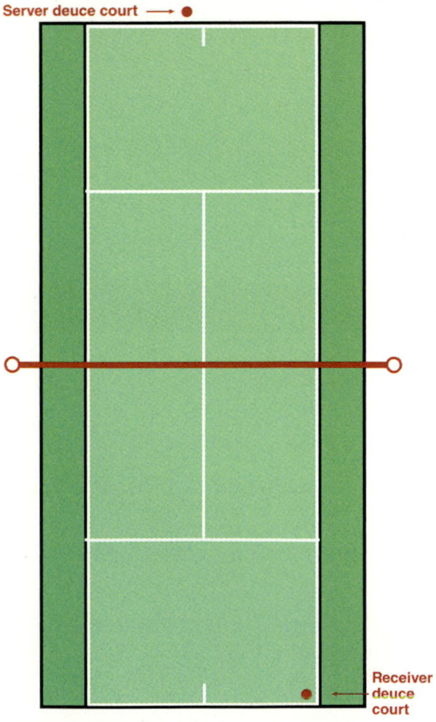

FIGURE 11.2 Serving and receiving positions.

Interpreting Tennis Rules

The tennis court has universal dimensions and terminology associated with it. Key terms include *baseline*, *center mark*, *backcourt*, *forecourt*, right *service court* (deuce), left *service court* (ad), *service line*, and *alley*. (See Figure 11.1.) The singles court size is 27′ × 78′ and the expanded doubles court size is 36′ × 78′. The net is 3′6″ high at the net supports and 3′ high at the center. The net height at the center is of particular importance, because a lower or higher height impacts the rally between two players (Figure 11.1).

The center net height used to be measured by placing one racket vertically at the center strap position and the other racket horizontally on top of the butt of the first racket's handle. Because most rackets today are oversized, the second string of the horizontal racket should be even with the top of the net for the net to be at the correct height. A more accurate means of measurement is to use a yardstick to measure the center net height.

Preplay Choices

At the beginning of a match, significant choices are to be made regarding who serves and receives. A decision on choice of service and side of court to begin play is made by spinning the racket or flipping a coin. To spin a racket, place the top of the racket head on the court. The opposing player calls either "up" or "down" to signify the position of the butt end of the racket when it falls to the court. The winner of the spin chooses, or requests the opponent to choose, the right to be the server or receiver. The player who doesn't have first choice then selects the end of the court to begin play. The choices may be reversed, with the winner of the spin choosing, or requesting the opponent to choose, the end to begin play, followed by the nonselecting player's choice of service or receiving serve.

This scenario might clarify the choices available: Player A wins the spin and states, "I will serve." Player B then states, "I will take the north side." A second scenario consists of Player A winning the spin and stating, "Your choice." Player B then states, "I will receive," followed by Player A's rejoinder, "I will take the north side." The point is that the first player has the option of choosing service, receipt of serve, or end of the court or of passing those choices to the opponent.

Serving and Receiving Positions

The first serve is always made from the deuce side to the deuce side. Once that point is completed, the serve is directed from ad court to ad court (Figure 11.2).

Order of Serve

In both singles and doubles play, the *order of serve* is a simple alternation of serves. A player must serve through a full game and then exchange service with the opponent at the conclusion of that game. In doubles, the situation is the same except that teams alternate serving following each game. If Team 1 serves the first game, Team 2 will serve game two, and the rotation will continue. Player A of Team 1 serves the first game, Player A of Team 2 serves the second game, Player B of Team 1 serves the third game, and Player B of Team 2 serves the fourth game. The sequence repeats throughout the set, with Player A of Team 1 serving in game five, etc.

Doubles Receiving Position

In doubles, the team decides who will receive in the deuce court and

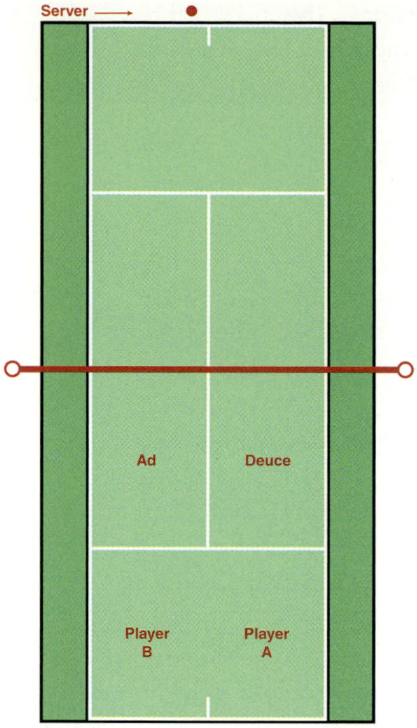

FIGURE 11.3 Doubles receiving position.

ad court. This remains the same throughout a set (Figure 11.3).

Changing Sides of the Court

Changing sides of the court has a significant effect on performance when playing outdoors. Without changing the side of court, one player often faces the sun or wind during play, giving the opponent an advantage. Rotation to opposite sides of the court occurs when the total number of games played is an odd number.

If Player A (or Team 1) serves from the north side of a court in game one, sides will be exchanged for game two. Player B (or Team 2) then serves from the north side of the court, followed by Player A (or Team 1) serving game three from the south end of the court. At the conclusion of game three, the players (or teams) again change sides of the court, with Player B (or Team 2) serving from the south side of the court in game four.

The sequence continues with players (or teams) exchanging sides of the court at the conclusion of the fifth, seventh, ninth, and eleventh, etc. total games played. At the end of a set, the players or teams change sides only if the total number of games is an odd number (such as 6–3, for a total of nine games). In singles, the rotation of server is continuous throughout play of a set. In doubles, the same principle applies, with the rotation of each team in order of service.

At the beginning of a new set, singles rotation continues as defined during the first set. This is also true regarding doubles play, but within a team the order of serve can be changed in a new set, and the positioning of the team when receiving may also be changed. Once changed, the order of serve and receive positions remains the same throughout that set.

Scoring

When viewed systematically, scoring is simple to understand. A tennis match is played in a sequence of points, games, sets, and match. It takes 4 points to win a *game* (provided that the margin for victory is 2 points). A player (or team) must win six games to win a *set,* with a winning margin of two games.

One exception to the rule is that if each player (or team) wins six games, a tie-breaker is played to determine the winner, the final score always 7–6—a margin of only one game for the victory. In most situations, the winner of the *match* is the winner of two of three sets (professional players on the men's tour play three of five sets in some tournaments).

Each point won by a player (or team) is assigned a term, as given in Table 11.1. Scores to complete a set are one of the following: 6–0, 6–1, 6–2, 6–3, 6–4, 7–5, or 7–6. If a set score reaches 5–5 in terms of games won, two more games must be played. If one player (or team) wins both games, the final score is 7–5. If the players (or team) split games, the score will be 6–6, and a tie-breaker will be played. Examples of a match score are 6–2, 7–5, or 6–3, 1–6, 6–4. The winning player's (or team) scores are always identified first in a match; consequently, the 1–6 score of the second set of the second match example indicates that the winner of the match lost the second set by a 6-to-1 game score.

Tie-Breakers

A *tie-breaker* is played only when a set is tied 6–6. There are several forms of tie-breakers, including what are called 7-, 9-, and 12-point tie-breakers. The 7-point tie-breaker is the most popular. The winner of the tie-breaker is the first player to win 7 points with a winning margin of 2 points. If the score in a tie-breaker

TABLE 11.1
Point Scoring

Point Number	Equivalent Term
First point	15
Second point	30
Third point	40
Fourth point	game (must win by two points)
No points	love
Tie score at 30–30 or beyond	deuce
After a tie at 3 points each—server leads by 1 point	advantage in (AD IN)
After a tie at 3 points each—receiver leads by 1 point	advantage out (AD OUT)

reaches 6–6 in number of points scored, the players must continue the game until one player has a winning margin of 2 points (e.g., 8–6, 9–7, 10–8, etc.). A 5–5 point score can still produce a winner at 7 points if one player wins the next 2 points.

The server for the first point of a tie-breaker is designated by the continued rotation of serve per the normal rotation. The first server serves only 1 point—from the *deuce service court*. The second server then begins the serve from the *ad service court*. This server serves one point from the ad service court and then one point from the deuce service court.

In singles, the service order now reverts to the first server, who begins service for 1 point from the ad service court and then moves to the deuce service court for the second point. The players exchange ends of court after a total of 6 points are played, with a continuation of the rotation.

In doubles play rotation, movement is the same as in singles except that four players are involved instead of two. This rotation in the tie-breaker is based on who is scheduled to serve by the normal rotation process. Player A of Team 1 serves point number 1 to the deuce service court. Player A of Team 2 serves 2 points—one from the ad service court followed by one from the deuce service court. Player B of Team 1 then serves points 1 and 2 from the respective ad and deuce service courts, and the rotation continues to Player B of Team 2, and so on. The tie-breaker singles and doubles rotations are presented in Table 11.2. Once the tie-breaker is completed, the server of the first game of the next set is the player who received the first serve of the first point of the tie-breaker.

Alternative Scoring

Alternative scoring is prevalent at various levels of play. There are eight-game pro sets, four-game short sets (first to win four games with a 2-point margin), and creative other game lengths designed for shorter play periods. ("No-Ad" scoring tends to be popular, because it speeds up play. The no-ad scoring sequence is specific to a 3–3 point tie, with the winner of the next point as the winner of a game.

In addition to alternative scoring in matches, in lieu of a third set, a 10-point tie-breaker (first to win 10 points with a 2-point margin) is sometimes used to break a 1–1 set score.

TABLE 11.2
Tie-Breaker Server Rotation

Singles

Player Number	Service Court to Serve To	Number of Points
1	Deuce Service Court	1
2	Ad Service Court	1
2	Deuce Service Court	1
1	Ad Service Court	1
1	Deuce Service Court	1
2	Ad Service Court	1
change sides of court		
2	Deuce Service Court	1
1	Ad Service Court	1
1	Deuce Service Court	1
etc.		

Doubles

Team No.	Player No.	Service Court to Serve To	Number of Points
1	A	Deuce Service Court	1
2	A	Ad Service Court	1
2	A	Deuce Service Court	1
1	B	Ad Service Court	1
1	B	Deuce Service Court	1
2	B	Ad Service Court	1
change sides of court			
2	B	Deuce Service Court	1
1	A	Ad Service Court	1
1	A	Deuce Service Court	1
etc.			

The Ball in Play

Every game other than a tie-breaker begins with a service to the right service court. The service point, both in a regular game situation and in a tie-breaker, allows a maximum of two opportunities to hit a legal serve. The one exception is a let, a serve that is hit in all ways legally except that the ball touches the net on its path to the service court. A let permits the server to repeat the serve, and any number of lets may be played in succession. Having identified a let as a serve to be repeated, it is important to point out that this rule may change over time. The likelihood is that a "let" some day may be played as a legal serve, and, in fact, at the college level a let is presently played as a "good" serve.

Once the ball is in play, a player must hit it over the net so that it lands in the opponent's court. During a rally, players may hit the ball on the bounce or during flight (return of serve requires the bounce of the ball in the service court). A point is lost when

1. a ball bounces twice before being returned,
2. a ball lands out of the court boundaries on the fly,
3. a ball hits the net and does not go over the net, or
4. two serves (excluding a let) in a row do not fall into the appropriate service court.

A serve that does not strike the appropriate service court is called a *fault*. Servers also fault by swinging and missing a service toss or by stepping on the baseline during the serve. Touching the service line on a serve is called a *foot fault*. Many players have the habit of touching the baseline in this manner, and legally that is not accepted. If a player strikes the ball and then comes down on the baseline, the serve is legal. When the foot touches the line while the racket is in contact with the ball or prior to hitting the ball, the serve is lost. In "friendly" play, foot faults usually are ignored because they are difficult to see. But the server has a responsibility to avoid the illegal foot position.

Rule Infractions

Tennis has numerous rule infractions and interpretations. Some of them are as follows.*

1. Hitting a volley prior to the ball crossing the net is a loss of point except when a ball crosses the net and backspin carries the ball back across the net, or the wind blows the ball back over the net.
2. A ball that strikes the player or the player's clothing carries a loss of point.
3. Throwing a racket at the ball carries the penalty of loss of the point.
4. If the ball strikes the net (excluding the serve) and continues on into the opponent's court, the ball is still in play.
5. If a doubles player hits the partner with the ball, the team loses the point.
6. An opposing player may not hinder an opponent by distracting the opponent; however, partners on a doubles team are allowed to talk to each other when the ball is directed to their side of the court.
7. A player hit by a ball prior to the ball striking the court loses that point even if the ball is going to land out of bounds.
8. After the conclusion of a tie-breaker, the first server of the next set is the player who did not serve first in the previously played set.

The beginning tennis player should treat the rules with respect and take them seriously so that the game will be enjoyable.

* A review of USTA's *The Code: The Player's Guide for Unofficiated Matches* is found in Appendix A, by permission of the United States Tennis Association, Publications Department, 70 West Red Oak Lane, White Plains, NY 10604.

POINTS to REMEMBER

INTERPRETING TENNIS RULES

1. On the spin of the racket, the winner has the choices of electing to serve or receive, side of court, or to pass the choice to the opponent.
2. The order of service is a simple alternation of serves after each game is played.
3. Players change sides of the court on uneven total number of games.
4. A serve that doesn't strike the appropriate court is called a *fault*.
5. A set score is the first to six games with a winning margin of two games.
6. A score of 6–6 requires a 12-point tie-breaker.
7. A tie-breaker is played to 7 points, with a winning margin of 2 points.

CHECKPOINTS

1. A ball that strikes the line of the court during play is considered
   a. a replay.
   b. out.
   c. in.
   d. none of the above.
2. Sides of the tennis court are changed by players after
   a. every third game.
   b. every odd total number of games accumulated by both players.
   c. every other game played.
   d. a player has an odd total number of games played.
3. Typically, an official legal score of a match is
   a. 6–3, 3–6, 6–5.
   b. 7–6, 3–6, 6–3.
   c. 5–6, 7–6, 7–5.
   d. 7–5, 5–7, 7–1.
4. Which of the following is not a legal score?
   a. Deuce
   b. Advantage In (Ad In)
   c. 15–love
   d. 45–15
5. A let is a
   a. serve that is hit legally but touches the net before falling into the opponent's service court.
   b. replay of a point when a call is considered in doubt.
   c. term used to say "take two."
   d. fault.
6. Hitting a volley shot while the ball is on the opponent's side of the court is considered
   a. loss of point.
   b. fair play.
   c. a replay.
   d. a mistake.
7. A tie-breaker is played
   a. when the game score is tied 5–5.
   b. when the game score is tied 6–6.
   c. any time there is a tie score in a game.
   d. until a player is ahead by 2 points.
8. It is poor etiquette to
   a. talk quietly on the court.
   b. not wear appropriate tennis clothing.
   c. throw a tennis racket in anger.
   d. all of the above.
9. If a ball is not observed to be in or out the reaction should be
   a. "out."
   b. "replay the point."
   c. "play a let."
   d. "good" or "in."
10. When the ball is in play during a rally and strikes the net, but goes into the opponent's side,
    a. the ball is in play.
    b. it is automatically a "let."
    c. the ball is out.
    d. play stops and two serves are rewarded to play the point over.

Answers to Checkpoints can be found on page 167.

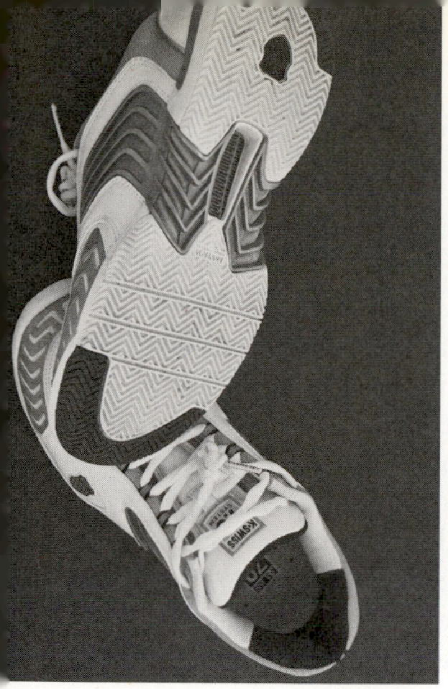

Photography by J.E. Bryant

12 Tennis Courts, Equipment Design, Tournament Competition, Tennis Perspective, and Resources

As your tennis participation expands, your skills and knowledge base will also improve and contribute to your continual development. This chapter covers how a court is designed, which tennis racket to select, how to get involved in tennis competition, a tennis perspective, and what additional resources are available.

The Tennis Court

Tennis court surfaces are of four types.

Grass Courts

Grass courts are traditional but have outlived their usefulness. Wimbledon is the only major professional tournament still played on a grass court. For normal play, the upkeep and expense involved in maintaining the surface are nearly prohibitive. As a result, few grass courts are found in the United States, and they are nearly extinct worldwide.

Soft Courts

Soft courts are popular throughout much of the world and east of the Mississippi River in the United States. The typical soft court is a *clay court*. Its surface provides a high bounce and a slow ball, which encourages long baseline rallies. The term *clay court* is descriptive of what used to be the surface composition of a claylike material and coarse sand. A number of other claylike surfaces include shale and synthetic composites that result in play similar to clay.

Today a "clay court" is composed of a two-layer base of crushed limestone with ⅛″ of brick dust or a one-layer base of crushed and firmly packed stone material called "fast-dry." The clay surface poses a maintenance problem when reasonable play conditions are desired, because it requires watering and rolling, but the more recent surfaces are easier to maintain.

Hard Courts

All-weather (*hard court*) surfaces are extremely popular in the United States. This is the surface with which most developing players are familiar. The surface may be composed of asphalt or cement topping, which contributes to ease of maintenance and cleaning. Courts with this surface are usually public, and they are easily recognized because they give a uniform, fast-bouncing action to the ball.

Synthetic Courts

The *synthetic surface* is another type of hard surface that many players have used on their college campuses. The synthetic court surface usually is composed of a series of granulated rubber particles pulled together with an epoxy resin sprayed with a polyurethane coating and laid on a porous foundation. The court is designed to play like a naturally made court, but it is free of maintenance and cleaning problems. The synthetic court is called the Mercury Grassphalts Court.

Another court surface, called a *carpet,* is used for indoor tournaments on the professional tennis tour. The carpet is laid over whatever existing surface is available, and that combination produces a fast court that encourages a serve-volley game.

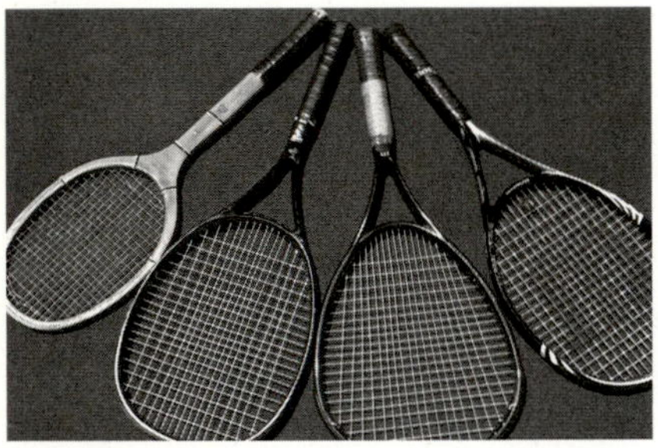

Photography by J. E. Bryant

PHOTO 12.1 Comparison of wood and composite wide-body rackets.

Court Specifications

Hard and synthetic courts are smoothed or roughened, depending on the amount of play and rally circumstances expected in a given geographical area. High-altitude locations tend to have a roughened surface to provide more opportunity for baseline play. Courts in low altitudes tend to have a smoother surface, because the density of the air allows for more rally situations.

When a high level of competition is projected, a tennis court is measured through a process called ITF surface pace setting in order to ensure a proper court speed. Regardless of which type of tennis court surface is used, there is one consistency and that is associated with the dimensions of the court. Dimensions are the same worldwide, at every play level.

Tennis Equipment

Tennis Rackets

At one time, tennis rackets were made of various woods, including ash or beech and combinations of perhaps sycamore, obeche, or mahogany. The wood racket was handcrafted, and the number of wood laminations indicated the quality of the racket. Wood rackets now are obsolete, replaced by modern technology's new materials (Photo 12.1).

Following wood rackets, tennis rackets were designed with metal and aluminum materials, but these, too, are all but obsolete. The tennis racket of the early 2000s was made of materials such as a polyurethane, carbon, Kevlar, fiberglass, graphite, and titanium. These materials provided more power with control, and reduced racket vibration and shock, and a lighter racket for quicker reaction for stroke readiness.

Present changes are related to how the frame of the racket is made. These rackets continue to include graphite but now use tungsten, basalt, carbon black, and silicon dioxide materials to reduce racket vibration and provide more control with both spin and

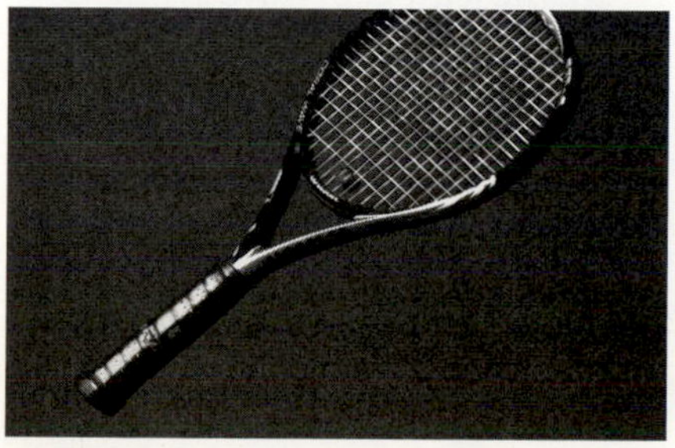

PHOTO 12.2 Hybrid racket.

speed, reduced racket vibration and shock, and a lighter racket for quicker reaction for stroke readiness.

Wide-Body and Extra-Long Rackets

Wide-body rackets emerged as a popular racket during the 1990s and early 2000s. They provided maximum power with increased control, and they bent less at contact, giving the ball more energy.

This technology has continued to evolve, producing a racket that is more elongated than any previous racket. These long-body *(extra-long) rackets* provided increased power, enhanced spin, and far more leverage when striking the ball. They enabled a player to reach balls hit wide to them, and because they were so light, they provided the player with the ability to move the racket more quickly in order to set up to hit a shot. The extra-long rackets (also called *stretch rackets*) typically are made of titanium and graphite, and they range from 27.5″ to 29″ in length.

The wide-body and extra-long rackets still exist, but the rackets of today are smaller, lighter, with an even larger sweet spot. Frames are made with different materials and even the strings have been redesigned to provide more of a catapult action when racket strings make contact with the ball.

Trends in Rackets—the Hybrid

The most recent technologically designed rackets are called *hybrids* or *tweeners* (Photo 12.2). They are called that since they are a blend of a beginner or intermediate player and a tournament player's racket. They have an increased sweet spot providing more surface to hit the ball. Their length is typically 27 inches. Hitting surface ranges from 90 to 118 square inches with most rackets at 100 square inches, and a racket weight of 10.5–11.5 ounces. These are rackets that include smaller grips than previously, generally sized at 4 1/4 to 4 3/8 inches. In addition the balance of these rackets are 3/8 to 1 inch head light which makes the racket easier to swing. In addition, some of these newly designed rackets have expanded the hitting zone of the racket by suspending the strings in the frame that puts more action on the ball when struck.

Hybrids are designed for beginning players (and most intermediate players) with a weight of approximately 10 ounces, length around 27.5 inches, head size of 102–118 square inches, and head light. Advanced players use hybrids that are 10.8–12.2 ounces in weight, have a 27-inch racket length, 90–98 square inches of head size, and are head light.

These lighter, smaller rackets enable the beginner to hit the ball with greater speed and make it easier to apply spin to their shots. Racket vibration is reduced, which reduces elbow shock, and allows the beginner, who typically has a shorter backswing, to apply increased velocity and spin to their shots ("Racket Guide," by B. Gray, *Tennis*, April 2010, p. 145).

Characteristics of Rackets

A *stiff racket* bends less on impact and offers less control and more power than a *flexible racket.* A flexible racket will provide more control but less power. Wide-body and extra-long rackets tend to be stiffer, thus providing more power.

Typically the beginner needs a racket with stiffness, to impart some power or zip to the ball. As skill is developed, more stiffness or more flexibility becomes a personal choice.

A flexible racket tends to reduce vibration and shock, which decreases the potential for developing *tennis elbow* (tendonitis). *Vibration* describes a lingering back-and-forth motion of the racket frame and strings after

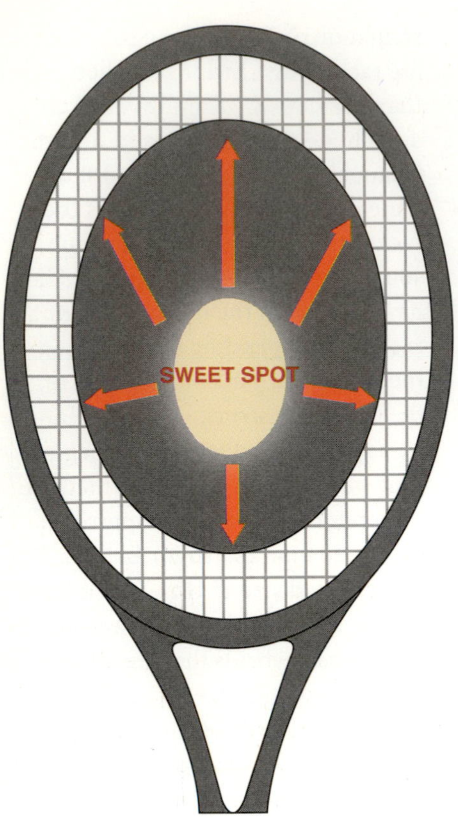

FIGURE 12.1 Sweet spot.

the ball has been hit. Torque from vibration then is transferred to the elbow. *Shock* describes the contact of string to ball, and when a ball is hit off-center, a subsequent twisting action also generates a torque action that is transferred to the elbow. In both cases, the transfer of shock or vibration to the elbow contributes to tendonitis of the elbow.

Other characteristics of a tennis racket—*power, control, feel, maneuverability, comfort, and stability*—are used in tennis publications and racket advertisements. Rackets also are characterized as head-light, balanced, and head-heavy. And they are light, semi-light, and medium in weight.

Sweet Spot

The ideal area for contact with the ball is called a sweet spot (Figure 12.1). It can be located below center, above center, elongated, or wide across center. Most sweet spots are found at center and above center, but they do vary. Sweet spots basically allow for a shot that is hit not quite on-center to still rebound effectively.

The larger the oversize racket, the larger is the sweet spot—and the more the chance for success. A stiffer racket stretches the sweet spot, and lowering the string tension increases a sweet spot's effectiveness ("Sweet Talk About the Sweet Spot," by S. Chirls, *Tennis,* June 1992, p. 77).

Grips

Conventional racket grips are measured from 4¼″ to 4⅜″. Grips are composed of several types of material, but a cushioned grip with a tacky feel that is perforated or embossed is recommended.

The conventional a grip should feel comfortable. Grip size is determined by a simple measure. Grasp the racket handle with an eastern forehand grip. When looking at your grip, there should be a space between the fingertips of your hand and the palm. If you can place the index finger of your nonracket hand snugly between the fingertips and the palm of the racket hand and the grip feels comfortable, you have a fit.

A trend is occurring regarding racket grips that is significantly different than the conventional grip. With the advent of tennis players using the semi-western grip smaller grips are being used. By using a smaller grip a player is able to generate more speed that translates into a faster ball flight and increased spin on the ball ("The Incredible Shrinking Grip," by B. Gray, *Tennis*, September 2009, p. 86).

Strings

Rackets are purchased unstrung if they are of reasonable quality. Tennis rackets are strung with gut or synthetic nylon strings. **Gut** is a high-quality string that has limited durability but great feel. Synthetic strings are designed to replace the feel of gut with a far more durable quality. A number of synthetic strings provide a combination of durability and holding their tension. There are four types: monofilaments, multifilaments, aramids, and polyester.

1. *Monofilaments*, also called *nylon solid core,* are composed of a single, solid-core string, encased in a thin outer cover. They are the most popular string for a tennis racket, for they hold their tension and provide both durability and playability. In addition, they are the least expensive synthetic string.
2. *Multifilaments* consist of thousands of individual fibers woven together to form one piece of a string. They absorb shock and provide an excellent "feel."
3. *Aramids*, sometimes called *hybrids*, are made of Kevlar or Technora, and they are the most

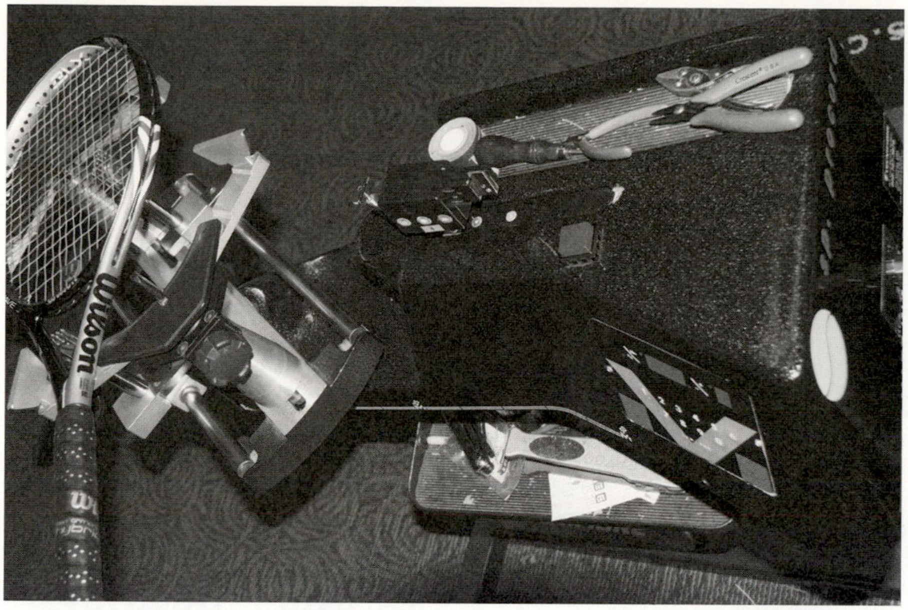

Photography by J. E. Bryant

PHOTO 12.3 Tennis stringer.

durable, but they do not provide much in the way of feel or power.

4. *Polyester* strings have become more popular, because they tend not to break. For the advanced player they take a little power off a shot, allowing the player to swing harder and still keep the ball in play ("Strings 101," *Tennis*, July 2004, pp. 90–91).

Racket strings also are defined by size, and when a racket is strung (Photo 12.3), the string is measured in amount of tension applied to the racket. *String size* is measured in gauge. A thinner string (e.g., 18-gauge) provides more feel and control, while a thicker 15-gauge has "less feel" but is more durable. *String tension* is measured in pounds of tension. The tension is usually identified in the 55- to 65-pound range, with 60 pounds a good starting point for a balanced tension. The higher the tension, the more control, but with less durability (string breaks). Lower tension enhances power.

Costs

Tennis rackets are expensive. So are strings. A high-performance tennis racket usually retails for $135–$300, and to string a racket is an added $20–$40. Based on this discussion regarding rackets, you have enough information to make a decision on what kind of racket to purchase. As a beginner you don't need a $300 racket. You don't even need a $135 racket. But you do need a racket that has as many qualities as possible that meet your needs and one that is within your price range.

Look for a racket with some flexibility (control) and a good feel but also one that provides power, since beginners typically have a short backswing and follow-through, creating limited swing velocity. A racket that provides a degree of stiffness, particularly with an oversize racket face, and is lightweight will assist in providing needed power. Check to determine what features the racket has that seem similar to what has been described, particularly the new hybrid racket. And check out the cost. Most sporting goods stores have "loaners," which allows you to try out the rackets. Take advantage of the loaner opportunity and play with different rackets. Pick one in your price range that meets your needs.

When you buy a racket, chances are that you also will have to have it strung, so apply the foregoing information to the choice of a string. You are best off with a monofilament string, but select one in your price range when you start out as a player.

Tennis Balls

A can of tennis balls ranges from $2 to $4 and lasts only 2 or 3 hours of play (if play is continuous and skillful). Discount stores and major sporting goods dealers often run specials for less than $2, but you should be aware that many types of tennis balls are sold at that price.

Regular-duty balls, with a tighter, thinner cover, tend not to "fluff" up.

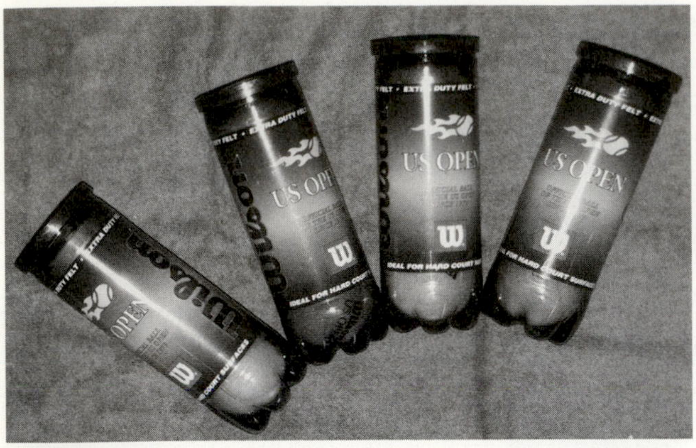

Photography by J. E. Bryant

PHOTO 12.4 Tennis balls.

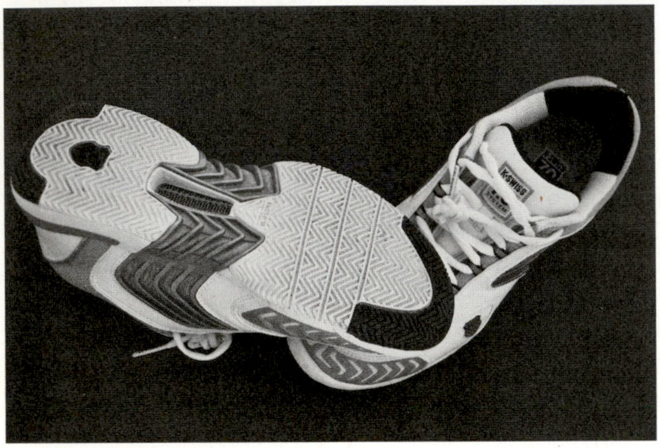

Photography by J. E. Bryant

PHOTO 12.5 Tennis shoes.

Extra-duty balls are thicker and more durable. Every beginner should look for premium and championship balls. An additional checkpoint for tennis balls is to be aware of "feel." For true bounce and longevity, balls should be a name brand. In the United States, three companies—Wilson, Penn, and Dunlop—make approved tennis balls. Each company sells several types. Dunlop balls play "hard," Penn balls are "softer," and Wilson balls are in between.

Tennis balls are made of molded rubber weighing between 1.975 and 2.095 ounces. Two cups are cemented together, covered with a wool material, and inflated with compressed air. They then are placed in a pressure-sealed container, ready to be used when you are ready to play with a new group of three tennis balls. Pressurized balls don't last as long as hard-core rubber tennis balls, but they are easier on elbows and they play with a true bounce (Photo 12.4).

There is a difference in ball bounce when playing at sea level and playing at 5,000 feet. Tennis balls designed for sea-level play bounce much higher at altitude, so a "high-altitude" ball allows for a bounce adjustment, and players who live at high altitudes should purchase only high-altitude balls.

Tennis Clothing

Selecting tennis shorts or skirt and a tennis top is up to the player. An investment of $10 for a pair of shorts and a tee-shirt to an expenditure in excess of $200 for designer tennis shorts and top is the range for purchase of clothing.

Tennis shoes (Photo 12.5) are a different matter expense-wise. They are never inexpensive. The tennis shoe is designed specifically for use on a tennis court and for the player's forward, backward, and lateral movement.

Tennis shoes are sized like regular shoes, and some tennis shoes also are measured in widths of wide or narrow. It is important that you consider your foot type when you select your tennis shoe. *Supinated feet* are characterized by high arches with a wide forefoot that requires a shoe with extra cushioning. *Pronated feet* indicate a flat foot, which requires extra support for the big toe area to prevent a rolling end effect of the foot. A *neutral foot* type means a player can wear almost any tennis shoe. Generally a tennis shoe must have a firm insole and a good arch support. The back portion of the shoe that rests against the Achilles tendon has to be soft and pliable, with an absorbent heel cushion. There should also be extra support under the arch and the medial (big toe). A tennis shoe also should have durability, be comfortable, have good traction, and be light weight, with men's shoes at about 14 ounces and women's shoes around 12 ounces ("Low or High Riders," by B. Gray, *Tennis*, May 2010, p. 56).

The toe of a tennis shoe is vulnerable to dragging and wearing out. Checking to determine how much abuse the toe of the shoe will take will help the player avoid a new purchase every 3 or 4 weeks. At the very least, you should check the flex point. Hold the shoe's heel firmly in one hand and press your other hand against the toe. The shoe should flex at the ball of the foot at its natural give point. If the tennis shoe fits, provides good support, has flexion, and won't wear out in a few weeks, it probably will cost $45 or more, but it is what a player ought to buy.

Tennis socks are not all that expensive, but they have to be selected carefully. You want a sock that leaves a little room for your toes, keeps your feet cool, moves moisture away from your skin to an outer layer of the cotton of the sock, and has a cushion for the soles of your feet. Look for a tennis sock that is made of cotton and has either a polyester fiber or a polyolefin fiber called Drylon to eliminate the excess sweat that contributes to blisters. Finally, to be fashionable, select either a low or below-the-calf-length sock that is white.

POINTS *to* REMEMBER

TENNIS COURTS, EQUIPMENT, AND CLOTHING

1. Tennis courts come in many surfaces, the most popular of which is either an all-weather court (hard court) or a synthetic hard court surface.
2. Beginners need to use a racket with a large face, of light weight, and defined as "stiff" but with some "feel" qualities.
3. Stiff rackets offer less control and more power, whereas flexible rackets provide more control and less power.
4. Rackets are rated on the qualities of control, maneuverability, vibration, weight, shock, comfort, and feel.
5. The most durable yet quality synthetic string (nylon solid core) designed for a tennis racket is a monofilament string.
6. Tennis strings are measured by their gauge size, and rackets are strung based on number of pounds of tension.
7. You can measure the fit of your tennis racket grip by placing your non-racket index finger in the space between the fingertips and the palm of your racket-hand grip, or use a smaller grip to provide speed and spin.
8. Check for flexion of a tennis shoe at the ball of the foot.
9. A tennis sock should be made of cotton with Drylon to eliminate excess sweat.

How to Get Started in Tennis Competition

A wide assortment of tennis tournaments takes place in the United States. Those that are of most interest to the beginning player are associated with recreation programs, college campus recreation programs, city tournaments, and club programs. There are tournaments for all types of players, from the novice who is just learning to hit a volley shot without ducking to a highly skilled player.

Tournaments come in several varieties: ladder tournaments, single-elimination or double-elimination tournaments, interclub tournaments, and social round-robin mixed doubles tournaments. Some are more competitive than others, and the player has to understand which are the more competitive and which are designed as recreational functions. With the proper perspective, all are fun to play.

Ladder tournaments are found in all situations, including most campus recreation programs. They allow players to play at their own level by challenging individuals of similar skill who are positioned higher on the ladder. *Club competition* is a highly competitive league type of play, in which records are kept and league standings are established. Rewards are given to the team finishing first and second in a league, with a team or teams advancing to another round of competitive play.

Many programs have single- and double-elimination tournaments with ratings, including novice, C, B, A, and open divisions. Most are sanctioned by the *United States Tennis Association* (USTA) and require membership in that organization to participate. Most USTA tournaments are identified by a rating scale, usually through the USTA National Tennis Rating Program. There also are age-division tournaments that have an open competition under 35 years of age, then age divisions, including 35 and over, 40 and over, 45 and over, 55 and over, 65 and over, and so on.

Most single- or double-elimination tournaments are played through a 3-day weekend, and a player may play five or six matches if play continues all the way to the championship. The number of matches depends on the size of a draw for the tournament (a draw is the number of entrants).

The USTA also sponsors a Tennis on Campus program designed specifically for college students who want to compete in tennis without the controls that an intercollegiate athletic program would require. This is a program presently participated in on over 500 college campuses and by 30,000 college students. It provides opportunities to compete on local campus, regionally with other colleges, in USTA Sectional Championships, and USTA National Championships. It is a coed-based program emphasizing social networking and competition. These programs are student driven with teams formed by an independent group of students or through college sport club or campus recreation programs. Internet contact for this program is www.tennisoncampus.com.

The *USTA National Rating Program* has become popular for rating players, not only for tournament play but also for social play, to help players identify their level of skill so that a match can be an equal competition. The rating scale is established from 1.0 through 7.0. The lower the rating classification, the closer to a beginner; the higher the rating, the closer to a professional player. The classification of 3.0 to 5.0 seems to be the typical club player rating and probably is a major first goal for a developing player. The beginner usually starts at the 1.0 through the 2.5 level and progresses rapidly through the early classifications. The rating program provides a descriptive version of each classification, and many tennis teachers now are able to use the rating objectively and systematically. The great thing is that you can rate yourself based on how you compare your skills with the NTRP rating categories. Appendix B gives you a view of the National Tennis Rating Program categories.

Tennis Perspective

Tennis across the World and Other Places

Tennis is played across the world. There are four major professional tennis events. The Australian Open in Melbourne, Australia, starts off the professional season each January. The French Open, played on clay courts at Roland Garos outside Paris, France, follows in the spring. Wimbledon, outside London, is played on grass less than a month later as a showcase event in front of royalty. The U.S. Open follows in late summer in Flushing Meadows, Queens, New York, as the feature American professional tennis event. These major events are well worth attending if you ever have the opportunity, and they are certainly events you should watch on television if you can't get there personally. One additional item related to all four events: Although identified as professional tournaments, part of each tournament is also for nonprofessional age-group players. For example, the junior age groups surface in these tournaments as future stars.

There are other professional world tennis events. Two that are important are the Davis Cup and the Federation Cup, both International Tennis Federation (ITF) events. The Davis Cup is an annual playoff competition between countries, with male professional players forming teams from their countries. The Federation Cup follows a similar concept for professional female players. Tennis at the Olympic Games is also an international event sanctioned by the ITF. In addition, the ITF sponsors the Paralympics, for disabled world tennis players, every four years. Then, as a major yearlong professional tennis competition, the ATP, men's professional tennis tour, and the WTA, women's professional tennis tour, engage in competition throughout the year, culminating with the identification of the top-ranked players based on point totals. The International Tennis Hall of Fame and Museum, located at Newport Casino, Newport, Rhode Island, is designed to preserve the history and legacy of tennis. This nonprofit institution enshrines the greatest tennis players and hosts professional tennis events on grass courts.

Professional tennis within the United States and throughout the world is also played at lower levels called *satellite tours*. Beyond these tours is World Team Tennis, the most sacrilegious and enjoyable professional tennis played. This is a 12-team league played in July of each year. It was invented by Billie Jean King, one of America's greatest female tennis players, who believed that tennis can be fun for fans. The league encourages boisterous behavior and cheering during play. Each team has a roster of four players, two men and two women, who compete in two singles matches, men's doubles, women's doubles, and mixed doubles. Players are allowed to substitute for each other, and the coach has the opportunity to challenge a line call by requiring a video replay on the sidelines. Matches are played, with the first to win five games declared the winner of a match; within each game, a no-ad scoring system (first to win four games) is used. The competition becomes even more exciting because the match scores are added together, resulting in a cumulative team match score. If in the last match the losing team wins the last game of the match, the teams are forced to engage in a tie-breaker. If the losing team wins that match, then a super tie-breaker is played to determine the winner of the overall team match.

Tennis also exists for the majority of nonprofessional players, who have varied skills. At the top level would be collegiate players, who may or may not be scholarship athletes but who represent their colleges and universities in formalized competition. Matches played at this level are well worth watching from a learning standpoint. They are also interesting because they are often played with scoring that ranges from standard scoring to eight-game sets and no-ad scoring. In some cases college competition can involve both the men's and women's teams in a cumulative-score setting.

The next step beyond the professional and collegiate levels consists of tennis players who play for the competition and enjoyment of the game. These are the majority of players. They are you. At this level there are several types of competition. One of them is informal tennis, which consists of a large portion of informal play. These are the "walk-on" games engaged in on college and public tennis courts throughout the country. Players simply bring a friend or friends and play, or they join others in "pickup" matches. Typically there is a system of some type that occurs on the courts with pickup matches. These may be as simple as finding and asking someone if he or she wants to play, or some elaborate plan that requires a process by which a "walk-on" eventually gets to play through some form of "pecking order."

Beyond informal play exists recreation-sponsored tennis events on college campuses and through local community recreation department programs. These programs exist in many forms, from ladder tournaments for various skill levels to single- and double-elimination tournaments. The play can be as low as novice level to a high level of NTRP rating of 4.5 or higher.

There is another sponsored form of tennis play opportunity: Club tennis exists for those who are willing to pay an annual membership fee to be part of a tennis club. Within a tennis club there are various levels of play, including participation in mixers, organized ladder competition, periodic club-sponsored tournaments, and open play. *Mixers* are tennis socials that involve players of various skill levels playing a variety of formats that usually include rotating partners and playing opponents within set periods of time. The nice part is that food and beverages are part of the atmosphere and whether the play is highly competitive or not, fun is a major part of the event. The other types of tournaments are far more conventional with an emphasis on competition. Club tennis also often sponsors interclub competition, with representative club members playing against other clubs. These competitions are often defined by NTRP ratings or an A, B, C level of play arrangement and are typically serious forms of play. The next higher level of tennis organization is connected to league play. The USTA sponsors and organizes a league program that involves in excess of 500,000 participants. This level involves a strong competitive component with a regular schedule of matches. Finally, come the sanctioned tournaments designed for the competitive player and sponsored by the USTA or other tennis-interested organizations. These tend to be weeklong age-group and open NTRP tournaments.

Tennis, indeed, is played across the world, by players of a variety of ability and skill levels. You are in the mix somewhere, and it is important that you analyze your skill level in order to play at a level that will provide you with enjoyment and an incentive to improve.

Tennis for the Ages

Tennis as a sport may very well go back as far as the 5th century, when Tuscany (Italy) villagers are said to have struck balls up and down the streets with their bare hands. There also seems to be evidence that monks as early as the 11th century were playing a form of handball within the walls of monasteries and schools. The monks traveled over those early centuries, innovating new rules and promoting the game through their enthusiasm and play. In fact, the game became so popular that the Pope banned the playing of the game.

By the 14th century this handball-type game had spread from the monasteries to the nobility in royal courts, but with an evolutionary twist. It was at that point that tennis, a game the English called *real tennis* and the French called *jeu de paume*, emerged. It was this game, played particularly in these two countries, that evolved from using bare hands, to gloves, to cords attached to the fingers of the player. From that point it didn't take long to invent a racket with a frame and then a handle. A ball was developed made of a cork core, covered in cloth, wound in string, and covered in felt. The balls were hand-stitched and used for about two weeks before falling apart. Play took place in the courtyards of castles using the nooks and crannies of the courtyard area. Nobles, including kings, enjoyed the game so much that many of them played the game competitively. Royalty, during the Tudor and Stuart periods (16th and 17th centuries), including Henry VII, Henry VIII, James I, Charles I, and Charles II, played the game, some with great enthusiasm and skill. In the 18th century, due primarily to the French Revolution, the French version of England's real tennis declined in popularity. In England there was also a brief decline, followed by royal support for the game in the late 18th century, the mid- and late 19th century, and on into the 20th century, with George IV, Edward VII, and George V all supporting the game. In 1876 the real tennis game was exported to the United States, where it was called *court tennis*, and to Australia in 1882 and called *royal tennis*.

This game of real tennis was the forerunner to lawn tennis, a game played on the lawns of England similar to present-day tennis. Tennis made the transition from real tennis in the mid-1850s and has continued to evolve and develop. In 1859 a Major Thomas Henry Gem of England played a game on a lawn surface, similar to today's game, that he and friends called *pelota*. By the early 1870s, several men, including a Dr. Frederick Haynes and Dr. A. Wesley Tomkins, went on to form a lawn tennis club in England, eventually forming original rules for the game. In 1873 Major Walter Clopton Wingfield developed a similar game derived from real tennis but played on lawns. His lawn surface was shaped like an hourglass and was played primarily by wealthy English people. From that beginning, tennis spread rapidly around the world, reaching American soil in 1874, allegedly played first on the lawn of Mary Ewing Outerbridge of Staten Island, New York. In the United States, tennis clubs were established quickly in the 1870s. The U.S. National Lawn Tennis Association (now the United States Tennis Association, or USTA) was formed in 1881 in order to standardize rules. The first U.S. Open followed quickly in that same year in Newport, Rhode Island. A U.S. National Women's Open came along in 1887, and the Davis Cup surfaced for world play by 1900. Other nations were developing their own tennis opens, all around the same time. In 1875 the Marylebone Cricket Club of Wimbledon (United Kingdom) replaced a croquet court with a lawn tennis court. This was immediately followed by significant rule changes that included a rectangular court with identical measurements to today. Other innovations included two serves per point played, and terminology including *deuce* and *advantage*. In 1877 the first world tennis championship was played, held in Wimbledon, and by 1884 women were permitted to play at Wimbledon. The French established the French Championships in 1891, although they limited play to French players. The French opened play to women in 1897, but it wasn't until 1927 that the "French residents only" rule was dropped. In 1905 the Australasian Championships (forerunner to the Australian Open) was played, with women participating by 1922. These four countries' early involvement with national championships have since evolved into the Grand Slam of Tennis, which is defined by worldwide championships known as Wimbledon, the French Open, the U.S. Open, and the Australian Open.

In 1950 the Pro Tour was founded by American Jack Kramer. It allowed elite players to play for financial return. The open era was initiated in 1968, allowing professional and amateur players to compete against one another. Tennis rules remained much the same from the late 1800s for nearly 100 years. It wasn't until 1970 that the tie-breaker was adopted. At Wimbledon, in 1971, the tie-breaker was introduced, with the caveat that when scores reached 8–8 in all sets but the last one there would be a tie-breaker played. In 1979 that tie-breaker rule at Wimbledon then changed to a 6–6 tie through all but the last set. This rule, influenced by television to speed up play and allowing for more structure in program planning, still exists today. Slowly but surely other rule changes followed, most relatively subtle.

The implement known as a tennis racket has evolved over the years. From the early real tennis game through to modern-day tennis, the racket has changed significantly. Ash rackets were used early on, and in 1930 they were replaced by laminated wood rackets. The first metal rackets appeared in 1967. Graphite and fiberglass rackets appeared in 1976; technology took over by the 1980s, with continual changes to the tennis racket as we know it today. Television surfaced in the 1960s, and with television both tennis advocates and new tennis enthusiasts began watching the game. During that same period, the tennis professional circuit developed to involve truly international players. Female tennis players gained equal pay for their play at the international level, and they have captured the interest of fans everywhere with their remarkable play.

Equipment has changed the game from a technological standpoint. So has television. The game, however, after the early centuries of evolution, has remained consistent for over a century. Tennis is now played by people of all ages with amazing skill. Yet the early players, even though limited by rudimentary equipment and cultural expectations that prevented equal opportunity, still performed at a high level, providing the basis for today's game.

Tennis Resources

Numerous textbooks, periodicals, videos, and the Internet are available to help you to learn to play tennis and to continue to develop skills and knowledge associated with the game. Also, tennis associations have been formed to promote the game in community and tennis club environments.

The USTA is the most well-known agency or organization, with the goal of promoting tennis at every level of play and competition. To play in sanctioned USTA tournaments, membership in the USTA is required. The same group sponsors the National Tennis Rating Program. The USTA also publishes USTA Magazine. Other publications produced by the USTA include general textbooks, material for group instruction and for teaching tennis, strategy material, program planning, tennis information, and rules/regulations.

Membership in the USTA is a small investment for the beginning player. The benefits for a serious player are excellent, and the organization really does function to promote tennis. The USTA membership address is: USTA/Membership Department/70 West Red Oak Lane/ White Plains, NY 10604.

The USTA also has sectional offices and state organizations. The major role of these groups is to promote tennis, which includes the sponsorship of tennis tournaments. With a USTA membership, the member receives newsletters from sectional and state organizations. The local, state, and sectional organizations also rate players and carry on the work of the USTA.

Tennis publications and the Internet provide a plethora of instructional materials for the avid tennis player. There are hundreds of tennis books on the market. Some are good, some not so good. If you are discriminating, you can be successful in selecting a tennis book to supplement this text, particularly if you look for a book that might take a specific area and present an in-depth coverage of a topic. The USTA also provides an excellent magazine, entitled *Tennis*. It comes with a USTA membership, or you can purchase it at a newsstand. The great thing about *Tennis* is that it covers skills, strategy, and countless additional topics, most of which will match your interests and needs.

The Internet is a reference source that will continually change, but it is a fascinating option for finding information and instructional help regarding tennis. If you are interested in information associated with tennis results and stories, the assortment of major choices include:

CBS.Sportsline (www:CBSsports.com)

CNN/SI (www:sportsillustrated.CNN.com)

ESPN. Sportszone (www:ESPN.go.com)

Foxsports (www:foxsports.com)

MSNBC-Sports (www.MSNbc.com)

Nando-Tennis (www:tennisisserved blogspot.com)

USA Today. Tennis (www:usatoday.com/sports/tennis/digest)

Tennis on Campus (www.tennisoncampus.com)

If you are interested in websites with instructional analysis, general tennis information, and new ideas regarding tennis try:

- *Welcome to Tennis One*
  www.tennisone.com

  An excellent tennis instructional site.

- *The Tennis Serve* Center Court for Tennis on the Internet
  www.tennisserver. com

  A newsletter website that is a great source for just about any instructional or informational item that might be of interest.

- *Tennis Links—The Ultimate Website*
  www.tennislinks.com

  An excellent source of tennis links for equipment, tournaments, and general tennis information.

- *International Hall of Fame*
  www.tennisfame.com

  Official site for the Tennis Hall of Fame.

- *United States Tennis Association*
  www.usta.com

  Official site for the USTA office; includes extensive information regarding membership, the organization, and countless tennis-related information.

- *International Tennis Federation*
  www.itftennis.com

  Includes information regarding tennis development, the Davis Cup, the Federation Cup, etc.

- *ATP*
  www.atptennis.com

  Covers the men's professional tennis tour.

- *WTA Tour*
  www.sonyericssonwatour.com

  Covers the women's professional tennis tour.

- *Davis Cup*
  www.daviscup.org

  Discusses men's international team play.

- *Fed Cup*
  www.fedcup.org

  Discusses international women's team play.

- *Intercollegiate Tennis Association*
  www.itatennis.com

  Represents the governing body of collegiate tennis.

- *NCAA*
  NCAASports.com

  This is the official site of NCAA tennis news and statistics.

- *College Tennis Online*
  CollegeTennisOnline.com/tennis/news.aspx

  Provides news articles information, and statistics regarding college tennis.

Television provides extensive coverage of major tennis events, including the Australian Open, the French Open, the U.S. Open, and Wimbledon. In addition, smaller tournaments surface on television, along with an occasional collegiate tennis competition. These are instructional, in the sense that, by watching skilled players, you can pick up new techniques, skills, and a feel for the game.

A final but important resource for a player who continues to develop after group instruction at the college/university level is a teaching professional. As an occasional review or to have technique analyzed, a teaching professional is of value. The professional should be able to present the mechanics of stroke execution in an interesting and informative way and should be able to analyze stroke mistakes.

Finding a teaching pro who is appropriate for you requires some effort. Look for teaching pros affiliated with tennis clubs who have credentials. What is their teaching background? Are they certified as a teaching professional? Do they come with good recommendations from former students?

Selecting the proper resources is important and must be done with some insight. A player needs to keep up with changes in tennis and to have enough knowledge to discuss tennis intelligently.

POINTS to REMEMBER

TENNIS COMPETITION AND RESOURCES

1. Be sure to read and identify the NTRP Rating Categories. Identify where you fit, and use that rating as a measure for improvement.
2. Once you have acquired a skill level at which you are comfortable, seek out a tennis tournament that fits your skill level.
3. Countless tennis resources are available. Refer to the discussion on tennis books, *Tennis* magazine, and website addresses to explore tennis on the Internet.

CHECKPOINTS

1. The tennis court surface used by most players is
   a. clay.
   b. grass.
   c. all-weather (hard court).
   d. synthetic.
2. A stiff racket has
   a. more control and less power than a flexible racket.
   b. more power and less control than a flexible racket.
   c. both more control and more power than a flexible racket.
   d. both less control and less power than a flexible racket.
3. A typical racket grip size ranges from
   a. $4\frac{1}{4}$ to $4\frac{5}{8}$ inches.
   b. $4\frac{3}{8}$ to $4\frac{7}{8}$ inches.
   c. $4\frac{1}{8}$ to $4\frac{7}{8}$ inches.
   d. $4\frac{1}{8}$ to $4\frac{3}{8}$ inches.
4. The sweet spot of a tennis racket can be found
   a. above center.
   b. in the center.
   c. wide across the center.
   d. all of the above.
5. Important characteristics to consider when buying tennis shoes include:
   a. Firm insole and good arch support.
   b. Absorbent heel cushion and a soft, pliable heel cup.
   c. Neither a nor b.
   d. Both a and b.
6. The most resilient, long-lasting, and inexpensive string used for a tennis racket is
   a. synthetic gut.
   b. gut.
   c. synthetic nylon.
   d. none of the above.
7. A player who is consistent when hitting medium-placed shots but not comfortable when trying for directionality, depth, or power is rated as
   a. a 2.5 player.
   b. a 3.0 player.
   c. a 3.5 player.
   d. a 4.0 player.
8. The USTA's major publication is
   a. *International Tennis Players.*
   b. *Tennis*.
   c. *Racquet*.
   d. *World Tennis*.
9. Other tennis resources besides magazines include:
   a. usta.com
   b. www.tennislinks.com
   c. itftennis.com
   d. All of the above
10. The real tennis game was the forerunner to
    a. royal tennis.
    b. handball in the 14th century.
    c. lawn tennis.
    d. all of the above.

Answers to Checkpoints can be found on page 167.

Appendix A

USTA's The Code: The Player's Guide for Unofficial Matches

Preface

When your serve hits your partner stationed at the net, is it a let, fault, or loss of point? Likewise, what is the ruling when your serve, before touching the ground, hits an opponent who is standing *back* of the baseline. The answers to these questions are obvious to anyone who knows the fundamentals of tennis, but it is surprising the number of players who don't know these fundamentals. All players have a responsibility to be familiar with the basic rules and customs of tennis. Further, it can be distressing when a player makes a decision in accordance with a rule and the opponent protests with the remark: "Well, I never heard of that rule before!" Ignorance of the rules constitutes a delinquency on the part of a player and often spoils an otherwise good match.

What is written here constitutes the essentials of *The Code*, a summary of procedures and unwritten rules that custom and tradition dictate all players should follow. No system of rules will cover every specific problem or situation that may arise. If players of good will follow the principles of *The Code,* they should always be able to reach an agreement, while at the same time making tennis more fun and a better game for all. The principles set forth in *The Code* shall apply in cases not specifically covered by the **ITF Rules of Tennis** and **USTA Regulations.**

Before reading this you might well ask yourself: Since we have a book that contains all the rules of tennis, why do we need a code? Isn't it sufficient to know and understand all the rules? There are a number of things not specifically set forth in the rules that are covered by custom and tradition only. For example, if you have a doubt on a line call, your opponent gets the benefit of the doubt. Can you find that in the rules? Further, custom dictates the standard procedures that players will use in reaching decisions. These are the reasons we need a code.

—Col. Nick Powel

Reprinted Courtesy of the USTA

Note: *The Code* is not part of the official ITF Rules of Tennis. Players shall tallow *The Code* in all unofficiated matches. Many of the principles also apply when officials are present. This edition of *The Code* is an adaptation of the original, which was written by Colonel Nicolas E. Powel.

Principles

1. *Courtesy.* Tennis is a game that requires cooperation and Courtesy from all participants. Make tennis a fun game by praising your opponents' good shots and by not:
   - Conducting loud postmortems after points;
   - Complaining about shots like lobs and drop shots;
   - Embarrassing a weak opponent by being overly gracious or condescending;
   - Losing your temper, using vile language, throwing your racket, or slamming a ball in anger; or
   - Sulking when you are losing.
2. *Counting points played in good faith.* All points played in good faith stand. For example, if after losing a point, a player discovers that the net was four inches too high, the point stands. If a point is played from the wrong court, there is no replay. If during a point, a player realizes that a mistake was made at the beginning (for example, service from the wrong court), the player shall continue playing the point. Corrective action may be taken only after a point has been completed.

   Shaking hands at end of the match is an acknowledgment by the players that the match is over.

The Warm-Up

3. *Warm-up is not practice.* A player should provide the opponent a 5-minute warm-up (ten minutes if there are no ballpersons). If a player refuses to warm up the opponent, the player

forfeits the right to a warm-up. Some players confuse warm-up and practice. Each player should make a special effort to hit shots directly to the opponent. (If partners want to warm each other up while their opponents are warming up, they may do so.)

4. *Warm-up serves and returns.* A player should take all warm-up serves before the first serve of the match. A player who returns serves should return them at a moderate pace in a manner that does not disrupt the Server.

Making Calls

5. *Player makes calls on own side of the net.* A player calls all shots landing on, or aimed at, the player's side of the net.
6. *Opponent gets benefit of doubt.* When a match is played without officials, the players are responsible for making decisions, particularly for line calls. There is a subtle difference between player decisions and those of an on-court official. An official impartially resolves a problem involving a call, whereas a player is guided by the unwritten law that any doubt must be resolved in favor of the opponent. A player in attempting to be scrupulously honest on line calls frequently will find himself keeping a ball in play that might have been out or that the player discovers too late was out. *Even so, the game is much better played this way.*
7. *Ball touching any part of line is good.* If any part of the ball touches the line, the ball is good. A ball 99% out is still 100% good.
8. *Ball that cannot be called out is good.* Any ball that cannot be called out is considered to have been good. A player may not claim a let on the basis of not seeing a ball. One of tennis' most infuriating moments occurs after a long hard rally when a player makes a clean placement and the opponent says; "I'm not sure if it was good or out. Let's play a let." Remember, it is each player's responsibility to call all balls landing on, or aimed at, the player's side of the net. If a ball can't be called out with certainty, it is good. When you say your opponent's shot was really out but you offer to replay the point to give your opponent a break, you are deluding yourself because you must have had some doubt.
9. *Calls when looking across a line or when far away.* The call of a player looking down a line is much more likely to be accurate than that of a player looking across a line. When you are looking across a line, don't call a ball out unless you can clearly see part of the court between where the ball hit and the line. It is difficult for a player who stands on one baseline to question a call on a ball that landed near the other baseline.
10. *Treat all points the same regardless of their importance.* All points in a match should be treated the same. There is no justification for considering a match point differently than the first point.
11. *Requesting opponent's help.* When an opponent's opinion is requested and the opponent gives a positive opinion, it must be accepted. If neither player has an opinion, the ball is considered good. Aid from an opponent is available only on a call that ends a point.
12. *Out calls corrected.* If a player mistakenly calls a ball "out" and then realizes it was good, the point shall be replayed if the player returned the ball within the proper court. Nonetheless, if the player's return of the ball results in a "weak sitter," the player should give the opponent the point. If the player failed to make the return, the opponent wins the point. If the mistake was made on the second serve, the Server is entitled to two serves.
13. *Player calls own shots out.* With the exception of the first serve, a player should call against himself or herself any ball the player clearly sees out regardless of whether requested to do so by the opponent. The prime objective in making calls is accuracy. All players should cooperate to attain this objective.
14. *Partners' disagreement on calls.* If one partner calls the ball out and the other partner sees the ball good, they shall call it good. It is more important to give your opponents the benefit of the doubt than to avoid possibly hurting your partner's feelings. The tactful way to achieve the desired result is to tell your partner quietly of the mistake and then let your partner concede the point. If a call is changed from out to good, the principles of **Code §12** apply.
15. *Audible or visible calls.* No matter how obvious it is to a player that the opponent's ball is out, the opponent is entitled to a prompt audible or visible out call.
16. *Opponent's calls questioned.* When a player genuinely doubts an opponent's call, the player may ask: "Are you sure of your call?" If

the opponent reaffirms that the ball was out, the call shall be accepted. If the opponent acknowledges uncertainty, the opponent loses the point. There shall be no further delay or discussion.

17. *Spectators never to make calls.* A player shall not enlist the aid of a spectator in making a call. No spectator has a part in the match.

18. *Prompt calls eliminate two chance option.* A player shall make all calls promptly after the ball has hit the court. A call shall be made either before the player's return shot has gone out of play or before the opponent has had the opportunity to play the return shot.

    Prompt calls will quickly eliminate the "two chances to win the point" option that some players practice. To illustrate, a player is advancing to the net for an easy put away and sees a ball from an adjoining court rolling toward the court. The player continues to advance and hits the shot, only to have the supposed easy put away fly over the baseline. The player then claims a let. The claim is not valid because the player forfeited the right to call a let by choosing instead to play the ball. The player took a chance to win or lose and is not entitled to a second chance.

19. *Lets called when balls roll on the court.* When a ball from an adjacent court enters the playing area, any player on the court affected may call a let as soon as the player becomes aware of the ball. The player loses the right to call a let if the player unreasonably delays in making the call.

20. *Touches, hitting ball before it crosses net, invasion of opponent's court, double hits, and double bounces.* A player shall promptly acknowledge when:
    - A ball in play touches the player;
    - The player touches the net or opponent's court while the ball is in play;
    - The player hits a ball before it crosses the net;
    - The player deliberately carries or double hits the ball; or
    - The ball bounces more than once in the player's court.

    The opponent is not entitled to make these calls.

21. *Balls hit through the net or into the ground.* A player makes the ruling on a ball that the player's opponent hits:
    - Through the net; or
    - Into the ground before it goes over the net.

22. *Calling balls on clay courts.* If any part of the ball mark touches the line on a clay court, the ball shall be called good. If you can see only part of the mark on the court, this means that the missing part is on the line or tape. A player should take a careful second look at any point-ending placement that is close to a line on a clay court. Occasionally a ball will strike the tape, jump, and then leave a full mark behind the line. This does not mean that a player is required to show the opponent the mark. The opponent shall not cross the net to inspect a mark. See **USTA Regulation IV.C.8.** If the player hears the sound of the ball striking the tape and sees a clean spot on the tape near the mark, the player should give the point to the opponent.

Serving

23. *Server's request for third ball.* When a Server requests three balls, the Receiver shall comply when the third ball is readily available. Distant balls shall be retrieved at the end of a game.

24. *Foot Faults.* The Receiver or Receiver's partner may call foot faults only after the Server has been warned at least once and the request for an official has failed. This call should be made only when the Receiver or Receiver's partner is absolutely certain and the foot faulting is so flagrant as to be clearly perceptible from the Receiver's side. The plea that a Server should not be penalized because the Server only just touched the line and did not rush the net is not acceptable. Habitual foot faulting, whether intentional or careless, is just as surely cheating as is making a deliberate bad line call.

25. *Service calls in doubles.* In doubles the Receiver's partner should call the service line, and the Receiver should call the sideline and the center service line. Nonetheless, either partner may call a ball that either clearly sees.

26. *Service calls by serving team.* Neither the Server nor Server's partner shall make a fault call on the first service even if they think it is out because the Receiver may be giving the Server the benefit of the doubt. There is one exception. If the Receiver plays a first service that is a fault and does not put the return in play, the Server or Server's partner may make the fault call. The Server and the Server's partner shall call out any second serve that either clearly sees out.

27. *Service let calls.* Any player may call a service let. The call shall be made before the return of serve goes out of play or is hit by the Server or the Server's partner. If the serve is an apparent or near ace, any let shall be called promptly.
28. *Obvious faults.* A player shall not put into play or hit over the net an obvious fault. To do so constitutes rudeness and may even be a form of gamesmanship. On the other hand, if a player does not call a serve a fault and gives the opponent the benefit of a close call, the Server is not entitled to replay the point.
29. *Receiver readiness.* The Receiver shall play to the reasonable pace of the Server. The Receiver should make no effort to return a serve when the Receiver is not ready. If a player attempts to return a serve (even if it is a "quick" serve), then the Receiver (or Receiving team) is presumed to be ready.
30. *Delays during service.* When the Server's second service motion is interrupted by a ball coming onto the court, the Server is entitled to two serves. When there is a delay between the first and second serves:
    - The Server gets one serve if the Server was the cause of the delay;
    - The Server gets two serves if the delay was caused by the Receiver or if there was outside interference.

    The time it takes to clear a ball that comes onto the court between the first and second serves is not considered sufficient time to warrant the Server receiving two serves unless this time is so prolonged as to constitute an interruption. The Receiver is the judge of whether the delay is sufficiently prolonged to justify giving the Server two serves.

Scoring

31. *Server announces score.* The Server shall announce the game score before the first point of the game and the point score before each subsequent point of the game.
32. *Disputes.* Disputes over the score shall be resolved by using one of the following methods, which are listed in the order of preference:
    - Count all points and games agreed upon by the players and replay only the disputed points or games;
    - Play from a score mutually agreeable to all players;
    - Spin a racket or toss a coin.

Hindrance Issues

33. *Talking during a point.* A player shall not talk while the ball is moving toward the opponent's side of the court. If the player's talking interferes with an opponent's ability to play the ball, the player loses the point. Consider the situation where a player hits a weak lob and loudly yells at his or her partner to get back. If the shout is loud enough to distract an opponent, then the opponent may claim the point based on a deliberate hindrance. If the opponent chooses to hit the lob and misses it, the opponent loses the point because the opponent did not make a timely claim of hindrance.
34. *Body movement.* A player may feint with the body while the ball is in play. A player may change position at any time, including while the Server is tossing the ball. Any other movement or any sound that is made solely to distract an opponent, including, but not limited to, waving the arms or racket or stamping the feet, is not allowed.
35. *Lets due to hindrance.* A let is not automatically granted because of hindrance. A let is authorized only if the player could have made the shot had the player not been hindered. A let is also not authorized for a hindrance caused by something within a player's control. For example, a request for a let because the player tripped over the player's own hat should be denied.
36. *Grunting.* A player should avoid grunting and making other loud noises. Grunting and other loud noises may bother not only opponents but also players on adjacent courts. In an extreme case, an opponent or a player on an adjacent court may seek the assistance of the Referee or a Roving Umpire. The Referee or official may treat grunting and the making of loud noises as a hindrance. Depending upon the circumstance, this could result in a let or loss of point.
37. *Injury caused by a player.* When a player accidentally injures an opponent, the opponent suffers the consequences. Consider the situation where the Server's racket accidentally strikes the Receiver and incapacitates the Receiver. The Receiver is unable to resume

play within the time limit. Even though the Server caused the injury, the Server wins the match by retirement.

On the other hand, when a player deliberately injures an opponent and affects the opponent's ability to play, then the opponent wins the match by default. Hitting a ball or throwing a racket in anger is considered a deliberate act.

When to Contact an Official

38. *Withdrawing from a match or tournament.* A player shall not enter a tournament and then withdraw when the player discovers that tough opponents have also entered. A player may withdraw from a match or tournament only because of injury, illness, or personal emergency. A player who cannot play a match shall notify the Referee at once so that the opponent may be saved a trip. A player who withdraws from a tournament is not entitled to the return of the entry fee unless the player withdrew more than six days before the start of the tournament.
39. *Stalling.* The following actions constitute stalling:
    - Warming up longer than the allotted time;
    - Playing at about one-third a player's normal pace;
    - Taking more than 90 seconds on the odd-game changeover; or more than 120 seconds on the set break.
    - Taking longer than the authorized 10 minutes during a rest period;
    - Starting a discussion or argument in order for a player to catch his or her breath;
    - Clearing a missed first service that doesn't need to be cleared; and
    - Excessive bouncing of the ball before any serve.

    A player who encounters a problem with stalling should contact an official. Stalling is subject to penalty under the Point Penalty System.
40. *Requesting an official.* While normally a player may not leave the playing area, the player may contact the Referee or a Roving Umpire to request assistance. Some reasons for visiting the Referee include:
    - Stalling;
    - Flagrant foot faults;
    - A medical timeout;
    - A scoring dispute; and
    - A pattern of bad calls.

    A player may refuse to play until an official responds.

Ball Issues

41. *Retrieving stray balls.* Each player is responsible for removing stray balls and other objects from the player's end of the court. A player's request to remove a ball from the opponent's court must be honored. A player shall not go behind an adjacent court to retrieve a ball, nor ask a player for return of a ball from players on an adjacent court until their point is over. When a player returns a ball that comes from an adjacent court, the player shall wait until their point is over and then return it directly to one of the players, preferably the Server.
42. *Catching a ball.* If a player catches a ball before it bounces, the player loses the point regardless of where the player is standing.
43. *New balls for a third set.* When a tournament specifies new balls for a third set, new balls shall be used unless all players agree otherwise.

Miscellaneous

44. *Clothing and equipment malfunction.* If clothing or equipment, other than a racket, becomes unusable through circumstances outside the control of the player, play may be suspended for a reasonable period. The player may leave the court after the point is over to correct the problem. If a racket or string is broken, the player may leave the court to get a replacement, but the player is subject to code violations under the Point Penalty System.
45. *Placement of towels.* Place towels on the ground outside the net post or at the back fence. Clothing and towels should never be placed on the net.

Appendix B

NTRP Rating Categories

Guidelines

The rating categories are generalizations about skill levels. You may find that you actually play above or below the category which best describes your skill-level, depending on your competitive ability. The category you choose is not meant to be permanent, but may be adjusted as your skills change or as your match play demonstrates the need for reclassification.

To place yourself:

A. Begin with 1.0. Read all categories carefully and then decide which one best describes your present ability level.
B. The rating categories are generalizations about skill levels. You should place yourself in the category that most closely matches your playing skill level. The ultimate test is in match play results.
C. When rating yourself assume you are playing against a player of the same gender and the same ability.
D. If you are undecided between two NTRP levels, you should place yourself in the higher level of play.
E. **Ultimately your true NTRP rating is based upon your match results,** so use match play history against players who have an established NTRP rating as a major indicator of your true NTRP level.

NTRP 1.0

This player is just starting to play tennis.

NTRP 1.5

This player has limited experience and is still working primarily on getting the ball over the net, has some knowledge of scoring but is not familiar with the basic positions and procedures for singles and doubles play.

NTRP 2.0

This player may have had some lessons but needs on-court experience; has obvious stroke weaknesses but is beginning to feel comfortable with singles and doubles play.

Forehand: Incomplete swing; lacks directional intent

Backhand: Avoids backhands; erratic contact; grip problems; incomplete swing

Serve/Return of Serve: Incomplete service motion; double faults common; toss is inconsistent; return of serve erratic

Volley: Reluctant to play net; avoids backhand; lacks footwork

Playing Style: Familiar with basic positions for singles and doubles play; frequently out of postion

NTRP 2.5

This player has more dependable strokes and is learning to judge where the ball is going; has weak coverage or is often caught out of position, but is starting to keep the ball in play with other players of the same ability.

Forehand: Form developing; prepared for moderately paced shots

Backhand: Grip and preparation problems; often chooses to hit forehand instead of backhand

Serve/Return of Serve: Attempting a full swing; can get the ball in play at slow pace; inconsistent toss; can return slow paced serves

Volley: Uncomfortable at net especially on the backhand side; frequently uses forehand racket face on backhand volleys

Special Shots: Can lob intentionally but with little control; can make contact on overheads

Playing Style: Can sustain a short rally of slow pace; weak court coverage; usually remains in the initial doubles position

NTRP 3.0

This player can place shots with moderate success, can sustain a rally of slow pace but is not comfortable with all strokes; lacks control when trying for power.

Forehand: Fairly consistent with some directional intent; lacks depth control

---

Backhand: Frequently prepared; starting to hit with fair consistency on moderate shots

Serve/Return of Serve: Developing rhythm; little consistency when trying for power; second serve is often considerably slower than first serve; can return serve with fair consistency

Volley: Consistent forehand volley; inconsistent backhand volley, has trouble with low and wide shots

Special Shots: Can lob consistently on moderate shots

Playing Style: Consistent on medium-paced shots; most common doubles formation is still one-up, one-back; approaches net when play dictates but weak in execution

NTRP 3.5

This player has achieved improved stroke dependability and direction on shots within reach, including forehand and backhand volleys, but still lacks depth and variety; seldom double faults and occasionally forces errors on the serve.

Forehand: Good consistency and variety on moderate shots; good directional control; developing spin

Backhand: Hitting with directional control on moderate shots; has difficulty on high or hard shots; returns difficult shots defensively

Serve/Return of Serve: Starting to serve with consistency and some power, developing spin; can return serve consistently with directional contol on moderate shots

Volley: More aggressive net play; some ability to cover side shots; uses proper footwork; can direct forehand volleys; controls backhand volley but with little offense; difficulty in putting volleys away

Special Shots: Consistent overhead shots within reach; developing approach shots, drop shots, and half volleys; can place the return of most second serves

Playing Style: Consistency on moderate shots with directional control; improved court coverage; starting to look for the opportunity to come to the net; developing teamwork in doubles

NTRP 4.0

This player has dependable strokes on both forehand and backhand sides; has the ability to use a variety of shots including lobs, overheads, approach shots and volleys; can place the first serve and force some errors; is seldom out of position in a doubles game.

Forehand: Dependable; hits with depth and control on moderate shots; may try to hit too good a placement on a difficult shot

Backhand: Player can direct the ball with consistency and depth on moderate shots; developing spin

Serve/Return of Serve: Places both first and second serves; frequent power on first serve; uses spin; dependable return of serve; can return with depth in singles and mix returns in doubles

Volley: Depth and control on forehand volley; can direct backhand volleys but usually lacks depth; developing wide and low volleys on both sides of the body

Special Shots: Can put away easy overheads; can poach in doubles; follows aggressive shots to the net; beginning to finish point off; can hit to opponent's weaknesses; able to lob defensively on setups; dependable return of serve

Playing Style: Dependable ground strokes with directional control and depth demonstrated on moderate shots; not yet playing good percentage tennis; teamwork in doubles is evident; rallies may still be lost due to impatience

NTRP 4.5

This player has begun to master the use of power and spins; has sound footwork; can control depth of shots and is able to move opponent up and back; can hit first serves with power and accuracy and place the second serve; is able to rush net with some success on serve in singles as well as doubles.

Forehand: Very dependable; uses speed and spin effectively; controls depth well; tends to overhit on difficult shots; offensive on moderate shots

Backhand: Can control direction and depth but may break down under pressure; can hit power on moderate shots

Serve/Return of Serve: Aggressive serving with limited double faults; uses power and spin; developing offense; on second serve frequently hits with good depth and placement; frequently hits aggressive service returns; can take pace off with moderate success in doubles

Volley: Can handle a mixed sequence of volleys; good footwork; has depth and directional control on backhand; developing touch; most common error is still overhitting

Special Shots: Approach shots hit with good depth and control; can consistently hit volleys and overheads to end the point; frequently hits aggressive service returns

Playing Style: More intentional variety in game; is hitting with more pace; covers up weaknesses well; beginning to vary game plan according to opponent; aggressive net play is common in doubles; good anticipation; beginning to handle pace

NTRP 5.0

Player has good shot anticipation; frequently has an outstanding shot or exceptional consistency around which a game may be structured; can regularly hit winners or force errors off of short balls; can successfully execute lobs, drop shots, half volleys, and overhead smashes; has good depth and spin on most second serves.

Forehand: Strong shot with control, depth, and spin; uses forehand to set up offensive situations; has developed a good touch; consistent on passing shots

Backhand: Can use backhand as an aggressive shot with good consistency; has good direction and depth on most shots; varies spin

Serve/Return of Serve: Serve is placed effectively with the intent of hitting to a weakness or developing an offensive situation; has a variety of serves to rely on; good depth, spin, and placement on most second serves to force weak return or set up next shot; can mix aggressive and off-paced service returns with control depth, and spin

Volley: Can hit most volleys with depth, pace, and direction; plays difficult volleys with depth; given opportunity, volley is often hit for a winner

Special Shots: Approach shots and passing shots are hit with pace and a high degree of effectiveness; can lob offensively; overhead can be hit from any position; hits mid-court volley with consistency; can mix aggressive and off-paced service returns

Playing Style: Frequently has an outstanding shot or attribute around which his game is built; can vary game plan according to opponent; this player is "match wise," plays percentage tennis, and "beats himself" less than the 4.5 player; solid teamwork in doubles is evident; game breaks down mentally and physically more often than the 5.5 player

NTRP 5.5

This player can execute all strokes offensively and defensively; can hit dependable shots under pressure; is able to analyze opponents' styles and can employ patterns of play to assure the greatest possibility of winning points; can hit winners or force errors with both first and second serves. Returns of serve can be an offensive weapon.

NTRP 6.0

This player has mastered all the above skills, has developed power and/or consistency as a major weapon; and can vary strategies and styles of play in a competitive situation. This player typically has had intensive training for national competition at junior or college levels.

NTRP 6.5

This player has has mastered all of the above skills and is an experienced tournament competitor who regularly travels for competition and whose income may be partially derived from prize winnings.

NTRP 7.0

This is a world class player.

Answer Key to Checkpoints

Chapter 1
1-a, 2-c, 3-d, 4-a, 5-a, 6-b, 7-d, 8-c, 9-b, 10-e

Chapter 2
1-b, 2-a, 3-c, 4-d, 5-d, 6-d, 7-a, 8-b, 9-c, 10-d

Chapter 3
1-d, 2-a, 3-a, 4-d, 5-c, 6-b, 7-c, 8-a, 9-d, 10-c

Chapter 4
1-d, 2-a, 3-a, 4-c, 5-d, 6-a, 7-a, 8-d, 9-c, 10-a

Chapter 5
1-c, 2-c, 3-a, 4-d, 5-a, 6-a, 7-c, 8-b, 9-d, 10-c

Chapter 6
1-a, 2-d, 3-c, 4-b, 5-a, 6-c, 7-d, 8-b, 9-d, 10-a

Chapter 7
1-a, 2-a, 3-b, 4-b, 5-c, 6-d, 7-a, 8-b, 9-a, 10-b

Chapter 8
1-a, 2-a, 3-c, 4-d, 5-c, 6-a, 7-c, 8-c, 9-b, 10-c

Chapter 9
Refer to the various skill drills in the chapter and your skill level in executing them

Chapter 10
1-d, 2 and 3—Refer to discussion regarding dynamic stretching, 4 and 5—Refer to discussion regarding static stretching under the heading "The Cool-Down," 6-a, 7-c, 8-a, 9-a, 10-c

Chapter 11
1-c, 2-b, 3-b, 4-d, 5-a, 6-a, 7-b, 8-d, 9-d, 10-a

Chapter 12
1-c, 2-b, 3-a, 4-d, 5-d, 6-c, 7-b, 8-b, 9-d, 10-c

Photo Credits

141: Reprinted courtesy of the USTA.
145: Printed with permission of the USTA.

Chapter One

1: top, Photography by Terrell Lloyd, assisted by Anna Symonds Myers **1:** lower right, Photography by Virginia Bryant **1:** inset, Photography by Virginia Bryant **2:** center left, Photography by Virginia Bryant **2:** center right, Photography by Virginia Bryant **2:** bottom left, Photography by Virginia Bryant **2:** bottom right, Photography by Virginia Bryant **3:** top right, Photography by Virginia Bryant **3:** top left, Photography by Virginia Bryant **3:** center right, Photography by Virginia Bryant **3:** center left, Photography by Virginia Bryant **3:** bottom right, Photography by Virginia Bryant **3:** bottom left, Photography by Virginia Bryant **5:** top center, Photography by Terrell Lloyd, assisted by Anna Symonds Myers **5:** top center, Photography by Terrell Lloyd, assisted by Anna Symonds Myers **5:** top right, Photography by Terrell Lloyd, assisted by Anna Symonds Myers **5:** center left, Photography by Terrell Lloyd, assisted by Anna Symonds Myers **6:** top left, Photography by Terrell Lloyd, assisted by Anna Symonds Myers **6:** bottom left, Photography by Terrell Lloyd, assisted by Anna Symonds Myers **7:** top left, Photography by Terrell Lloyd, assisted by Anna Symonds Myers **7:** top center, Photography by Terrell Lloyd, assisted by Anna Symonds Myers **7:** top right, Photography by Terrell Lloyd, assisted by Anna Symonds Myers **8:** top left, Photography by Terrell Lloyd, assisted by Anna Symonds Myers **8:** top center, Photography by Terrell Lloyd, assisted by Anna Symonds Myers **8:** top right, Photography by Terrell Lloyd, assisted by Anna Symonds Myers **9:** top left, Photography by Virginia Bryant **9:** top center, Photography by Virginia Bryant **9:** top right, Photography by Virginia Bryant

Chapter Two

13: top left, Photography by Terrell Lloyd, assisted by Anna Symonds Myers **14:** inset, Photography by Virginia Bryant **14:** top left, Photography by Terrell Lloyd, assisted by Anna Symonds Myers **14:** top center, Photography by Terrell Lloyd, assisted by Anna Symonds Myers **14:** top right, Photography by Terrell Lloyd, assisted by Anna Symonds Myers **15:** top center, Photography by Virginia Bryant **15:** top right, Photography by Virginia Bryant **15:** bottom left, Photography by Virginia Bryant **15:** top left, Photography by Terrell Lloyd, assisted by Anna Symonds Myers **16:** top left, Photography by Terrell Lloyd, assisted by Anna Symonds Myers **16:** top center, Photography by Terrell Lloyd, assisted by Anna Symonds Myers; inset photo by Virginia Bryant **16:** top right, Photography by Terrell Lloyd, assisted by Anna Symonds Myers; inset photo by Virginia Bryant **18:** top center, Photography by Virginia Bryant **18:** center left, Photography by Terrell Lloyd, assisted by Anna Symonds Myers **18:** center, Photography by Terrell Lloyd, assisted by Anna Symonds Myers **18:** top left, Photography by Terrell Lloyd, assisted by Anna Symonds Myers; inset photo by Virginia Bryant **19:** top left, Photography by Virginia Bryant **19:** top center, Photography by Terrell Lloyd, assisted by Anna Symonds Myers **19:** top right, Photography by Terrell Lloyd, assisted by Anna Symonds Myers **20:** inset, Photography by Virginia Bryant **20:** top left, Photography by Terrell Lloyd, assisted by Anna Symonds Myers **20:** top center, Photography by Terrell Lloyd, assisted by Anna Symonds Myers **20:** top right, Photography by Terrell Lloyd, assisted by Anna Symonds Myers **22:** inset, Photography by Virginia Bryant **22:** top left, Photography by Terrell Lloyd, assisted by Anna Symonds Myers **22:** top center, Photography by Terrell Lloyd, assisted by Anna Symonds Myers **22:** top right, Photography by Terrell Lloyd, assisted by Anna Symonds Myers **24:** top left, Photography by Terrell Lloyd, assisted by Anna Symonds Myers **24:** top center, Photography by Terrell Lloyd, assisted by Anna Symonds Myers **24:** bottom left, Photography by Terrell Lloyd, assisted by Anna Symonds Myers **24:** bottom center, Photography by Terrell Lloyd, assisted by Anna Symonds Myers **25:** top left, Photography by Virginia Bryant **25:** bottom left, Photography by Virginia Bryant **25:** center right, Photography by Virginia Bryant **25:** top right, Photography by Virginia Bryant **25:** center left, Photography by Virginia Bryant **26:** top left, Photography by Virginia Bryant **26:** top right, Photography by Virginia Bryant **26:** center left, Photography by Virginia Bryant **26:** center right, Photography by Virginia Bryant **27:** top left, Photography by Terrell Lloyd, assisted by Anna Symonds Myers; inset photo by Virginia Bryant **27:** top center, Photography by Terrell Lloyd, assisted by Anna Symonds Myers; inset photo by Virginia Bryant **27:** top right, Photography by Terrell Lloyd, assisted by Anna Symonds Myers; inset photo by Virginia Bryant **28:** bottom left, Photography by Terrell Lloyd, assisted by Anna Symonds Myers; inset photo by Virginia Bryant **28:** bottom center, Photography by Terrell Lloyd, assisted by Anna Symonds Myers; inset photo by Virginia Bryant **28:** bottom right, Photography by Terrell Lloyd, assisted by Anna Symonds Myers; inset photo by Virginia Bryant **29:** top left, Photography by Terrell Lloyd, assisted by Anna Symonds Myers **29:** top center, Photography by Terrell Lloyd, assisted by Anna Symonds Myers **29:** top right, Photography by Terrell Lloyd, assisted by Anna Symonds Myers **29:** bottom left, Photography by Terrell Lloyd, assisted by Anna Symonds Myers **29:** bottom center, Photography by Terrell Lloyd, assisted by Anna Symonds Myers **29:** bottom right, Photography by Terrell Lloyd, assisted by Anna Symonds Myers; inset photo by Virginia Bryant **30:** top left, Photography by Terrell Lloyd, assisted by Anna Symonds Myers; inset photo by Virginia Bryant **30:** top right, Photography by Terrell Lloyd, assisted by Anna Symonds Myers; inset photo by Virginia Bryant **30:** top center, Photography by Terrell Lloyd, assisted by Anna Symonds Myers; inset photo by Virginia Bryant

Chapter Three

35: inset, Photography by Virginia Bryant **35:** top left, Photography by Terrell Lloyd, assisted by Anna Symonds Myers **35:** bottom right, Photography by Terrell Lloyd, assisted by Anna Symonds Myers **36:** top left, Photography by Terrell Lloyd, assisted by Anna Symonds Myers **36:** center,

Photography by Terrell Lloyd, assisted by Anna Symonds Myers **36:** center left, Photography by Terrell Lloyd, assisted by Anna Symonds Myers **37:** top left, Photography by Virginia Bryant **37:** top right, Photography by Virginia Bryant **37:** top center, Photography by Virginia Bryant **38:** top left, Photography by Terrell Lloyd, assisted by Anna Symonds Myers **38:** top center, Photography by Terrell Lloyd, assisted by Anna Symonds Myers **38:** top right, Photography by Terrell Lloyd, assisted by Anna Symonds Myers **38:** bottom left, Photography by Terrell Lloyd, assisted by Anna Symonds Myers **38:** bottom center, Photography by Terrell Lloyd, assisted by Anna Symonds Myers **39:** center, Photography by J.E. Bryant **41:** center left, Photography by Terrell Lloyd, assisted by Anna Symonds Myers **42:** top left, Photography by Terrell Lloyd, assisted by Anna Symonds Myers **42:** top right, Photography by Terrell Lloyd, assisted by Anna Symonds Myers **42:** top center, Photography by Terrell Lloyd, assisted by Anna Symonds Myers **42:** bottom left, Photography by Terrell Lloyd, assisted by Anna Symonds Myers **42:** bottom right, Photography by Terrell Lloyd, assisted by Anna Symonds Myers **42:** bottom center, Photography by Terrell Lloyd, assisted by Anna Symonds Myers **44:** top left, Photography by Terrell Lloyd, assisted by Anna Symonds Myers **44:** top center, Photography by Terrell Lloyd, assisted by Anna Symonds Myers **44:** top right, Photography by Terrell Lloyd, assisted by Anna Symonds Myers **44:** top center, Photography by Terrell Lloyd, assisted by Anna Symonds Myers **45:** inset, Photography by Virginia Bryant **45:** top left, Photography by Terrell Lloyd, assisted by Anna Symonds Myers **45:** top right, Photography by Terrell Lloyd, assisted by Anna Symonds Myers **45:** bottom center, Photography by Terrell Lloyd, assisted by Anna Symonds Myers **45:** bottom right, Photography by Terrell Lloyd, assisted by Anna Symonds Myers **45:** bottom center, Photography by Terrell Lloyd, assisted by Anna Symonds Myers **45:** bottom left, Photography by Terrell Lloyd, assisted by Anna Symonds Myers

Chapter Four

49: top left, Photography by Terrell Lloyd, assisted by Anna Symonds Myers **50:** top left, Photography by Terrell Lloyd, assisted by Anna Symonds Myers **50:** bottom left, Photography by Terrell Lloyd, assisted by Anna Symonds Myers **50:** bottom center, Photography by Terrell Lloyd, assisted by Anna Symonds Myers **50:** bottom right, Photography by Terrell Lloyd, assisted by Anna Symonds Myers **51:** top left, Photography by Terrell Lloyd, assisted by Anna Symonds Myers **51:** top center, Photography by Terrell Lloyd, assisted by Anna Symonds Myers **51:** top right, Photography by Terrell Lloyd, assisted by Anna Symonds Myers **52:** top left, Photography by Terrell Lloyd, assisted by Anna Symonds Myers **52:** top center, Photography by Terrell Lloyd, assisted by Anna Symonds Myers **52:** top right, Photography by Terrell Lloyd, assisted by Anna Symonds Myers **54:** top left, Photography by Terrell Lloyd, assisted by Anna Symonds Myers **54:** top center, Photography by Terrell Lloyd, assisted by Anna Symonds Myers **54:** top right, Photography by Terrell Lloyd, assisted by Anna Symonds Myers **54:** center left, Photography by Terrell Lloyd, assisted by Anna Symonds Myers **54:** center, Photography by Terrell Lloyd, assisted by Anna Symonds Myers **55:** top left, Photography by Terrell Lloyd, assisted by Anna Symonds Myers **55:** top right, Photography by Terrell Lloyd, assisted by Anna Symonds Myers **56:** top left, Photography by Terrell Lloyd, assisted by Anna Symonds Myers **56:** top right, Photography by Terrell Lloyd, assisted by Anna Symonds Myers **57:** top right, Photography by Terrell Lloyd, assisted by Anna Symonds Myers **57:** top left, Photography by Terrell Lloyd, assisted by Anna Symonds Myers

Chapter Five

59: top left, Photography by Terrell Lloyd, assisted by Anna Symonds Myers **60:** inset, Photography by Virginia Bryant **60:** bottom left, Photography by Terrell Lloyd, assisted by Anna Symonds Myers **61:** top left, Photography by Terrell Lloyd, assisted by Anna Symonds Myers **61:** bottom center, Photography by Terrell Lloyd, assisted by Anna Symonds Myers **61:** bottom center, Photography by Terrell Lloyd, assisted by Anna Symonds Myers **61:** bottom right, Photography by Terrell Lloyd, assisted by Anna Symonds Myers **62:** top left, Photography by Terrell Lloyd, assisted by Anna Symonds Myers **62:** top right, Photography by Terrell Lloyd, assisted by Anna Symonds Myers **62:** top center, Photography by Terrell Lloyd, assisted by Anna Symonds Myers **65:** inset, Photography by Virginia Bryant **65:** top left, Photography by Terrell Lloyd, assisted by Anna Symonds Myers **65:** top center, Photography by Terrell Lloyd, assisted by Anna Symonds Myers **65:** top right, Photography by Terrell Lloyd, assisted by Anna Symonds Myers **65:** bottom left, Photography by Terrell Lloyd, assisted by Anna Symonds Myers **65:** bottom center, Photography by Terrell Lloyd, assisted by Anna Symonds Myers **65:** bottom right, Photography by Terrell Lloyd, assisted by Anna Symonds Myers **66:** inset, Photography by Virginia Bryant **66:** top right, Photography by Terrell Lloyd, assisted by Anna Symonds Myers **66:** top center, Photography by Terrell Lloyd, assisted by Anna Symonds Myers **66:** top right, Photography by Terrell Lloyd, assisted by Anna Symonds Myers **66:** bottom left, Photography by Terrell Lloyd, assisted by Anna Symonds Myers **66:** bottom center, Photography by Terrell Lloyd, assisted by Anna Symonds Myers **66:** bottom right, Photography by Terrell Lloyd, assisted by Anna Symonds Myers **67:** top left, Photography by Terrell Lloyd, assisted by Anna Symonds Myers **67:** top center, Photography by Terrell Lloyd, assisted by Anna Symonds Myers **67:** top right, Photography by Terrell Lloyd, assisted by Anna Symonds Myers **67:** bottom left, Photography by Terrell Lloyd, assisted by Anna Symonds Myers **67:** bottom center, Photography by Terrell Lloyd, assisted by Anna Symonds Myers **67:** bottom right, Photography by Terrell Lloyd, assisted by Anna Symonds Myers **68:** top left, Photography by Terrell Lloyd, assisted by Anna Symonds Myers **68:** top right, Photography by Terrell Lloyd, assisted by Anna Symonds Myers **68:** bottom right, Photography by Terrell Lloyd, assisted by Anna Symonds Myers **68:** bottom left, Photography by Terrell Lloyd, assisted by Anna Symonds Myers **69:** top right, Photography by Terrell Lloyd, assisted by Anna Symonds Myers **69:** bottom right, Photography by Terrell Lloyd, assisted by Anna Symonds Myers **69:** bottom left, Photography by Terrell Lloyd, assisted by Anna Symonds Myers **69:** top right, Photography by Terrell Lloyd, assisted by Anna Symonds Myers

Chapter Six

73: top left, Photography by Terrell Lloyd, assisted by Anna Symonds Myers

Chapter Seven

81: top left, Photography by Terrell Lloyd, assisted by Anna Symonds Myers **83:** top left, Photography by Terrell Lloyd, assisted by Anna Symonds Myers **86:** center left, Photography by Terrell Lloyd, assisted by Anna Symonds Myers **89:** center left, Photography by Terrell Lloyd, assisted by Anna Symonds Myers **91:** top left, Photography by Terrell Lloyd, assisted by Anna Symonds Myers

Chapter Eight

95: top left, Photography by Terrell Lloyd, assisted by Anna Symonds Myers **96:** top left, Photography by Terrell Lloyd, assisted by Anna Symonds Myers **97:** top left, Photography by Terrell Lloyd, assisted by Anna Symonds Myers **97:** top right, Photography by Terrell Lloyd, assisted by Anna Symonds Myers **97:** center left, Photography by Terrell Lloyd, assisted by Anna Symonds Myers **98:** top left, Photography by Terrell Lloyd, assisted by Anna Symonds Myers **99:** top left, Photography by Terrell Lloyd, assisted by Anna Symonds Myers **99:** center left, Photography by Terrell Lloyd, assisted by Anna Symonds Myers

Chapter Nine

105: top left, Photography by Terrell Lloyd, assisted by Anna Symonds Myers **107:** top left, Photography by Terrell Lloyd, assisted by Anna Symonds Myers **107:** top right, Photography by Terrell Lloyd, assisted by Anna Symonds Myers **108:** top left, Photography by Terrell Lloyd, assisted by Anna Symonds Myers **108:** top center, Photography by Terrell Lloyd, assisted by Anna Symonds Myers **108:** top right, Photography by Terrell Lloyd, assisted by Anna Symonds Myers **109:** top left, Photography by Terrell Lloyd, assisted by Anna Symonds Myers **109:** top right, Photography by Terrell Lloyd, assisted by Anna Symonds Myers **110:** top left, Photography by Terrell Lloyd, assisted by Anna Symonds Myers **110:** center right, Photography by Terrell Lloyd, assisted by Anna Symonds Myers **110:** center left, Photography by Terrell Lloyd, assisted by Anna Symonds Myers **110:** top right, Photography by Terrell Lloyd, assisted by Anna Symonds Myers **111:** top left, Photography by Terrell Lloyd, assisted by Anna Symonds Myers **111:** top right, Photography by Terrell Lloyd, assisted by Anna Symonds Myers **112:** top left, Photography by Terrell Lloyd, assisted by Anna Symonds Myers **112:** center left, Photography by Terrell Lloyd, assisted by Anna Symonds Myers **112:** bottom center, Photography by Terrell Lloyd, assisted by Anna Symonds Myers **112:** bottom left, Photography by Terrell Lloyd, assisted by Anna Symonds Myers **113:** top left, Photography by Terrell Lloyd, assisted by Anna Symonds Myers **113:** bottom left, Photography by Terrell Lloyd, assisted by Anna Symonds Myers **113:** top right, Photography by Terrell Lloyd, assisted by Anna Symonds Myers **113:** center left, Photography by Terrell Lloyd, assisted by Anna Symonds Myers **113:** center right, Photography by Terrell Lloyd, assisted by Anna Symonds Myers **114:** top left, Photography by Terrell Lloyd, assisted by Anna Symonds Myers **115:** top left, Photography by Terrell Lloyd, assisted by Anna Symonds Myers **115:** center left, Photography by Terrell Lloyd, assisted by Anna Symonds Myers **115:** top right, Photography by Terrell Lloyd, assisted by Anna Symonds Myers

Chapter Ten

117: top left, Photography by Terrell Lloyd, assisted by Anna Symonds Myers **118:** top left, Photography by Terrell Lloyd, assisted by Anna Symonds Myers **118:** bottom right, Photography by Terrell Lloyd, assisted by Anna Symonds Myers **118:** bottom left, Photography by Terrell Lloyd, assisted by Anna Symonds Myers **118:** right, Photography by Terrell Lloyd, assisted by Anna Symonds Myers **119:** top left, Photography by Terrell Lloyd, assisted by Anna Symonds Myers **119:** bottom center, Photography by Terrell Lloyd, assisted by Anna Symonds Myers **119:** top center, Photography by Terrell Lloyd, assisted by Anna Symonds Myers **119:** bottom left, Photography by Terrell Lloyd, assisted by Anna Symonds Myers **119:** top right, Photography by Terrell Lloyd, assisted by Anna Symonds Myers **121:** top left, Photography by Terrell Lloyd, assisted by Anna Symonds Myers **121:** bottom left, Photography by Terrell Lloyd, assisted by Anna Symonds Myers **121:** top right, Photography by Terrell Lloyd, assisted by Anna Symonds Myers **121:** center right, Photography by Terrell Lloyd, assisted by Anna Symonds Myers **122:** top left, Photography by Terrell Lloyd, assisted by Anna Symonds Myers **122:** bottom center, Photography by Terrell Lloyd, assisted by Anna Symonds Myers **122:** center left, Photography by Terrell Lloyd, assisted by Anna Symonds Myers **122:** center, Photography by Terrell Lloyd, assisted by Anna Symonds Myers **122:** bottom left, Photography by Terrell Lloyd, assisted by Anna Symonds Myers **122:** top center, Photography by Terrell Lloyd, assisted by Anna Symonds Myers **123:** bottom left, Photography by Terrell Lloyd, assisted by Anna Symonds Myers **124:** bottom left, Photography by Terrell Lloyd, assisted by Anna Symonds Myers

Chapter Eleven

133: top left, Photography by J. E. Bryant **134:** top left, Photography by Virginia Bryant **134:** center left, Photography by Virginia Bryant **135:** top left, Photography by J. E. Bryant **135:** center left, Photography by J. E. Bryant

Chapter Twelve

143: top left, Photography by J. E. Bryant
144: top left, Photography by J. E. Bryant
145: top left, Photography by J. E. Bryant
147: top left, Photography by J. E. Bryant
148: top left, Photography by J. E. Bryant
148: center left, Photography by J. E. Bryant

Glossary of Terms

Ad: Advantage of one point to the server or receiver in a tie game.

Ad in: Advantage to the server.

Ad out: Advantage to the receiver.

Ad service court: The left service court.

Aerial game: Overhead smashes and defensive and offensive lobs as part of the total tennis game.

Aerobic: Literally, "with oxygen."

Alley: Space on the court between singles and doubles sidelines.

American twist service: Serve that has a reverse sidespin applied to the ball.

Anaerobic: The release of energy without using oxygen.

Anxiety: Mental pressure that reduces physical performance.

Approach shot: A groundstroke hit inside the baseline toward the net.

Australian doubles: A two-player alignment in doubles that places the net player in a position perpendicular from server to the net.

Backcourt: Area of the tennis court defined between service court back line and baseline. Extends beyond baseline for purpose of understanding the concept of standing in that area to return a groundstroke.

Backhand: Balls hit on the nonracket side of the body.

Ballistic movement: Physically moving the body to prepare for a match.

Baseline: The end of the court, located 39 feet from the net.

Center mark: The division line on the baseline that separates the right side from the left side of the court.

Center strap: The strap that anchors the middle of the net to the court at a 3-foot height.

Chop: An exaggerated slice stroke.

Closed face: Position of the racket face as it is turned down toward the court.

Complex overhead: Includes a scissors kick as the player jumps to hit the ball.

Control: The measure of how effectively the racket permits the player to place the ball on various shots.

Conventional doubles: Two players in a doubles match who are positioned as one up (at net), one back (at baseline).

Close in: Move in on the net following an approach shot, an overhead, or a volley.

Cool-down: Cooling off the body in a sequential, logical order upon finishing a tennis match.

Cross-court: Hitting the ball at an angle across the width of the court, with the net as the central boundary.

Defensive lob: A ball hit to give the defending player a chance to recover from an opponent's offensive shot.

Deuce: A tie score in games at 40–40 or beyond.

Deuce service court: The right-side service court.

Dink shot: A sidespin drop shot hit at an angle from the net to the other side of the court.

Division-line theory of play: The division of the court between the opponent's position and the other player's position that provides an equal distance to reach a forehand or a backhand shot.

Double fault: Serving two illegal serves during one service point.

Down the line: A shot hit down a sideline in a direct line from the player.

Drive: A ball hit with force.

Drop shot: A ball hit from a groundstroke position that barely clears the net and dies on the opponent's side of the court.

Drop volley: Same shot as drop shot but from a position of hitting the ball before it bounces on the court.

Dump shot: A push action that guides the ball to an open area beyond the opponent's side of the court.

Dynamic stretch: A stretch of muscle groups through a ballistic range of motion.

Eye–hand coordination: The coordination between visual observation and hand reaction.

Etiquette: Rules of behavior on a tennis court.

Fault: An illegally hit serve.

Feel: The general kinesthetic sense of how a racket feels in the hand of the player.

Flat serve: A serve hit with little spin and with a basically flat trajectory.

Flexible racket: A tennis racket that has more control and less power.

Focus: The ability to concentrate on seeing and hitting the ball while eliminating outside influences.

Foot fault: An illegal serve due to a foot's touching the baseline before or at contact with the ball.

Forecourt: Area of the tennis court between the net and the service court line.

Forehand: Balls hit on the racket side of the body.

Game: First player to win 4 points with a winning margin of 2 points.

Groundstroke: The act of hitting a ball following the bounce of the ball on the court.

Gut: Type of racket string.

Half-volley: A ball hit immediately following the bounce on the court.

Homebase: The position assumed by a player who prefers to play from the baseline and rally.

Hybrid racket: A blend of an intermediate and beginner's tennis racket characterized as a lighter and smaller racket that provides more speed and spin to the ball.

Ladder tournament: A challenge form of tournament often played in club tennis.

Let: A point played over because of interference or a serve replayed because of an otherwise legal serve touching the net.

Lob: A ball hit up over the net player, driving that player back away from the net.

Long-body: An extra-long racket.

Loop: A groundstroke backswing action that is defined by a high backswing position to contact with the ball.

Love: A zero score.

Match: The best two of three sets in most play situations.

Moonball: A lofted topspin shot intended to change the pace of a rally; halfway between a lob and a groundstroke.

Net play: Generally, offensive play near the net, with volley shots and approach shots characteristic of the shots hit.

No-Man's-Land: The area on the court between the service court line and baseline where a player should never set up to begin a rally.

Nonracket shoulder: The shoulder of the arm on which the racket is not grasped (right-hand player's nonracket shoulder is the left shoulder).

Nonracket side of the body: The same description as for nonracket shoulder, but refers to the whole side of the body (right-handed player's left side of the body).

Offensive lob: A lofted shot hit deep to opponent's baseline, with topspin ball action used to chase opponent away from the net.

Open racket face: Position of racket face as it is turned up to the sky.

Orthodox overhead: An overhead that requires no foot position exchange.

Overhead stroke: An offensive throwing action stroke similar to a serve in motion but delivered at the net, back to the baseline.

Pace: A ball hit with the same consistency, usually with some degree of velocity.

Percentage tennis: A philosophical strategy based on forcing the opponent to make the error rather than one's hitting all winning shots.

Playability: A subjective measure of how the racket responds in general during play.

Power: Also described as a "sweet spot," the measure of the "power zone" of the racket.

Punching action: Hitting the ball with little backswing or follow-through.

Racket face: The strings of the racket as they face the oncoming ball during a stroke sequence.

Racket head: The total racket area, including the string and the material around the face.

Racket shoulder: The shoulder of the arm with which the player grasps the racket.

Racket side of the body: Same description as for the racket shoulder but including the whole side of the body.

Rally: Sustained play of a point, usually associated with hitting only groundstrokes from the baseline area; never refers to hitting a ball on the fly, as in a volley.

Ready position: The foundation position a player assumes prior to initiating a stroke in tennis. Term is usually used as a ready position for a groundstroke or a volley shot.

Return of serve: The act of hitting a ball back off a serve.

Service court: Area of court for placement of a serve.

Service court line: The line that is the base of the service courts and that is parallel to the net and baseline.

Set: Represents the winning of six games with a margin of two games, or winning by a score of 7–5 or 7–6.

Sidespin: Spin action imparted on a tennis ball so that the ball will land on the court and kick away from the person hitting the ball; ball is hit on the backside portion to give the sidespin effect.

Slice: A ball hit with sidespin.

Social doubles: Tennis played in a friendly atmosphere, with a player alignment usually of one up, one back.

Stability: Ability of a racket to resist the twisting motion when the ball is hit off-center.

Static stretching: A stretch that places the muscle in a fixed position, typically used in a cool-down phase.

Stiff racket: A tennis racket that has less control and more power.

Strategy: The planning of an attack when competing against another player or a doubles team.

Stretch racket: An extra-long racket or long-body racket.

Stretch warm-up: Static stretching of muscle groups to prepare for a match.

Sweet spot: Surface area of the racket face that provides a functional rebound area as the ball strikes the racket at contact.

Swinging action: A groundstroke movement that represents the motor pattern of swinging as in a baseball bat swing.

Throwing action: A serving or overhead motion used to strike a tennis ball that represents a throwing pattern as in throwing a baseball.

Timing: The coordinated effort of hitting a ball at the right synchronized point.

Topspin: A ball hit with an overspin rotation action.

Topspin serve: A serve that has a forward or overspin rotation applied to the ball; end result is a high-bouncing, quick rebound from the tennis court.

Tweener racket: Another term for hybrid racket.

Underspin: A ball hit with backspin rotation; the ball will have a tendency to float and slow down when striking the tennis court.

USTA: United States Tennis Association.

Volley: A shot hit before the ball bounces on the court.

Vibration: The measure of how well a racket absorbs vibration at contact with the ball.

Warm-up: Physically preparing for a tennis match by working the muscles and stretching.

Index

Note: Italic page numbers indicate photos and figures.